DOING MORE GOOD THAN HARM: THE EVALUATION OF HEALTH CARE INTERVENTIONS

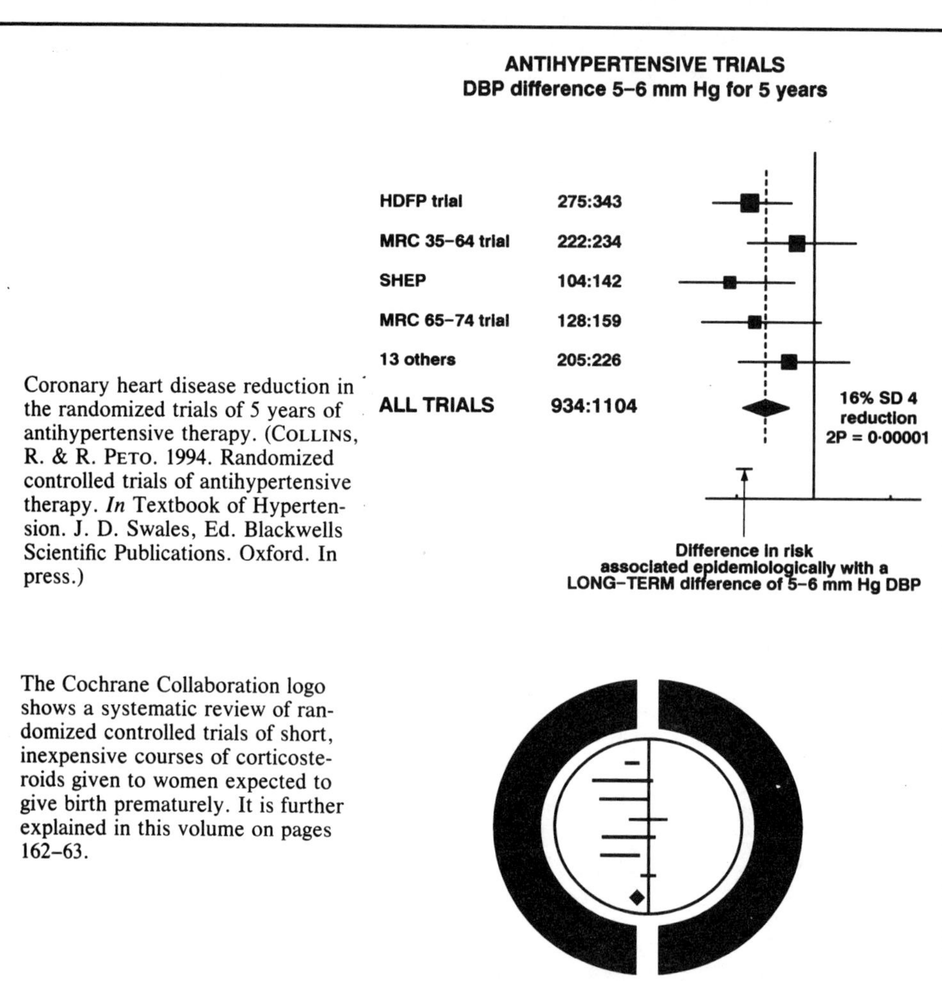
ANTIHYPERTENSIVE TRIALS
DBP difference 5–6 mm Hg for 5 years
HDFP trial
275:343
MRC 35–64 trial
222:234
SHEP
104:142
MRC 65–74 trial
128:159
13 others
205:226
ALL TRIALS
934:1104
16% SD 4 reduction
2P = 0·00001
Difference in risk associated epidemiologically with a LONG–TERM difference of 5–6 mm Hg DBP

ANNALS OF THE NEW YORK ACADEMY OF SCIENCES
Volume 703

DOING MORE GOOD THAN HARM: THE EVALUATION OF HEALTH CARE INTERVENTIONS

Edited by Kenneth S. Warren and Frederick Mosteller

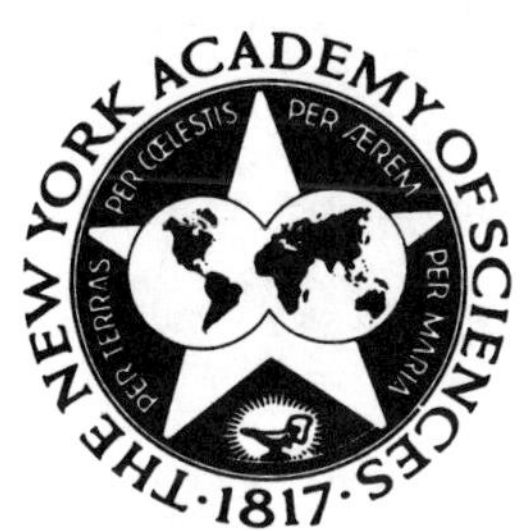

The New York Academy of Sciences
New York, New York
1993

Library of Congress Cataloging-in-Publication Data

Doing more good than harm : the evaluation of health care interventions / edited by Kenneth S. Warren and Frederick Mosteller.
    p. cm.—(Annals of the New York Academy of Sciences ; v. 703)
    "This volume is the result of a conference . . . held by the New York Academy of Sciences and the L. W. Frohlich Charitable Trust on March 22–25, 1993, in New York, N.Y."—Contents p.
    Includes bibliographical references and index.
    ISBN 0-89766-833-2. —ISBN 0-89766-834-0 (pbk.)
    1. Medical care—Evaluation—Congresses. I. Warren, Kenneth S.
II. Mosteller, Frederick, 1916–   . III. New York Academy of Sciences.
IV. L. W. Frohlich Charitable Trust. V. Series.
Q11.N5 vol. 703
[RA399.A3]
500 s—dc20
[362.1]
                                          94-2873
                                          CIP

BiC/PCP
Printed in the United States of America
ISBN 0-89766-833-2 (cloth)
ISBN 0-89766-834-0 (paper)
ISSN 0077-8923

ANNALS OF THE NEW YORK ACADEMY OF SCIENCES

Volume 703
December 31, 1993

DOING MORE GOOD THAN HARM: THE EVALUATION OF HEALTH CARE INTERVENTIONS[a]

Editors and Conference Organizers
KENNETH S. WARREN AND FREDERICK MOSTELLER

CONTENTS

Preface. *By* KENNETH S. WARREN and FREDERICK MOSTELLER.   xi

Part I. Introduction

All Effective Treatment Could Be Free. *By* KENNETH S. WARREN   1

Doing More Good Than Harm. *By* WILLIAM A. SILVERMAN   5

Some Evaluation Needs. *By* FREDERICK MOSTELLER   12

Part II. Types of Evidence

Observational Evidence. *By* CHARLES H. HENNEKENS and
    JULIE E. BURING   18

Can We Learn Anything from Small Trials? *By* DAVID L. SACKETT and
    DEBORAH J. COOK   25

Doing Good Before There's Harm. *By* WILLIAM L. ROPER and
    STEPHEN B. THACKER   33

Large-Scale Randomized Evidence: Large, Simple Trials and Overviews
    of Trials.[b] *By* RICHARD PETO, RORY COLLINS, and RICHARD GRAY . .

Part III. Observational Methods: Major Achievements and Future Potential

On the Proper Use of Clinical Trials. *By* HENRY GREENBERG.   41

Regional Organization for Outcomes Research. *By* GERALD T.
    O'CONNOR, STEPHEN K. PLUME, and JOHN E. WENNBERG   44

[a] This volume is the result of a conference entitled Doing More Good Than Harm: The Evaluation of Interventions held by the New York Academy of Sciences and the L.W. Frohlich Charitable Trust on March 22–25, 1993 in New York, New York.
[b] This paper can be found on page 314.

Outcomes Research, PORTs, and Health Care Reform. *By* JOHN E.
WENNBERG, MICHAEL J. BARRY, FLOYD J. FOWLER, and
ALBERT MULLEY 52

Use of Claims Data to Monitor Patients over Time: Acute Myocardial
Infarction as a Case Study. *By* BARBARA J. MCNEIL 63

Using Scientific Information to Improve Quality of Health Care. *By*
ROBERT H. BROOK 74

Patient Outcomes Research Teams: Examples from a Study on Knee
Replacement. *By* DEBORAH A. FREUND, BARRY P. KATZ, and
CHRISTOPHER M. CALLAHAN 86

Part IV. Randomized Trials: Major Achievements and Future Potential

Randomized Control Trials and Meta-Analyses in Gastroenterology:
Major Achievements and Future Potential. *By* THOMAS C.
CHALMERS and JOSEPH LAU 96

Randomized Trials in Perinatology: Major Achievements and Future
Potential. By ADRIAN GRANT 107

General Discussion: I 119

**Part V. Combining Evidence: Reviews, Overviews,
and Meta-Analyses**

The Science of Reviewing Research. *By* ANDREW D. OXMAN and
GORDON H. GUYATT 125

Publication Bias: The Problem That Won't Go Away. *By* KAY DICKERSIN
and YUAN-I MIN. 135

Collaborative Worldwide Overviews of Randomized Trials. *By*
PETER SANDERCOCK 149

The Cochrane Collaboration: Preparing, Maintaining, and Disseminating
Systematic Reviews of the Effects of Health Care. *By*
IAIN CHALMERS 156

Part VI. Disseminating Evidence

Panel Discussion 1. 166

Dissemination of Medical Information: A Journal's Role. *By*
JEROME P. KASSIRER 173

NIH Consensus Conferences: Dissemination and Impact. *By*
JOHN H. FERGUSON 180

Bringing the News to the Public: The Role of the Media.
By LAWRENCE K. ALTMAN 200

Some Problems in Applying Evidence in Clinical Practice. *By*
R. BRIAN HAYNES 210

Diffusion, Dissemination, and Implementation: Who Should Do What?
By JONATHAN LOMAS.. 226

General Discussion: II... 238

Part VII. Using Evidence

Education

Introduction to the Panel on Education. *By* HENRY WALTON............ 242

Using Evidence to Teach Effective Use of Health Interventions. *By*
HAROLD C. SOX, JR. 245

Public Health Education. *By* JULIO FRENK 250

Using Evidence to Teach Clinical Epidemiology. *By* ARTURO MORILLO .. 255

Continuing Education for Medical Practice. *By* DENNIS K. WENTZ 257

Panel Discussion 2... 261

Utilization

The Clinical Efficacy Assessment Program of the American College of
Physicians. *By* JOHN R. FEUSSNER and LINDA JOHNSON WHITE..... 268

Using Evidence for Utilization Management: An HMO Manager's
Perspective. *By* STEPHEN C. SCHOENBAUM 272

The Role of Evidence in the Approval of Pharmaceuticals. *By*
JERE E. GOYAN... 275

Panel Discussion 3... 278

Financing

Health Care Reform in the United States: The Contribution of Health
Services Research to the Debate. *By* KAREN DAVIS............... 287

Using Evidence: The Role of Foundations. *By* BARBARA STOCKING 291

Financing Medical Effectiveness Research: Role of the Agency for
Health Care Policy and Research. *By* J. JARRETT CLINTON......... 295

Panel Discussion 4... 298

____

Guest Lecture: Alternative Medicine. *By* JOSEPH J. JACOBS 304

Summation of the Conference. *By* SIR RICHARD DOLL 310

Large-Scale Randomized Evidence: Large, Simple Trials and Overview
of Trials. *By* RICHARD PETO *et al*................................. 314

Index of Contributors 341

Financial support was received from:

Major funders
- THE COMMONWEALTH FUND
- THE L. W. FROHLICH CHARITABLE TRUST
- THE ROBERT WOOD JOHNSON FOUNDATION

Supporters
- NIH—AGENCY FOR HEALTH CARE POLICY AND RESEARCH
- SANDOZ PHARMACEUTICAL CORPORATION

Contributors
- GLAXO INC. RESEARCH INSTITUTE

To

THOMAS C. CHALMERS

A Meta-Analyst for All Seasons

Preface

KENNETH S. WARREN

*The Picower Institute for Medical Research
350 Community Drive
Manhasset, New York 11030*

FREDERICK MOSTELLER

*Technology Assessment Group
Harvard School of Public Health
677 Huntington Avenue
Boston, Massachusetts 02115*

A revolution in the quality and efficiency of health care is in the making. The rational design of diagnostics, drugs, and vaccines made possible by molecular biomedical science, in conjunction with statistical methods designed to eliminate bias in the evaluation of these interventions, will dramatically change health care delivery by the turn of the century and beyond. By then, the backlog in unevaluated interventions will be greatly reduced, and new interventions will be evaluated properly and expeditiously. Then, to update Archie Cochrane's memorable phrase of the 1930s, "All effective treatment might be free."

The theme of the conference *Doing More Good Than Harm* was described in its program as follows:

> Until this century, doctors and other health workers had little in the way of effective care to offer the sick. With few exceptions, such as vaccination and digitalis, clinical care was largely ineffective or actually harmful. Since the 1930s, however, a variety of effective pharmaceutical and other interventions have been developed and introduced. Some of these have represented important advances; many have not. Acknowledgement of medicine's potential for doing harm as well as good has led to the development and refinement of methods for considering evidence on the effectiveness of interventions. Escalating costs have now made such evidence essential for coping with the economics of health and medical practices. The purpose of this conference is to consider the strengths and weaknesses of the principal means of evaluating interventions: these range from consensus among "distinguished physicians" to rigorously organized trials and overviews of related trials.

At the end of the conference Sir Richard Doll asked us to "consider first the scientific overviews that were introduced by Tom Chalmers and Richard Peto, which have been turned into a tool for reassessing objectively the whole edifice of medical practice by Iain Chalmers." This statement was particularly appropriate since this New York Academy of Sciences conference, the third in the L. W. Frohlich *Science and the Human Prospect* Award series, honored Richard Peto and Iain Chalmers as "scientists whose singular achievements in research hold significant, direct promise for major improvements of human life, the promotion of human survival and the creation of new economic or educational opportunities." Two points of consensus related to both obtaining and disseminating reliable information on interventions occurred at the conference. The crucial importance of minimizing both systematic and random errors by obtaining large-scale randomized evidence as emphasized by Richard Peto was accentuated by the demand in the discussion period for early randomization of patients for new interventions. When the Chairman queried the audience on the advisability of this idea, the response was virtually unanimous. The reaction to Iain Chalmers' description of The Cochrane Collaboration, a burgeoning worldwide network preparing, maintaining, and disseminating systematic reviews on the effects of health care interventions, was nothing less than enthusiastic.

Sir Richard Doll's summation of the conference concluded: "the principal issues raised [were] the relative roles of meta-analyses, or as I prefer to call them, overviews, and large-scale, simple, randomized clinical trials. . . . I conclude that we have need for both because they provide the only techniques for making small advances in the treatment of common conditions and, in the current state of scientific development, it is only small advances that we can generally hope to make. . . . The few subjects of primary interest with which we have been concerned, if taken to heart by the profession and by those responsible for providing medical care, will ensure that the conference marks a turning point in the history of medicine."

All Effective Treatment Could Be Free

KENNETH S. WARREN

Vice President for Academic Affairs
The Picower Institute for Medical Research
350 Community Drive
Manhasset, New York 11030

and

Department of Medicine
New York University
New York, New York 10016

Archie Cochrane wrote, "when I was a medical student in London in the 1930s
. . . there was to be some rally about the possibility of a National Health Service
in some London suburb, and I decided to go alone with my own banner. After
considerable thought I wrote out my slogan: ALL EFFECTIVE TREATMENT MUST
BE FREE. I had a deep inner feeling that this was absolutely right: although I doubt
very much if I would have passed a viva on the meaning of 'effective'! The slogan,
I regret to say, was a flop, but I still thought it had something."[1]

Sixty-three years later, I too think that Archie Cochrane had something, and
so does the National Health Service of the United Kingdom, which has just
developed The Cochrane Centre as a laboratory for its new Research and Development Programme. The purpose of such a facility was succinctly described by
Cochrane in 1979: "It is surely a great criticism of our profession that we have not
organized a critical summary, by specialty or subspecialty, adapted periodically, of
all relevant randomized controlled trials (RCTs)."[2] The RCT, which remains the
gold standard for the evaluation of interventions, was first used in the 1940s by
Sir Austin Bradford Hill to evaluate the treatment of tuberculosis.[3] Methods have
been refined since then, and the two Frohlich Awardees—Richard Peto and Iain
Chalmers—have each played a significant role in this process. Richard Peto has
developed large-scale, multi-center randomized controlled trials for the study of
chronic diseases, and has developed statistical methods for combining RCTs via
meta-analysis (e.g., the Mantel–Haenszel–Peto method). Iain Chalmers has
produced the first medical textbook based on RCTs and meta-analyses,[4] and is
the founding director of The Cochrane Centre (the initial unit of the global Cochrane
Collaboration).

Through my work in medical information science and international clinical
epidemiology I became involved with both Peto and Chalmers. I have long believed
that obtaining clinical information from databases of the medical literature such
as MEDLINE is a time-consuming and inexact process.[5] This led some years ago
to discussions with Iain Chalmers and others to produce an electronic database
of RCTs and meta-analyses which would specifically answer physician's clinical
queries. My work in epidemiology, largely in the developing world, taught me the
importance of medical economics and the setting of priorities for health care
initiatives in financially constrained parts of the world.[6] It has now become all
too apparent that the economics of health care is a crucial matter for the rich
countries as well as the poor.

1

In many of his elegant essays Lewis Thomas, a biomedical scientist and belletrist, has described the appalling status of medical therapy in the past. He movingly depicted George Washington's death from therapeutic bleeding for a fever and sore throat; his last words were, "Pray take no more trouble about me. Let me go quietly."[7] One hundred years later, the situation was essentially unchanged, as grapically described in "1911 Medicine," Thomas' essay on his father's medical training at Columbia University. "Paper after paper recounts the benefits of bleeding, cupping, violent purging, the raising of blisters by vesicant ointments, the immersion of the body in either ice water or intolerably hot water. . . . Endless lists [were provided] of botanical extracts cooked up and mixed together under the influence of nothing more than pure whim." Just about that time Sir William Osler prescribed "therapeutic nihilism" by claiming that "most of the medicines in common use were **more likely to do harm than good**." A generation later, as recorded in his essay "1937 Internship," Thomas observed that hospitals were "simply custodial." "Whether you survived or not depended on the natural history of the disease itself. Medicine made little or no difference."[8]

Another historical testimony to the ineffectiveness of medical interventions was provided by Thomas McKeown, professor of Social Medicine of the University of Birmingham, England. In detailed studies of data from 1838 to 1970 from England and Wales, McKeown revealed marked declines in mortality in tuberculosis prior to the advent of chemotherapy and BCG vaccination, in pertussis and measles prior to the availability of vaccines, and in scarlet fever before antibiotics. In his great monograph, *The Modern Rise of Population*, he claimed that "The increase of population is attributable not to an increase in fertility but to a decline in mortality," which was due essentially to a reduction of deaths from infectious diseases, as a result of "improvements in the environment."[9]

McKeown made a crucial mistake in that he extrapolated his conclusions from historical data from the United Kingdom to the developing world of today by proclaiming that "Medical measures of immunization and treatment were relatively ineffective; they were also unnecessary." There seems to be little question, however, that the development of "unequivocal successes,"[7] as Lewis Thomas termed them, since about 1940, particularly antibiotics and vaccines, has had an enormous effect on infant and child mortality and, consequently, life expectancy on a global level. While inexpensive antibiotics were rapidly disseminated throughout the world, the use of other low-cost measures has occurred at a slow rate. In 1979 a cost-effective strategy for decreasing infant and child mortality called "selective primary health care," which focussed particularly on vaccines, oral rehydration therapy, and breast feeding, was suggested.[6] This proposal was implemented several years later by UNICEF's great "Children's Revolution" initiative.[10]

There is no question that a crucial factor in the changes in infant and child mortality and life expectancy was "improvements in the environment," as McKeown suggested. The outcome was described in a conference in 1985 called Good Health at Low Cost, which validated the notion that countries with minimal per capita gross national products could have excellent life expectancies. Thus, denizens of China, Sri Lanka, and Kerala State in India, with GNPs per capita of about $300, had life expectancies of about 65 years, and that for Costa Rica, with a GNP of $1,300, was over 70.[11] At that time a citizen of Saudi Arabia, with a GNP of $12,200, close to that of the United States, had a life expectancy of 56. It was then found that major determinants of these figures were good primary health care and primary educational systems. A further indication that high-tech, high-cost modern medical interventions have little effect on mean life expectancies is provided by Lynn Payer's description of the strikingly different application of interventions in France, Germany, Great Britain, and the United States, all of the citizens of which have life expectancies of about 76.[12]

The World Bank's annual World Development Report for 1993[13] opens with: "Over the past forty years life expectancy has improved more than during the entire previous span of human history. In 1950 life expectancy in developing countries was forty years; by 1990 it had increased to sixty-three years." Global life expectancy is now sixty-five!

A vast, sanctioned establishment of alternative (traditional) medicine exists in China. India has Ayurvedic medicine, for which "Western medicine" is the alternative. In the United Kingdom it is a well known fact that many members of the Royal Family, among others, have an interest in alternative medicine. For the United States, a recent study has examined alternative, unconventional, unorthodox forms of medicine, including relaxation techniques, chiropractic, massage, spiritual healing, herbal medicine, megavitamin therapy, energy healing, hypnosis, homeopathy, acupuncture, and folk remedies. It was found that there were an estimated 425 million visits to unconventional therapists in 1990, which exceeded all visits to primary care physicians (388 million). Expenditures on unconventional therapy cost approximately $13.7 billion, of which $10.3 billion was out-of-pocket. This can be compared with $12.8 billion spent out-of-pocket for all hospitalizations in the United States.[14] Under political pressure by the Congress, the National Institutes of Health has just set up a program to evaluate alternative treatment. This initiative, if carried out with the proper rigor, would actually provide a major opportunity for studying the efficacy of other forms of intervention.

In conclusion, countries with little by way of financial and technical resources and very low expenditures on health care are rapidly moving towards the life expectancies of countries with great wealth and vast technical resources. Wealthy countries with totally different medical and health cultures all have approximately the same life expectancies. Vast amounts of money are being spent on alternative treatments, which are bereft of scientific basis and remain unevaluated as to efficacy. Moreover, as demonstrated in *Effective Care in Pregnancy and Childbirth,*[4] only 35 percent of the 283 interventions examined were demonstrably beneficial; of the remainder, 22 percent were found to do more harm than good. In spite of the dearth of present evidence, the State of Oregon attempted to develop a health plan that would not reimburse for ineffective or questionable therapies in order to provide more equitable health care. This pioneering approach, which the *Wall Street Journal* has described as "an unprecedented way to expand basic medical coverage to all people living in poverty,"[15] has just been approved for implementation by the new administration of the national government. The rate at which interventions are now being evaluated by a variety of methods, which themselves will be evaluated at this conference, is constantly accelerating.

In conclusion, to return to Archie Cochrane's slogan, we can now say that when we have achieved a critical mass of evaluations of all therapies, conventional and unconventional, it may well be that *all effective and appropriate treatment could be both freely available and free of charge.*

REFERENCES

1. COCHRANE, A. L. 1989. Effectiveness and Efficiency: Random Reflections on Health Services. British Medical Journal. Cambridge University Press. Cambridge.

2. The Cochrane Centre (brochure). 1992. National Health Service Research and Development Programme. Oxford.

3. DANIELS, M. & A. B. HILL. 1952. Chemotherapy of pulmonary tuberculosis in young adults. An analysis of the combined results of three Medical Research Council trials. Br. Med. J. **1:** 1162– .

4. CHALMERS, I., M. ENKIN & M. J. N. KEIRSE. 1989. Effective Care in Pregnancy and Childbirth. Oxford University Press. Oxford.

5. WARREN, K. S. 1993. Health information technology for the third millennium: The legacies of Charles Darwin, Charles Babbage and Adam Smith. *In* Medical Technology for the Third Millennium. The Royal Society. London. In press.

6. WALSH, J. A. & K. S. WARREN. 1979. Selective primary health care: An interim strategy for disease control in developing countries. N. Engl. J. Med. **301:** 967–974.

7. THOMAS, L. The Fragile Species. Charles Scribner's Sons. New York.

8. THOMAS, L. 1983. The Youngest Science. The Viking Press. New York.

9. McKEOWN, T. 1976. The Modern Rise of Population. Academic Press. New York.

10. GRANT, J. P. 1982. The State of the World's Children, 1982–83. UNICEF/Oxford University Press. Oxford.

11. HALSTEAD, S. B., J. A. WALSH & K. S. WARREN. 1985. Good Health at Low Cost. The Rockefeller Foundation. New York.

12. PAYER, L. 1988. Medicine and Culture. Viking Penguin. New York.

13. 1993. World Development Report 1993: Investing in Health. World Bank/Oxford University Press. Oxford.

14. EISENBERG, D. N., R. C. KESSLER, C. FOSTER, F. E. NORLOCK, D. R. CALKINS & T. L. DELBANCO. 1993. Unconventional medicine in the United States: Prevalence, costs, and patterns of use. N. Engl. J. Med. **328:** 246–252.

15. STOUT, H. 1993. Oregon's revised Medicaid proposal is expected to win Clinton's approval. The Wall Street Journal **221:** A12.

Doing More Good Than Harm

WILLIAM A. SILVERMAN[a]

Department of Pediatrics
Columbia University
College of Physicians & Surgeons
New York, New York 10032

> *No people do so much harm as those who*
> *go about doing good.*
> —BISHOP MANDELL CREIGHTON

In 1939, when I was a medical student, my professor of pharmacology showed the class a bottle of Prontosil (the German sulfonamide drug just coming into wide use in the United States). "Gentlemen," he said, "this will work. And do you know why it will work?" [*dramatic pause*] "Because it's red!" These skeptical words about the hope for anything more than a placebo effect of this first of the modern antibacterial drugs and, in fact, all the lectures in pharmacology I attended, reflected an attitude of "therapeutic nihilism." The usual teaching in American medical schools more than 50 years ago was, in essence, "Don't just do something, stand there!"

The nihilistic point of view had been introduced to the United States about 125 years ago by Oliver Wendell Holmes,[1] as a reaction to medicine's long-standing and unbridled use of horrendous treatments. These included bleeding, purging, cupping, and blistering; the use of prescriptions containing mercury, arsenic, bismuth, endless varieties of botanical substances, and an incredible number of bizarre substances like lizard's blood, crocodile dung, and fly specks. Holmes studied in France and was influenced by Pierre Louis of Paris, who pioneered in the use of numerical methods to evaluate claims of benefit for treatments (Louis demonstrated that copious and repeated exsanguinations were of no value in the treatment of pneumonia). In 1860, Holmes told American doctors that they were doing more harm than good, and that nearly all drugs then in use should be ". . . thrown into the sea, where it would be better for mankind and all the worse for the fishes." In the latter part of the 19th century the trend away from exuberant treatment in Europe was led by Josef Skoda in Vienna, who said, "While we can diagnose and describe illness, we dare not expect by any manner of means to cure it" (only God performs miracles, was the implication).

The "do nothing" advice, to allow nature to take its course, did not sit well with American doctors, who had a long tradition of activism. Payer has pointed out[2] that medical aggressiveness in this country, as far back as pre-Revolutionary times, reflected the character of the early frontiersmen. Anything was possible in the vast new land, it was argued, "if only the natural environment, with its extremes of weather, poisonous flora and fauna, and the unfriendly native-Americans, could be conquered." Similarly, Doctor Benjamin Rush, a signer of the Declaration of Independence, held that American doctors were misguided to place "undue reliance upon the powers of nature in curing disease." He urged practitioners and patients alike to be "heroic, bold, courageous, manly, and patriotic."

---

[a] Address for correspondence: 90 La Cuesta Drive, Greenbrae, California 94904.

5

Rush advised copious bleeding until four-fifths of the body's blood had been removed. "Americans are tougher than Europeans," he said,[3] and "American diseases are, correspondingly, tougher than mild European diseases; to cure Americans will require uniquely powerful doses [of drugs] administered by heroic American physicians." In early 19th-century Louisiana, Duffy has noted,[4] Creole doctors believed that the role of the doctor was to assist nature in making a cure. But Anglo-American doctors followed the teaching of Benjamin Rush: they scorned the healing power of nature and firmly believed in direct, drastic intervention. "When confronted by a sick patient, [the activists] gathered their purges and emetics, [bared] their lancets, and charged the enemy, prepared to bleed, purge and induce vomiting until the disease was conquered."

By the beginning of the present century, William Osler and his colleagues at Johns Hopkins had turned the teaching of medicine in this country away from mindless heroics. Lewis Thomas writes[5] that his father, who was a medical student in 1901, was given the Oslerian message: most remedies in common use were likely to do more harm than good, and "there were only a small number of genuinely therapeutic drugs—digitalis and morphine the best of all." Although surgery prospered in the early decades of this century, with the improvement of anesthesia and aseptic technique, general medicine in the United States shifted away from treatment to diagnosis: "the recognition of specific illness, if possible through an understanding of the natural history of disease." Thomas remembers that when he was a medical student, in 1933, "treatment of disease was the most minor part of the curriculum, almost left out altogether." Leading medical schools taught that a physician should be able to make an accurate diagnosis, a fairly reliable prediction of the course of an illness, and, most importantly, a doctor should "stand by" as a compassionate family friend and advisor. Sir Luke Fildes' famous painting[6] *The Doctor* provided a widely admired image of the caring physician in the conservative era. It depicted a physician sitting at the bedside of a dying child. The doctor is shown leaning forward, chin cupped in hand, with a kindly, puzzled expression on his face—but doing absolutely *nothing*!

The therapeutic explosion following World War II did away with any notion that doctors would remain observers, sitting passively at the bedside of the sick and dying. Miracles brought about by penicillin, streptomycin, polio vaccine, and the steroids led to a soaring optimism, accompanied by feverish activity. It was clear that things would never be the same again.

Since I can speak firsthand about the revolution that took place in treatment of sick newborn infants, I will focus on this field of activity. (A similar upheaval was, of course, shaking up all of medicine.) I can recall, for example, the arrival of penicilin in 1945,[7] when it was in very short supply in the United States and was first made available for the experimental treatment of congenital syphilis. We assembled eight very sick neonates with florid lesions of the disease in an isolation ward at The Babies Hospital in New York. The new drug was given to all of these infants, and the results were apparent almost immediately. Spirochetes disappeared from the skin and mucous membrane lesions within hours; in a day or two, all of the infants were miraculously improved. The results were strikingly different from anything ever seen by experienced pediatricians. The implied "yes/ no" form of our question at the outset of this trial was answered to our complete satisfaction: Penicillin "works" in the treatment of congenital lues! No thought was given to the need for parallel observations in a comparable group of conventionally treated syphilitic infants (concurrent controls receiving neo-arsphenamine) to develop a probabilistic argument (a point-estimate of the size of the favorable effect that might be expected in future treatment, and calculation of a confidence interval to indicate the imprecision of the point-estimate based on the small experience with eight babies). Additionally, the spectacular results of penicillin reinforced a "magic-bullet–like mentality": there was preoccupation with a solitary target—the hoped-for benefit of treatment. The narrow view overlooked the ever-present risk of injury by "friendly fire" in medical warfare: there are usually multiple, and, too often, harmful effects of treatment. And there was little thought about the need for large numbers of observations to provide an estimate of the size of the risk of such unexpected injuries.

In the first heady years of optimism, many well-meaning innovations were introduced for the treatment of neonates with an enthusiastic (and uncritical) "let's try it and see" mind-set. For instance, prematurely born infants were placed in high concentrations of oxygen for prolonged periods to reduce the known risk of hypoxic brain damage, potent hormones were used to speed up their growth, synthetic vitamin K was used to prevent hemorrhagic disease of the newborn, new antibiotics were used to prevent serious infection, a series of devices and drugs were introduced to treat the highly lethal respiratory distress syndrome, bolus infusions of sodium bicarbonate were used in the management of asphyxiated neonates—this list could go on and on.[8] There was virtually no appreciation of the crucial importance of concurrent control study design when, as was so often the case, the new treatment did not bring about immediate and invariable "slam-bang" effects of the kind seen in the penicillin-for-syphilis experience. One hapless scenario was re-enacted over and over: an exciting proposal, based on findings in preclinical studies; a leap to widespread clinical application; belated recognition of the possibility of disastrous complications; and evaluation by controlled clinical trial, if it took place at all, long after the unevaluated treatment was in general use. We can see now, in hindsight, that immature human patients have played a risk-taking role, not unlike the function assigned to canaries carried underground by coal miners. Repeated treatment disasters involving the highly vulnerable babies have given early warning to all of medicine: The practice of adopting treatments for widespread use before they are subjected to rigorous comparative trials is very dangerous!

The postwar rush to introduce powerful new treatments here in the United States stands in sharp contrast to the more deliberate pace that was first forced on, and then chosen by Britain. For example, when streptomycin, developed in the United States in 1944, became freely available here for the treatment of tuberculosis, the experts were well aware of the difficulties in evaluating therapies for the highly variable, pulmonary form of the disease. Armitage has pointed out[9] that two experienced American workers had written quite explicitly about the need, in such studies, for untreated controls selected by "the toss of a coin." But, inexplicably, when the same authors reported their first use of streptomycin for pulmonary tuberculosis in the United States, their conclusions were based entirely on results in an *un*controlled case series.

At the same time (1946), Britain[10] was able to buy only a small amount of streptomycin, because of an acute shortage of funds in that country's Exchequer after the war. Bradford Hill and coworkers in the Medical Research Council decided that "a part of the small supply of streptomycin would best be employed in a rigorously planned investigation with concurrent controls." At the conclusion of this landmark randomized clinical trial (RCT), the need for a control group was "underlined by the finding that impressive clinical improvement was seen in some of the patients treated by bed-rest alone." But there was little doubt about an additional positive effect attributable to streptomycin: the mortality was reduced by one-half in the drug-treated group (within 12 months of enrollment, 24 deaths occurred among 52 patients randomized to bed-rest, compared with 12 deaths among 55 patients in the bed-rest-plus-streptomycin arm of the trial). And, very importantly, serious limitations of streptomycin treatment were also clearly revealed (bacterial resistance to the drug and concomitant worsening of the disease occurred in 18 of the 55 patients in the streptomycin-treated group; toxic effects on the vestibular apparatus were recorded in 36 patients receiving streptomycin).

After this convincing demonstration of the power of the RCT format to provide quantitative information concerning the efficacy and safety of a new treatment, Bradford Hill's group conducted a series of pathfinding controlled trials. "Together they represent the product," Armitage has written, "of what might be called the 'British school' of medical trials." (The distinctive features of the trials in Britain have been, from the start, a simple design, minimum collection of data, focus on a clear, prestated outcome of interest, and low budget; furthermore, the trials have been conducted with very little departure from everyday medical care.) In 1971, almost a quarter-century after the streptomycin trial, Cochrane[11] hailed the importance of "the critical step forward which brought an experimental approach into clinical medicine." He also commented on the relatively slow spread of the approach outside of Britain. "If some . . . index as the number of RCTs per 1000 doctors per year were worked out," he wrote, "and the map of the world shaded according to the level of the index (black being the highest), one would see the UK in black, and scattered black patches in Scandinavia, the USA, and a few other countries; the rest would be nearly white."

Hart has called attention[12] to an important influence that shaped the British experience in the modern era: the National Health Service in that country has been relatively isolated from the market pressures of the "medical-industrial complex" (Arnold Relman's term). As a result, Hart emphasizes, clinical procedures have been developed more cautiously and more skeptically than in the United States, where the market influences favoring rapid acceptance are quite powerful.

In recent years, the number of RCTs conducted throughout the world has multiplied, and the format has been accepted widely as the gold standard for comparing proposed treatments with the accepted routine. As Kassirer observed recently,[13] "We rely on such clinical experiments extensively, because most advances in therapy are not dramatically so much better that they can be accepted without a trial. . . . Most new treatments are only marginally better than existing [interventions]."

Another modern development has also increased the difficulties of determining the extent to which innovations do more good than harm: chronic illness has replaced acute disease as the principal concern in the United States and in other developed countries. For example, as "half-way technologies" (Lewis Thomas's term) prolong lives, more patients live with disability and disease. This country now spends an estimated[14] 80 percent of its health care resources for medical management of, and research on, chronic illness. Increasingly, questions about the outcome of a new treatment have shifted from "Does the new intervention prolong life?" to the more difficult question, "Do treated patients live better?" We are confronted with a dilemma faced by all who set out to study complex phenomena: Should we record what we can measure easily and with minimum error (duration of life), or measure what we think is directly relevant with the highest accuracy possible (quality of life)? In medicine, we often find ourselves in the position of the drunk who dropped his key in a dark hallway and was observed looking for it under the street lamppost: "The light is better here," he explained.

For instance, prior to the mid-1960s, the respiratory distress syndrome (RDS) of the newborn was known as a "three-day disease": mortality in affected infants was high and virtually all deaths occurred in the first three days of life. RDS-affected babies who lived improved rapidly after the third day of life and rarely suffered any complications. The technological transformation of this disorder in recent years is a fairly good example of the increasing complexities in the evaluation of potent new treatments. When mechanical aids to ventilation were introduced in the treatment of RDS in the 1960s, survival of smaller and smaller neonates increased, but the clinical course in many of the survivors was dramatically different than in the past. Now, oxygen dependency and other symptoms of chronic lung disease appeared: supportive treatment was required for weeks and months after birth. The present-day conundrum is this: What is the most relevant outcome of interest in new treatments for this and other life-prolonging measures that have increased the rate of survival of extremely small and seriously malformed babies? And, equally puzzling, particularly in our multicultural country, is the question of who has the authority to define the outcome used to judge whether more good has been done than harm—the state, the doctor, or the parents?

The problems in relying on the state to provide a definition of "success indicators" are not unique to medicine. Heilbroner points out[15] that a prominent cause in the collapse of the Soviet economic system was the simplistic approach to the measurement of the outcomes of central economic planning. For many years targets were given in physical terms—for example, so many numbers or tons of nails. If the output was determined by number, factories produced huge numbers of pin-like nails; if by weight, smaller numbers of very heavy nails. The satiric magazine *Krokodil* once ran a cartoon, Heilbroner notes, depicting a factory manager proudly displaying his record output—a single gigantic nail suspended from a crane.

Even the most cynical humorists in this country were unable to find anything amusing about the Reagan administration's authoritarian actions in the 1980s to impose a federal definition of the "success" of neonatal rescue.[16] So-called "Baby Doe" regulations were promulgated requiring life-prolonging treatment of all neonates without regard to the future quality of life for extremely premature infants or neonates with severe impairments. Notices of the government's pronouncements were posted in all hospitals, and "Baby Doe squads" were readied to conduct on-the-spot investigations of all allegations charging discriminatory nontreatment. Although this outlandish witch-hunt was struck down by the courts, the threat lingers on in the form of amendments in the Federal Child Abuse Act that define withholding of "medically indicated" treatment as a form of child abuse and neglect. Even though the regulations have not been enforced, many neonatologists have concluded that a new legal standard for medical action is now in place.[17]

The medical campaign to prolong the life of every newborn infant, irrespective of degree of immaturity, severity of malformation, or social circumstance of the family, is, I suggest, a unique experiment. This form of social and biological engineering has never before been tried in all of the several million-or-so years of human existence. The survival rate of marginally viable infants has soared, but this crude "body count" is a very misleading indication that we have done more good than harm with all-out medical efforts. What happens, we need to ask, when the dedicated actions of teams of neonatologists to rescue "losers" in the game of reproductive roulette is not matched by an equal dedication on the part of parents or the state when the babies are sent home? We need to see the folly of ignoring the disparity between unlimited medical action to prolong life in the weeks immediately after birth, and, later, the total lack of supporting care of vulnerable, often unwanted, infants living in unsanitary housing, amidst the social chaos of violence and crime in inner city slums. Parents of high-risk neonates are often impoverished, in their teens, unschooled and often unmarried; they often have dramatically unstable personal lives, and many are drug-addicted. Are our inventions, to paraphrase Thoreau, but improved means to an unimproved end?

It is extremely contentious to question the results of the concerted program for neonatal salvage that has become a $5-billion industry in this country.[18] But I am obliged to point out that the initial orders in the medical war to reduce neonatal mortality were, in effect, "Ready! Fire! . . . Aim!"[19] The aggressive campaign was mounted without consulting parents or the community at large about how to define "success." Additionally, the growing number of interventions available in neonatal medicine and the complexity of mixed medical and social consequences of these actions have made it more difficult than ever to make decisions about treatments.

The first requirement for rational decisions in the face of uncertainty is assessing the probabilities that specified events will occur after proposed courses of action. Since RCTs provide the most objective estimates of the size of effects after alternative interventions, it would seem to follow that summaries of this evidence, in the form of overviews (meta-analyses), should be used to develop uniform-practice policies to ensure that we will do more good than harm. But the choice between alternative treatments is not a value-free judgment; the *preferences* for different outcomes of those whose lives are directly affected, parents and families, are anything but uniform.

There is a similar problem in the attempts to develop uniform-practice policies in all fields of medicine.[20] As a result, there are many questions about the level of demand for the plethora of new treatments developed in recent years. Faced with alternatives, Wennberg has asked,[21] "What choices would patients make, if they were fully informed of their options, and if the probabilities of the various outcomes were presented to them comprehensively?" The question recognizes the inherent limit in the ability of doctors to determine vicariously what outcomes patients value most. "The only way to find out what patients want," Wennberg argues, "is to ask them." And there is every reason to expect, he adds, that the probabilities of various outcomes estimated from results of trials in which treatments are allotted in random order, will not be the same as outcome probabilities generated in preference trials (patients choose treatments based on the outcomes they prefer).

It is hard to escape the conclusion that practice policies must not take the form of rigid rules if they are to be responsive to individual patients' needs. Human values, attitudes about the meaning of life, are not the same for everyone, sick or well; and these values and attitudes are not necessarily the same for any one person at different times in her or his life.

Current explorations of ways and means to engage patients in medical decision-making,[22] an outcomes-based approach that takes into account patient preferences, are quite fascinating. I suggest that these preference studies should be watched with interest at this particular time by all of medicine, because we have come to a confusing crossroads in the long journey from therapeutic nihilism to present-day aggressive medical action. In the nihilistic era the doctor seen in Fildes painting was unarmed, but highly respected. Paradoxically, faith in these now heavily armed healers seems to be fading, at the very time they have become highly effective. Many patients and their families are confused and frightened about where they are being taken by teams of dispassionate medical technocrats. The severest critics charge that the perfection of means and the confusion of goals have made medical activities dangerously fanatical. (Fanaticism, Santayana once noted, consists in redoubling your efforts after forgetting your aims).

The crisis in confidence I have described need not be disabling. There is a crucial distinction between religious faith and faith in medicine's "vertical reasoning" (the belief that disordered mechanisms accounting for each disease state can be traced continuously from the molecular to the social level of biological organization[23]). Unlike biblical proclamations, medicine's claims are not carved in stone—doctors' conjectures are susceptible to *refutation*.[24]

REFERENCES

1. HOLMES, O. W. 1888. Medical Essays, 1842–1882. Houghton Mifflin, Boston, MA.
2. PAYER, L. 1988. Medicine & Culture: Varieties of Treatment in the United States, England, West Germany, and France. Penguin Books. New York.
3. PERNICK, M. 1983. The calculus of suffering in nineteenth-century surgery. Hastings Center Rep. April: 26–36.
4. DUFFY, J. 1976. The Healers: A History of American Medicine. McGraw-Hill. New York.
5. THOMAS, L. 1983. The Youngest Science. Viking. New York.
6. TREUHERZ, J. 1987. Hard Times: Social Realism in Victorian Art. Lund Humpheries. London.
7. SILVERMAN, W. A. 1992. Foreword. *In* Effective Care of the Newborn. J. C. Sinclair & M. Bracken, Eds. Oxford University Press. Oxford, England.
8. SILVERMAN, W. A. 1980. Medical inflation. Persp. Biol. Med **23** (Summer): 617–636.
9. ARMITAGE, P. 1992. Bradford Hill and the randomized controlled trial. Pharm. Med. **6:** 23–37.
10. HILL, A. B. 1990. Memories of the British streptomycin trial in tuberculosis. Contr. Clin. Trials **11:** 77–79.
11. COCHRANE, A. L. 1971. Effectiveness and Efficiency. The Nuffield Provincial Hospitals Trust.
12. HART, J. T. 1992. Two paths for medical practice. Lancet **340:** 772–775.
13. KASSIRER, J. P. 1992. Clinical trials and meta-analysis. What do they do for us? N. Engl. J. Med. **327:** 273–274.
14. WENGER, N. K., M. E. MATTSON, C. D. FURBERG & J. ELLISON, Eds. 1984. Assessment of Quality of Life in Clinical Trials of Cardiovascular Therapies. LeJacq. Washington, DC.
15. HEILBRONER, H. 1990. Reflections: After communism. The New Yorker (September 10): 91–100.
16. GERRY, M. H. & M. NIMZ. 1987. The federal role in protecting Babies Doe. Issues Law Med. **2:** 339–377.
17. KOPELMAN, L. M., T. G. IRONS & A. E. KOPELMAN. 1988. Neonatologists judge the "Baby Doe" regulations. N. Engl. J. Med. **318:** 677–683.
18. WINSLOW, R. 1992. Infant health problems cost business billions. Wall Street Journal: (May 1).
19. WONG, E. T. & T. L. LINCOLN. 1983. Ready! fire! . . . aim! An inquiry into laboratory test ordering. JAMA **250:** 2510–2513.
20. EDDY, D. M. 1990. Clinical decision making: From theory to practice. Practice policies—what are they? JAMA **263:** 877–880.
21. WENNBERG, J. E. 1990. Outcomes research, cost containment, and the fear of health care rationing. N. Engl. J. Med. **323:** 1202–1204.
22. WENNBERG, J. E. 1990. What is outcomes research? *In* Medical Innovation at the Crossroads, Volume I: Modern Methods of Clinical Investigation. A. C. Gelijns, Ed. National Academy Press. Washington, DC.
23. BLOIS, M. S. 1988. Medicine and the nature of vertical reasoning. N. Engl. J. Med. **318:** 847–851.
24. POPPER, K. R. 1965. Conjectures and Refutations: The Growth of Scientific Knowledge. Harper and Row. New York.

Some Evaluation Needs[a]

FREDERICK MOSTELLER

Technology Assessment Group
Department of Health Policy and Management
Harvard School of Public Health
677 Huntington Avenue
Boston, Massachusetts 02115

WHY NOW?

The beginning of a new administration in Washington is a good time for us to stop and think about our progress. We need to evaluate our methods for assessing health care interventions. The occasion coincides with a moment when Congress has requested its Office of Technology Assessment to review the methods of assessing medical interventions. Simultaneously, the Agency for Health Care Policy and Research is reviewing its procedures and considering what new directions may be helpful in its future work. Let us then discuss some of what is happening now or has gone on and ask what else may be needed.

One purpose of this conference is to review our progress in making assessments. Whether we call what we do technology assessment, effectiveness research, outcomes research, or cost–benefit analysis, the purposes of the scientific enterprise represented at this meeting are to improve the quality of care, get more payoff for the dollars spent, and to improve our system of evaluation. For example, we will be looking forward especially to information about the Patient Outcomes Research Teams, or PORTs, which should yield new insights into shaping future evaluation programs. Recently I heard Dr. Wennberg speak of clinical trials as a spectrum of tools and techniques rather than as a single method, a concept that will be explained further at this meeting. He has been emphasizing that satisfying patient preference is one of the most important goals of health care. And, of course, we have all seen the impressive video approach (in which patients view a videotape of other patients reporting *their* outcomes with or without surgery) to the problem of managing benign prostatic hypertrophy. To what extent does this approach need to be extended to other areas of medicine?

I have been especially impressed with the variety of methods used by Dr. Wennberg and his colleagues. They studied area variation in usage of operations as a way of appreciating what conditions needed more firm information about good treatment.[1] They used claims data to find out about deaths and reoperations after prostatectomy.[2] They found that deaths and reoperations were more frequent than had been previously understood. Then, to find out about other outcomes, the team interviewed patients before and after prostatectomy.[3] They found that nearly all patients with severe symptoms had improvements, and among all patients 4 percent had persistent incontinence and 5 percent impotence after surgery. Patients differed greatly in how much they were troubled by their conditions, and this is one reason why patient preference has become such a leading issue in prostatectomy work. What I want to emphasize, however, (as I have earlier[4]) is

[a] This project is supported by Grant No. HS 05936 from the Agency for Health Care Policy and Research, U.S. Public Health Service.

that this group uses many different methods to carry out evaluations and that this multiplicity has led to substantial changes in thinking and new directions in the management of conditions.

My question then to those who have been involved in the PORTs is: To what extent has multiplicity of methods contributed to findings in your research; has multiplicity been unnecessary, useful, or essential? In other words, how has it mattered?

CLINICAL TRIALS

Many papers on evaluation begin with the idea that randomized trials are our best method of assessing interventions, and then they continue with a *but. . . .* What might we say about clinical trials if there were no *but*? As of this moment the most important fact I know is that the Oxford group under the direction of Iain Chalmers succeeded in cataloging and following all the clinical trials, randomized or quasi-randomized, on effective care in pregnancy and childbirth. They did this by registering all trials and keeping track of them, by forming task forces which assembled the data, and by carrying out systematically dozens of meta-analyses of these trials. They also prepared a two-volume work called *Effective Care in Pregnancy and Childbirth* (ECPC).[5] They have also a shorter *Guide to ECPC*.[6] Associated with that publication, they also produced a database with the information from the trials, and they have been updating and distributing the information from the trials.

It had been a dream of Archie Cochrane's to have all the randomized trials from medicine organized and analyzed and updated. The opportunity to do this stands now as a challenge to medicine. It took a long time to carry this work out for ECPC, perhaps 15 years, and so if it is to be done for medicine as a whole, we cannot expect it to be carried out quickly; but with the example of ECPC before us, we can hope that much might be done in the next decade. Can we organize the clinical trial information for all of medicine and make it readily available for practitioners?

In the preparation of ECPC, it is important to recognize that the published work not only collected data from randomized and quasi-randomized trials, but also that it included quantitative information from many other sources such as epidemiologic studies, laboratory work, and even studies of a medical sociological sort, often examining the satisfaction of the patient.

One major problem is to develop and find funding for such an international cooperative program to carry this out for medicine as a whole. A second problem is to gain the cooperation of medical scholars to help with the work. I am sure that Iain Chalmers has with his colleagues begun to develop a plan for such a program, and I expect to hear more about the plans at this meeting.

It is important that the findings from the trials be organized and analyzed because there are too many trials for us to expect individuals to be able to assemble them and analyze them. Thousands of trials are published each year. When collections of trials bear on the same clinical question, it is too much to expect that the outcomes will all be so similar as not to need analysis and interpretation. Therefore we need to have these data collected and analyzed and their results put into a form that clinicians can readily appreciate and use.[7] The process has the further advantage that it tells us what treatments have been appraised convincingly and what have not.

Among the practical questions that require attention are how often updating is needed and what sort of updating it is to be. Medical practice as a whole changes with time, so that a given summary at one time may no longer be as appropriate later. For instance, more and more surgery now is being done on an outpatient basis. Will summaries of trials need to be changed substantially because of such changing practices?

I regard this effort as of major importance and as a truly international development rather than a national effort for the United Kingdom alone. I therefore feel that one important outcome from this period should be an effort to make Archie Cochrane's dream come true: We must find a way to organize and disseminate all the randomized and quasi-randomized trials in medicine and develop a plan for updating their findings.

FIRMS

A second important development, though not yet implemented on a large scale in this country, is that of firms.[8,9] The idea of firms, as I understand it, is for a care-giving institution such as a hospital to form itself into two or more equivalent parallel organizations. They are equivalent in the sense that they have about the same composition in number of beds, nursing staff, residents, and senior physicians and specialists. Patients entering the institution are assigned to the firms at random. We have therefore an arrangement that offers equivalent facilities in each firm within an institution.

The firms offer ways of making studies that can improve care. Hospital policies can be compared by assigning different policies to the different firms. Neuhauser[10] notes that the "approach needs to be embedded in a culture of continuous evaluation and improvement." The firm approach then makes possible the use of the idea of the randomized trial for general evaluation. And it has the advantage that it deals with patients as they appear and so has the possibility of carrying out effectiveness research in the sense of dealing with all patients or average patients rather than highly selected patients, as often occurs in efficacy research. Similarly it uses the physician and staff of the institution rather than an elite subset of them.

Some institutions that have developed such firms are the Regenstreif Medical Center, Indianapolis; Brook Army Medical Center; University Hospitals of Cleveland; Worcester Memorial Hospital; Henry Ford Medical Center, Detroit; Harborview Hospital, Seattle; and the St. Louis Veterans Administration hospital.

Neuhauser[10] points out that firms research has addressed such topics as promoting preventive efforts, lab tests, X-ray usage, test usage, patient education, and staff and patient satisfaction.

Because firms are set up in parallel, the opportunity for reduced costs for randomized trials is already built into the system. When several institutions with firms join together, they have the capability of carrying out multi-center trials. Because the institutions usually do not have equivalent information systems, that may require further development. On the other hand the VA system does have a nationally uniform system and so it represents a special opportunity for developing and using firms.

My feeling is that one reason for the *buts* in connection with RCTs is the need to have a major organization for each trial. If we had many firms and if they had comparability in the data that they gathered, then research in health care and medicine could go forward more smoothly and less expensively. Before sample survey organizations were widespread, it was difficult to take a national sample. Now it is relatively easy. If firms were widespread, experimentation could be much more routine. This seems to me to be a movement that deserves support.

LARGE SIMPLE TRIALS

A third development, which is being pressed by Richard Peto, is the large simple trial. It has advantages that he will describe, but it especially offers the opportunity to do more subgroup analysis than we usually can get from trials of modest size.

ECONOMIC ANALYSIS

Aside from access to care, almost all current attention to the health care problem in the United States deals with costs. The economics of treatments and procedures can be studied by the example of the Oregon medical proposal, in which about 700 condition-treatment pairs were to be ordered in a treatment package according to their quantitative cost-effectiveness.[11] A telephone survey was used to let the public help with the ordering. The community clinicians gave information about the outcomes from each pair, the public indicated preferences for health states through a telephone survey, and then an estimate was made of the condition-treatment pair's net benefit. Meanwhile the pairs were assigned to one of 17 service categories, and the categories were ranked by the Health Service Commission. Within the categories, the pairs were ranked according to net benefit.

The purpose of the ordering was to decide which condition-treatment pairs should be covered in the Oregon program. One would start at the top with the most cost-effective pairs and continue covering until the money ran out. After the condition-treatment pairs had been arranged according to essentially a formula, the Commission reviewed the list and concluded that the ordering was unsatisfactory. They therefore rearranged it into an order that they found more reasonable on the basis of their subjective impressions. In the re-ranking, more than half the pairs moved by at least 25 ranks, and about a quarter moved by at least 100 ranks out of the 700. When completed it was estimated that the program would be able to cover slightly fewer than 600 of the 700 items.

One feature of the program that caused criticism was that the plan did not have a minimum program that would be delivered. Another was that there would be considerable difference between the current Medicaid program and the one Oregon was proposing. There are also issues as to whether participants could sue if their needs were not being met, as they could under federal legislation. Also it was not clear whether Oregon could meet its financial responsibilities and therefore whether the federal government would have to take over shortfalls. The latest version of the plan has been approved and we will learn from its experience.

Any attempt to carry out cost reductions or capping total costs of health care will need clear measures of costs and benefits, if not in the form used in the Oregon effort, then in some other.

It is my impression that we do not have as much detail as we need on the costs of care for episodes of illness.

When Adams *et al.*[12] looked into situations where randomized trials had been done over a 22-year period, only 121 of about 50,000 randomized trials included economic analyses. I am not going to argue that a randomized trial of interventions is necessarily the best circumstance to get economic information, but I want to note that the rate of economic analysis is very low. Indeed searching separately for economic articles these investigators found 3,737 such articles using costs and other economic terms. The intersection had 778 articles, of which only 121 gave information adequate to study the economic means used to get some cost-effectiveness information.

When Adams and co-workers analyzed a sample of the studies they often found the economic analyses disappointing. Their article makes it sound as if guidelines for economic analyses are needed if we are to use the data in redesigning the health care system. Although there is an elaborate system for estimating Diagnosis Related Groups (DRGs), DRGs are not especially oriented to choosing which condition-treatment pairs should be covered by insurance and which not. I assume that as the financial pressure on the health system increases, some pairs traditionally covered will be covered less often and that we will need better ways of comparing benefits and costs to help with the development of a program that is generally regarded as fair.

Although the program of this conference is not especially tuned to this issue, we do need an improved political process for considering how to develop an effective, affordable, and seemingly fair system. Thus we need to develop better cost information and we need to associate it with benefits purchased. And in improving our health care system we need a process for the political debate that will lead the nation to regard the new plan as reasonably fair.

SUMMING UP CONTRIBUTIONS TO QUALITY OF LIFE

In the last few years I have been working with Drs. John Bunker and Howard Frazier to try to appreciate the benefits of medicine. We have divided the benefits into three areas, two dealing with possible extensions of life and one dealing with quality of life. The two dealing with extension of life relate to prevention and to cure. The third, on quality of life, deals with relief of pain or other acute or chronic conditions and restoration of function as well as ability to carry out various activities. Without going into details, the idea of extension of life has some simple aspects such as being roughly additive. Essentially we try to assess what benefits medicine gives us in return for the total health bill. As you know, much of medicine is not devoted very directly to life-saving, but to improving comfort, convenience, and function. When we try to write down the benefits from improved quality of life, we are hampered because there seem to be so many categories of benefit. We need some way of adding up, at least grossly, what these benefits amount to if we are to appreciate what we have been given.

When we merely produce lists such as so many million headaches relieved, so many operations carried out painlessly, so many chronic pains relieved, and so on, it is hard to bring any overall comprehension to the benefits. Our discussion above of prostate operations noted that degree of benefit perceived by the patients depended on their previous states. Although I may be searching for a "will o' the wisp," I feel we do need some better ways of communicating benefits.

For example, in medicine many of the five patient office visits per year (the U.S. national average) are primarily to get reassurance that some symptom does not represent a life-threatening situation. Often such assurance can be given, or so I am told. We understand that the diagnosis reduces anxiety even when the news is bad. How can we summarize this reduction in anxiety as part of the benefit of the national medical program?

Although I am familiar with measures of utility and of quality-of-life years, I am not persuaded that these ideas can communicate well the benefits being delivered for quality of life, even though perhaps they can be delivered for each situation separately. Because so much of health care is dedicated to improvement in quality of life, we need better ways of summarizing accomplishments toward this goal.

CODA

During the conference we will discuss and compare many methods of assessment. To put such discussion in context, let me remind you of a comment the economist Alfred Marshall is said to have made, "We are never so right as when defending our own methods and never so wrong as when attacking those of others."

REFERENCES

1. WENNEBERG, J. & A. GITTELSOHN. 1973. Small area variations in health care delivery. Science. **182:** 1102–1108.
2. WENNBERG, J. E., N. ROOS, L. SOLA *et al.* 1987. Use of claims data systems to evaluate health care outcomes: Mortality and reoperation following prostatectomy. JAMA **257:** 933–936.
3. FOWLER, F. J, JR., J. E. WENNBERG, R. P. TIMOTHY, M. J. BARRY, A. G. MULLEY, JR. & D. HANLEY. 1988. Symptom status and quality of life following prostatectomy. JAMA **259:** 3018–3022.
4. MOSTELLER, F. 1990. Improving research methodology: An overview. *In* Research Methodology: Strengthening Causal Interpretations of Non-experimental Data. L. Sechrest, E. Perrin & J. Bunker, Eds.: 221–230. U.S. Department of Health and Human Services, Public Health Service, Agency for Health Care Policy and Research.
5. CHALMERS, I., M. ENKIN & M. J. M. C. KEIRSE, Eds. 1989. Effective Care in Pregnancy and Childbirth. Oxford University Press. Oxford.
6. ENKIN, M., M. J. M. C. KEIRSE & I. CHALMERS. 1989. A guide to effective care in pregnancy and childbirth. Oxford University Press. Oxford.
7. ANTMAN, E. M., J. LAU, B. KUPELNICK, F. MOSTELLER & T. C. CHALMERS. 1992. JAMA **268:** 240–248.
8. Office of Medical Applications of Research, National Institutes of Health. 1990. Health Care Delivery Research Using Hospital Firms: Workshop Summary, April 30–May 1. Bethesda, MD: USPHS, NIH, OMAR.17.
9. 1991. Proceedings. Medical Care (July supplement).
10. NEUHAUSER, D. 1992. Progress in firms research. Int. J. Technol. Assess. Hlth. Care **8:** 321–324.
11. U.S. Congress, Office of Technology Assessment. Evaluation of the Oregon Medicaid Proposal. May 1992. OTA-H-531 U.S. Government Printing Office. Washington, DC.
12. ADAMS, M. E., N. T. McCALL, D. T. GRAY, M. J. ORZA & T. C. CHALMERS. 1992. Economic analysis in randomized control trials. Medical Care. **30:** 231–243.

Observational Evidence

CHARLES H. HENNEKENS AND JULIE E. BURING

Division of Preventive Medicine
Harvard Medical School
Brigham and Women's Hospital
Boston, Massachusetts 02215-1204

Observational studies make a critical contribution to the totality of evidence that permits the evaluation of risks and benefits of interventions.[1] As has often been the case, advances in medical knowledge proceed on several fronts, optimally simultaneously. First, basic researchers provide unique and crucial information on mechanisms that explain why a particular intervention averts premature death or disability. Second, clinicians provide enormous benefits to patients through advances in diagnosis and treatment and, in addition, formulate hypotheses from their own clinical experiences—that is, their case reports and case series. Finally, epidemiologists and biostatisticians formulate hypotheses from descriptive studies and test hypotheses in observational studies, either case-control or cohort, or, where necessary, in randomized trials, to answer the unique and crucial question of whether a particular intervention can prevent premature death or disability.

In evaluating the effects of an intervention, basic research has the unique advantage of precision, afforded by its ability to achieve virtually complete control of exposures, environment, and even genetics. On the other hand, results may differ so greatly from those that apply to free-living humans as to render them of questionable direct relevance. The inability to predict the applicability of findings from a particular species of animals to humans was underscored by John Cairns, who wrote: "Who could have guessed that *Homo sapiens* would share with the humble guinea pig the unenviable distinction of being incapable of synthesizing ascorbic acid, or share with armadillos a susceptibility to the bacterium that causes leprosy, or that intestinal cancer usually occurs in the large intestine of humans and the small intestine of sheep?"[2]

Another major concern about the extrapolation of the findings of animal studies to humans relates to differences in dosages and routes of administration. For example, animal experiments clearly indicated that Canadian rats fed daily the equivalent of 15 gallons of saccharin-containing beverages developed bladder cancer. However, observational studies of humans that followed showed no increase in bladder cancer for adults consuming usual amounts of saccharin-containing diet foods and beverages.[3]

While the findings from animals are limited in their ability to provide a reliable quantitative estimate of human risk, their precision provides crucial information to set priorities for epidemiologic research. Unfortunately, however, while epidemiology has the unique advantage of direct relevance to free-living humans, it also has the unique and troubling disadvantage of far greater imprecision. Unlike basic research, epidemiology is crude and inexact, since even careful observations on free-living humans can rarely take place under the rigidly controlled conditions possible in a laboratory. The results of a single observational study provide reliable evidence of whether there is a valid statistical association, but support for a judgment of causality derives from consideration of a number of studies that use different methods at various times in a variety of geographic or cultural settings and among different populations, and that yield consistent evidence.

Epidemiologic studies can be either descriptive (case reports, case series, correlational studies and cross-sectional surveys) or analytic (observational studies, either case-control or cohort, and randomized trials). Descriptive studies are primarily useful for the formulation of hypotheses, while analytic studies are useful for hypothesis-testing. Observational studies are often criticized because of their potential for bias—case-control studies because of the selection of individuals into the study and in their recall of prior events, and cohort studies because of losses-to-follow-up. Nonetheless, even at worst, observational studies, if well-designed and -conducted, will contribute importantly relevant information to a totality of evidence which provides a firm rationale for testing in randomized trials. At best, such observational studies can provide reliable evidence to test hypotheses. Indeed, many, if not most, exposure-disease relationships have been well established from observational evidence, sometimes well ahead of an understanding of biologic mechanisms.

For example, in 1950 Doll and Hill in the United Kingdom[4] and Wynder and Graham in the United States[5] conducted case-control studies clearly establishing a valid association between smoking and lung cancer. Doll and Hill went on to examine this question further in a prospective cohort study of British doctors,[6] and after a decade of follow-up, reported results consistent with the earlier case-control studies. Since the biggest impact of these findings was, in fact, on the behavior of the British doctors themselves, after a second decade of follow-up,[7] Doll and Peto were able to evaluate the effect of smoking cessation on decreasing risks of lung cancer as well as to quantitate the greater importance of duration than dose. On the basis of the totality of evidence, which included their case-control study, in 1950 Doll and Hill judged smoking to be a cause of lung cancer, but at that time postulated arsenic as a possible etiologic factor.[4] In 1964 the U.S. Surgeon General also judged smoking a definite cause of this disease,[8] still years before there was any clear understanding of the actual mechanism of alterations in DNA by initiators or promoters of cancer.

Thus, while basic research and theoretic speculations are crucial to identify mechanisms which may explain causal or preventive factors, direct answers to the question of whether factors play a causal or preventive role must come from straightforward observation of what actually happens in human populations.

There are a number of situations in which observational studies are particularly advantageous. The first relates to the evaluation of interventions that require long duration. An example of this is the evaluation of the treatment of mild to moderate hypertension in decreasing risk of coronary heart disease (CHD). Observational studies consistently demonstrated an approximately 40% increased risk of stroke and a 25–30% increased risk of CHD associated with a 6 mm Hg increase in diastolic blood pressure. Individual randomized trials of drug therapy for mild to moderate hypertension, defined as diastolic blood pressure between 90–105 mm Hg, yielded evidence of clear benefits as regards stroke, but inconsistent results for CHD. By the late 1980s, 14 randomized trials of drug therapy in 37,000 subjects had been conducted. An overview, or meta-analysis, showed that a decrease of 6 mm Hg in diastolic blood pressure significantly reduced stroke by 42% and myocardial infarction (MI) by 14%.[9] This decrease in MI seen in the randomized trials was about half the 25–30% reduction predicted from observational studies conducted over decades. This difference may well have been due to chance, but also could have been due to the fact that stroke risk immediately decreases after lowering of blood pressure levels, while risk of MI may be influenced by prolonged effects of hypertension on more chronic processes of atherogenesis. Observing the full impact of blood pressure lowering on MI risk, therefore, may require far longer than the usual three to five years of treatment in a randomized trial. Finally, there are cardiotoxic effects of chlorthiazide diuretics, the first-line class of drug used in most of these trials. These agents raise low-density lipoprotein (LDL) cholesterol by 5 percent, which could, at least in theory, increase risk of myocardial infarction about 10–15%. Thus, observational evidence is crucial to understanding the effects of exposures requiring long durations.

Another particular strength of observational studies lies in evaluating associations where the relative risk (RR) is moderate to large in size—greater than 1.5. For example, the finding that regular, lifelong smokers are at 15–20 times greater risk of lung cancer than nonsmokers has been reliably detected in observational studies, both case-control and cohort. Observational studies also provided reliable evidence that duration is more important than dose in lung cancer risk, and that smoking cessation lowers lung cancer risk to a level about midway between that of continuing smokers and never-smokers, with the effect begining 2–5 years after cessation and reaching a maximum benefit after 8–10 years.[10]

Similarly, the finding that current cigarette smokers have about 80% increased risk of CHD has been consistently demonstrated in a large number of case-control and cohort studies conducted over the last 30 years in a wide range of cultural settings and involving millions of person-years of observation.[11] Observational studies have further demonstrated that, for CHD risk, the amount currently smoked is more important than duration, and that cardiovascular disease risk reduction begins almost immediately upon cessation, with risks approaching those of never-smokers within several years, even among the elderly.[12] Nevertheless, smoking was not judged to be a causal factor in the etiology of CHD until far later than the judgment that smoking caused lung cancer.[13]

This may have been due, in part, to a lack of understanding of the biologic mechanisms responsible for an increase in CHD risk due to smoking, but also to the far smaller relative risk of CHD compared with lung cancer for smokers. As the relative risk gets smaller, there is increasing concern in observational studies that some factor other than the exposure being evaluated may actually explain all or part of the finding. For example, cigarette smokers may have other characteristics or lifestyle practices that independently affect their risk of CHD. Information can be collected on any potential confounding variables known to the investigator and then used in the data analysis to adjust for any impact of these factors. However, there can be no adjustment for unknown confounding variables.[1]

When a large effect is seen, such as with smoking and lung cancer, the amount of uncontrolled confounding may affect the magnitude of the relative risk estimate, making it, for example as high as 25 or as low as 10. However, it is unlikely that it would change the conclusion that there is a strong relationship between smoking and lung cancer. Even in the case of smoking and CHD, uncontrolled confounding may mean that the observed effect is as small as a relative risk of 1.6 or as large as a relative risk of 2.0, instead of the relative risk of 1.8 most consistently seen in observational studies. That range of uncertainty, however, will not materially affect the conclusion that current cigarette smoking clearly increases the risk of CHD. On the other hand, when the most plausible effect size is 20% to 30%, as is the case with many promising interventions, a small amount of uncontrolled confounding could mean the difference between a relative risk of 0.8, which indicates a 20% decreased risk, 1.0, which indicates no effect, or even 1.2, which suggests a 20% increased risk. For this reason, reliable inferences about interventions likely to confer only small to moderate benefits can emerge only from large-scale randomized trials.

By allocating subjects to the exposure of interest at random, clinical trials eliminate the confounding that may be introduced in observational studies by self-selection. The unique strength of randomized trials is that, if the sample is large enough, on average the two study groups will be comparable with respect not only to those confounding variables known to the investigators, but also to any unknown factors that might be related to risk of the disease. Thus, randomized trials achieve a degree of control of confounding that is simply not possible with any observational design strategy, and thus allow for the testing of small effects that are beyond the ability of observational studies to detect reliably.

Although observational studies are not the optimal strategy to detect small to moderate effects, their findings are often used to generate hypotheses or provide useful leads to be tested in randomized trials. For example, the possible role of beta-carotene in the chemoprevention of cancer has been extensively examined in case-control studies as well as in dietary and blood-based cohort studies.[14] The available observational evidence has provided strong support for the hypothesis that beta-carotene may reduce cancer risk, with particularly consistent findings for lung cancer. But while additional observational studies would certainly contribute to the totality of evidence, regardless of the number or size of such investigations or even the consistency of their findings, they would never be able to answer reliably whether beta-carotene reduces human cancer risk, since those whose diets are rich in beta-carotene may have other characteristics or lifestyle factors that independently decrease their risk of cancer. Moreover, the magnitude of the impact of such uncontrolled or uncontrollable confounding is likely to be as large as the postulated beneficial effect of beta-carotene on cancer risk. Observational evidence, however, has been crucial to the initiation of a number of large-scale trials to evaluate this hypothesis reliably. At present, ongoing trials are testing beta-carotene in cancer chemoprevention in a wide variety of populations, including Finnish men at high risk due to smoking history, poorly nourished Chinese men and women at high risk, and well-nourished American male physicians and female nurses at usual risk.[15]

Observational evidence has also provided sufficient promising evidence to support the conduct of randomized trials of antioxidant vitamins in the reduction of risk of cardiovascular disease. In basic research, antioxidants have been shown to inhibit oxidation of LDL cholesterol, the particularly atherogenic form of cholesterol, providing a mechanism for a possible benefit on cardiovascular disease. Several analytic blood-based and prospective cohort studies have now been carried out to explore this hypothesis, and their findings, while not wholly consistent, provide support for a possible role of antioxidant vitamins in cardiovascular disease.[16] As with cancer studies of beta-carotene, these observational data cannot definitively evaluate this hypothesis, but do provide a solid basis for examining this question in randomized controlled trials.[17]

A similar situation exists with respect to the possible role of aspirin on risks and benefits of cardiovascular disease in apparently healthy women. In secondary prevention among those with prior cardiovascular disease, as well as in the setting of acute MI, randomized trials have clearly demonstrated benefits of aspirin in both men and women.[18] In primary prevention, however, the randomized trial data are limited to two trials in men. Taken together, their results demonstrate a clear benefit of aspirin with regard to risk of a first MI,[19] although the data remain inconclusive on stroke and vascular mortality. In women, the currently available epidemiologic data on aspirin in primary prevention consist of four observational studies whose findings, not surprisingly, are inconsistent.

Specifically, the Boston Collaborative Drug Surveillance Program included two case-control studies involving a total of 776 patients hospitalized with acute MI.[20] Of these, 92 were women admitted for a first MI. For those reporting regular aspirin use, there was a 26% reduction in risk, a relative risk of 0.74. Most recently, a benefit was also reported in a subgroup analysis of aspirin use and cardiovascular disease from the Nurses' Health Study.[21] The Nurses' Health Study analysis was based on the experience of more than 87,000 participants free of diagnosed CHD and stroke at baseline. Those reporting the use of one to six aspirin tablets per week experienced a relative risk of MI of 0.75 compared with women not taking aspirin. However, no benefit of aspirin was apparent for women taking 7–14 or 15 or more aspirin tablets per week. A study of more than 22,000 residents of a California retirement community in 1989 reported a reduction in risk of MI for regular users of aspirin in men, but not women (RR = 1.06). Moreover, the risk of ischemic heart disease was elevated in women (RR = 1.7).[22] Finally, in the parent American Cancer Society Study—whose offspring study has reported a benefit of aspirin in colon and other cancers—an analysis that included more than 550,000 women found no apparent benefit of aspirin on death rates for CHD in men or women, with a relative risk of CHD death of 1.13 for women who selected themselves for regular aspirin use.[23]

Again, the serious limitation of such studies, regardless of the large sample sizes of women in the Nurses' Health Study and the American Cancer Society Study, is their observational design, in which there was self-selection of aspirin use, which may introduce modest, but uncontrollable, bias and confounding. To be able to distinguish the effect of the agent under study from that of other, unidentified differences between the groups when attempting to evaluate small to moderate benefits, the only reliable design strategy is a randomized trial of adquate sample size.[1]

On the basis of these observational data on aspirin and coronary heart disease in women, as well as those on beta-carotene with cancer and cardiovascular disease, a randomized trial is currently being conducted to evaluate these hypotheses. The Women's Health Study is a randomized, double-blind, placebo-controlled $2 \times 2 \times 2$ factorial trial evaluating the risks and benefits of low-dose aspirin (100 mg every other day, supplied by Miles Laboratories) as well as the antioxidant vitamins beta-carotene (50 mg every other day, supplied as Lurotin by BASF) and vitamin E (600 IU every other day, supplied by the Natural Source Vitamin E Association) on cardiovascular disease and cancer in healthy women.[24]

In conclusion, some investigators who conduct observational studies maintain that there is little need for trials, which they claim are overused and overemphasized. Similarly, clinical trialists occasionally state that the only way to answer reliably any research question is to perform a randomized trial. In fact, each discipline, and every research strategy within a discipline, contributes importantly relevant and complementary information to a totality of evidence upon which rational clinical decision-making and public policy can be reliably based. In this context, observational evidence has provided and will continue to make unique and important contributions to this totality of evidence upon which to support a judgment of proof beyond a reasonable doubt in the evaluation of interventions.

ACKNOWLEDGEMENT

We are indebted to Michael Jonas for his assistance.

REFERENCES

1. HENNEKENS, C. H. & J. E. BURING. 1987. Epidemiology in Medicine. Little, Brown. Boston, MA.
2. CAIRNS, J. 1985. The treatment of diseases and the war against cancer. Sci. Am. **253:** 51.
3. MORRISON, A. S. & J. E. BURING. 1980. Artificial sweeteners and cancer of the lower urinary tract. N. Engl. J. Med. **302:** 537.
4. DOLL, R. & A. B. HILL. 1950. Smoking and carcinoma of the lung. Br. Med. J. **2:** 739.
5. WYNDER, E. L. & E. A. GRAHAM. 1950. Tobacco smoking as a possible etiologic factor in bronchiogenic carcinoma. A study of 684 proved cases. JAMA **143:** 329.
6. DOLL, R. & A. B. HILL. 1964. Mortality in relation to smoking: Ten years' observations of British doctors. Br. Med J. **1:** 1399–1410; 1460–1467.
7. DOLL, R. & R. PETO. 1976. Mortality in relation to smoking: 20 years' observations on male British doctors. Br. Med. J **2:** 1525–1536.
8. U.S. DEPARTMENT OF HEALTH, EDUCATION AND WELFARE. 1964. Smoking and Health. Report of the Advisory Committee to the Surgeon General of the Public Health Service. PHS Publication No. 1103. Government Printing Office. Washington DC.
9. COLLINS, R., R. PETO, S. MACMAHON, P. HEBERT, N. H. FIEBACH, K. A. EBERLEIN, N. QIZILBASH, J. O. TAYLOR & C. H. HENNEKENS. 1990. Blood pressure, stroke and coronary heart disease, Part II: Effects of short-term reductions in blood pressure—An overview of randomised drug trials in an epidemiological context. Lancet *335:* 827–838.
10. DOLL, R. & R. PETO. 1978. Cigarette smoking and bronchial carcinoma: Dose and time relationships among regular smokers and lifelong non-smokers. J. Epidemiol. Community Health **32:** 303–313.
11. HENNEKENS, C. H., J. BURING & S. L. MAYRENT. 1984. Smoking and aging in coronary heart disease. *In* Smoking and Aging. R. Bosse & C. Rose, Eds.: 95–115.
12. LACROIX, A. Z., J. LANG, P. SCHERR, R. B. WALLACE, J. CORNONI-HUNTLEY, L. BERKMAN, J. D. CURB, D. EVANS & C. H. HENNEKENS. 1991. Smoking and mortality among older men and women in three communities. N. Engl. J. Med. **324:** 1619–1625.
13. U.S. DEPARTMENT OF HEALTH AND HUMAN SERVICES. 1983. The Health Consequences of Smoking: Cardiovascular Disease. A Report of the Surgeon General. Office on Smoking and Health. Rockville, MD.
14. BURING, J. E. & C. H. HENNEKENS. 1993. Retinoids and carotenoids. *In* Cancer: Principles & Practice of Oncology. V. T. DeVita, Jr., S. Hellman & S. Rosenberg, Eds. J. B. Lippincott. Philadelphia.
15. GREENWALD, P., D. W. NIXON, W. F. MALONE, G. H. KELLOFF, N. R. STERN & K. M. WITKIN. 1990. Concepts in cancer chemoprevention research. Cancer **65:** 1483–1490.
16. GAZIANO, J. M., J. E. MANSON, J. E. BURING & C. H. HENNEKENS. 1992. Dietary antioxidants and cardiovascular disease. *In* Beyond Deficiency: New Views on the Function and Health Effects of Vitamins. H. E. Sauberlich & L. J. Machlin, Eds. Ann. N.Y. Acad. Sci. **669:** 249–259.
17. STEINBERG, D. & WORKSHOP PARTICIPANTS. 1992. Antioxidants in the prevention of human atherosclerosis: Summary of the proceedings of a National Heart, Lung, and Blood Institute Workshop: September 1991, Bethesda, MD. Circulation **85:** 2338–2344.
18. HENNEKENS, C. H., J. E. BURING, P. SANDERCOCK, R. COLLINS & R. PETO. 1989. Aspirin and other antiplatelet agents in the secondary and primary prevention of cardiovascular disease. Circulation **80:** 749–756.
19. HENNEKENS, C. H., R. PETO, G. B. HUTCHISON & R. DOLL. 1988. An overview of the British and American aspirin studies. N. Engl. J. Med. **318:** 923–924.
20. BOSTON COLLABORATIVE DRUG SURVEILLANCE GROUP. 1974. Regular aspirin intake and acute myocardial infarction. Br. Med. J. **1:** 440–443.
21. MANSON, J. E., M. J. STAMPFER, G. A. COLDITZ, W. C. WILLETT, B. ROSNER,

F. E. SPEIZER & C. H. HENNEKENS. 1991. A prospective study of aspirin use and primary prevention of cardiovascular disease in women. JAMA **266:** 521–527.
22. PAGANINI-HILL, A., A. CHAO, R. K. ROSS & B. E. HENDERSON. 1989. Aspirin use and chronic diseases: A cohort of the elderly. Br. Med. J. **299:** 1247–1250.
23. HAMMOND, E. C. & L. GARFINKEL. 1975. Aspirin and coronary heart disease: Findings of a prospective study. Br. Med. J. **2:** 269–271.
24. BURING, J. E. & C. H. HENNEKENS FOR THE WOMEN'S HEALTH STUDY RESARCH GROUP. 1992. The Women's Health Study: Summary of the study design. J. Myocardial Ischemia **4:** 27–29.

DISCUSSION

DR. ALAN MORRIS (*LDS Hospital, Salt Lake City, Utah*): That was a nice review, and I appreciate the distinction you made between the controls available in the laboratory setting and the imprecision characteristic of work in humans. I would just point out that there is one arena in which controls are now becoming quite readily available, at least in certain centers, and that is in the hospitalized patient in the critical care environment, in which the utilization of electronic databases has provided a means for reliable data capture. Furthermore, the introduction of computerized protocol control of decision making has provided a means of controlling the process of care. In one center such a protocol has been used now for about 45,000 hours of around-the-clock control of life support in critically ill people. These critically ill patients are particularly resource-consumptive because of the enormous cost of their care. So I would add that category of subject to your comments about clinical research in general and would point out that this circumstance may provide a means of introducing more laboratory characteristics into human research.

DR. C. H. HENNEKENS (*Brigham and Women's Hospital, Boston, Mass.*): You've made a very important point with respect to both advancing knowledge through epidemiologic research as well as trying to understand mechanisms from populations of the kind you've mentioned. Nevertheless, alternative explanations for any particular hypothesis derive from the roles of chance, bias, and confounding factors, although such databases as you've mentioned offer the opportunity to minimize the role of chance because of the very large sample size. And perhaps one can get a good handle on confounding factors because of the number and nature of the variables collected. But we still have to be concerned about modest or uncontrollable biases in such designs as well.

Can We Learn Anything from Small Trials?

DAVID L. SACKETT AND DEBORAH J. COOK

Fellowship Program in General Internal Medicine
Department of Medicine
McMaster University
Hamilton, Ontario L8V 1C3, Canada

INTRODUCTION

The overriding objective of therapeutic research is to get the most patients on the best treatment the soonest. The task of disseminating evidence regarding appropriate therapy and ensuring its application in health care is an heroic one and the measures taken to do so are discussed elsewhere in this volume by Brian Haynes and Jonathan Lomas.

This paper will address the strategies and tactics of deciding upon the best therapy, and attempt to answer the question of whether we can learn anything about that best therapy from small clinical trials. And we believe that the answer to that question is "yes" and that three useful things can be learned from small clinical trials. First, we can learn that "the emperor has no clothes" when small trials cause us to challenge conventional, but untested clinical wisdom. Second, because the important number in any trial is the number of events, and not the number of study patients, some small trials are so definitively positive that they can identify the best therapy on their own. And third, small trials, even when individually inconclusive, can be appraised and synthesized in scientific overviews and meta-analyses, which proffer greater credibility than a single huge trial of size similar to the sum of the small ones.

The trials we are referring to here are methodologically rigorous randomized trials, not studies with sub-experimental design such as cohort or case-control studies. In generating guides for the clinician to ensure appropriate health care delivery, all trials of the former type, large and small, need to be considered. These are key to deciding on the best therapy, as we have learned from both bitter and sweet prior experience.

What rules of evidence ought to apply when expert committees meet to generate recommendations for the clinical management of patients? Should only the thoroughly validated results of randomized clinical trials be admissible in order to avoid or minimize the application of useless or harmful therapy? Or, to maximize the potential benefits to patients (including those possible from unproved remedies), ought a synthesis of the experiences of experienced clinicians form the basis for such recommendations?

Ample precedent exists for the latter approach even when attempts are made to replace it.[1] However, for the following reasons, the non-experimental evidence that forms the recalled experiences of seasoned clinicians will tend to overestimate efficacy:

1. Favorable treatment responses are more likely to be recognized and remembered by clinicians when their patients comply with treatments and keep follow-up appointments. However, there are already five documented instances in which compliant patients in the placebo groups of randomized trials exhibited far more favorable outcomes (including survival) than their noncompliant companions.[2-7] Because high compliance is therefore a marker for better outcomes, even when treatment is useless, our uncontrolled clinical experiences often will cause us to conclude that compliant patients must have been receiving efficacious therapy.
2. Unusual patterns of symptoms (such as transient ischemic attacks) or signs (such as high blood pressure measurements) and extreme laboratory test results, when they are reassessed a short time later, tend to return toward the more usual, normal result.[8] Because of this universal tendency for regression toward the mean, any treatment (regardless of its efficacy) that is initiated in the interim may appear efficacious.
3. Routine clinical practice is never "blind," as both patients and their clinicians know when active treatment is under way. As a result, both the placebo effect (which has shown, for example, that angina pectoris can be relieved by mock internal mammary ligation[9]) and the desire of patients and clinicians for success can cause both parties to overestimate efficacy. The overestimate may in part be a consequence of bias in the interpretation of diagnostic tests which indicate whether patients have had an adverse outcome (such as a deep venous thrombosis as assessed by venography).

For the preceding reasons, the "consensus" approach based upon uncontrolled clinical experience risks precipitating the widespread application of treatments that are useless or even harmful. These same treatments are much less likely to be judged efficacious in double-blind, randomized trials than in uncontrolled case series of unblinded, "open" comparisons with contemporaneous or historical series of patients; hence the maxim: "Therapeutic reports with controls tend to have no enthusiasm, and reports with enthusiasm tend to have no controls."

Furthermore, for their results to be valid and clinically useful, scientific standards must be met by both large and small randomized trials. The clinician who uses the medical literature to help in patient care first identifies the specific question, then searches and retrieves a relevant article, and proceeds to critically appraise it. In assessing both the credibility and the clinical application of a therapy article, efficient users of the medical literature ask the following:

(1) *Are the results valid?*
  i. Was the assignment of patients randomized?
  ii. Was complete follow-up achieved?
  iii. Were patients and the health team masked to treatment allocation?
  iv. Were the groups comparable?
  v. Were non-experimental treatments equal?
(2) *How big was the treatment effect?*
(3) *What are the implications for the patient at hand, and for patients in general?*
  i. Were all clinically relevant outcomes considered?
  ii. To whom are the results generalizable?
  iii. What are the expected results of the intervention?

Having reviewed the guidelines available to evaluate a clinical trial, and having affirmed the need for rigorous randomized trials, regardless of size, we see that the stage is set for us to consider the three circumstances under which we *can* learn something from small trials.

LESSONS FROM THE SMALL TRIAL

First, sometimes small trials, even trials that are too small, prompt us to question conventional but untested therapeutic wisdom. The example we will give here involves the internal mammary artery. Now used with considerable success as a conduit in coronary artery bypass grafting, this vessel also was the object of surgical attention 40 years ago in efforts to combat intractable angina pectoris.

Nicely documented by Ernest Barsamian, the simple ligation of the internal mammary artery (a very safe operation, easily performed using local anesthesia) had repeatedly been followed not only by symptomatic, but also by electrocardiographic and treadmill improvements in more than three-quarters of the patients who underwent the procedure.[10] This procedure gained popularity throughout Europe and North America until skeptics challenged it with hard science.

When Fish and his colleagues, hypothesizing that its apparent efficacy was a placebo effect, told preoperative patients that the procedure was experimental, had no physiologic basis, and was of uncertain benefit, the rate of improvement fell to less than 20 percent.[11] The death blows to this procedure were dealt by two simultaneous trials in which the operation proceeded to the key step of placing a loose ligature around the isolated internal mammary artery, at which point a random half were tied off and the other half left alone.[9,12] When the sham-operated patients fared as well as those whose arteries were tied off, the state of the emperor's new clothes was apparent to all and the procedure was rapidly abandoned.

Although conducted to answer an important clinical question, and used to justify the need for randomized trials of coronary bypass two decades later, these two "negative" trials contained a grand sum of only 35 patients. In fact, to rule out even a 50 percent reduction in intractable angina, each of them should have contained more than that number of patients per treatment arm. Too small to be conclusive on their own, these studies forced the rethinking of the biologic rationale for the operation and led to its abandonment.

Second, because the important number in any trial is the number of events, not the number of study patients, some small trials give such definitively positive results that they identify the best therapy on their own. A useful example here is the first of the landmark U.S. Veterans Administration hypertension trials, in which patients with initial diastolic blood pressures between 115–129 mm Hg were randomly allocated to placebo or stepped care with active antihypertensive drugs.[13] It took just a year and a half, with only 70 patients on placebo and just 73 on active therapy, to demonstrate a statistically significant difference in major morbidity and mortality of 39 percent in the former group and 3 percent in the latter. Such combinations of high event rates on placebo and large risk reductions on active therapy are not common, but when they coexist, can be sufficient to demonstrate the best therapy in a small trial. And, of course, clinical trialists often seek to replicate this happy state of affairs by adjusting eligibility criteria so that only high-risk, highly responsive patients are admitted to a trial, sacrificing generalizability for power.

Finally, small trials, even when individually inconclusive, can serve as the basis for convincingly conclusive overviews and meta-analyses that have greater credibility than a large trial of similar size to their sum. This is best shown in reviewing the operation of large consensus development groups. For example, every 3 to 4 years a group of clinicians and other scientists gathers under the auspices of the American College of Chest Physicians to review and generate recommendations on the use of antithrombotic agents.[14] Each conference begins with a review of the reasons behind the previously noted statement: "Therapeutic reports with controls tend to have no enthusiasm, and reports with enthusiasm tend to have no controls."

Then the conference goes beyond this rigid view and recognizes that

> The foregoing discussion should not be misinterpreted as constituting a mandate for discarding the large body of uncontrolled observations by clinicians who have used these agents in an effort to halt the progression and complications of thromboembolism. For some of the disorders under consideration here, randomized control trials have not yet been carried out (nor, because of overwhelming evidence of efficacy from cohort studies, are they likely to be conducted), and the only information base for generating some of the recommendations comes from systematic clinical observations.
>
> What this does mean, however, is that it is important, whenever possible, to base firm recommendations (and especially those involving risk to patients) on the results of rigorously controlled investigations and to be much more circumspect when recommendations rest only on the results of uncontrolled clinical observations.

The limited place of the small randomized trial was recognized at the first such conference by its position in a hierarchy of levels of evidence. Thus, when summarizing what was known about the therapy of a given clinical entity, the participants began by specifying the level of evidence that was being used in each case, according to the following classification[a]:

Level I: Randomized trials with low false-positive (α) and low false-negative (β) errors (high power). By "low false-positive (α) error" is meant a "positive" trial that demonstrated a statistically significant benefit from experimental treatment. By "low false-negative (β) error (high power)" is meant a "negative" trial that demonstrated no effect of therapy, yet was large enough to exclude the possibility of a minimally important benefit (that is, had very narrow 95% confidence intervals, the upper end of which was less than the minimum clinically important benefit, thereby excluding any improvement due to the test treatment). The minimally important benefit, in this context, defines the smallest difference in function that a patient and clinician agree to be worth the risks and trouble of offering and accepting the treatment.[15] The elements of a valid and useful randomized trial were those already summarized above.

Level II: Randomized trials with high false-positive (α) and/or high false-negative (β) errors (low power). By "high false-positive (α) error" is meant a trial with an interesting positive trend that is not statistically significant. For example, five of the six early trials of the use of aspirin after myocardial infarction generated positive, but statistically nonsignificant trends favoring aspirin. By "high false-negative (β) error (low power)" is meant a "negative" trial that concluded that therapy was not efficacious, yet there was a real possibility of a clinically important benefit because the trial had very wide 95% confidence intervals on the effect of

---

[a] Levels III-V describe non-experimental evidence from contemporaneous and non-contemporaneous cohort studies and case series, and will not be further considered here.

experimental therapy. For example, several trials of anticoagulants in completed thrombotic stroke concluded that such treatment was ineffective when, in fact, the confidence intervals on the treatment effect they observed ranged from virtually eliminating subsequent deterioration and death to doubling the risk of these outcomes. In this situation, the 95% confidence interval includes the minimally important benefit, and clearly the strength of inference is lower than would be the case for Level I studies.

Primary studies are often limited by inadequate sample size, which leaves negative studies open to large false-negative (β) errors (in which important differences that actually exist may be missed). Moreover, even positive studies, when small, will generate such wide confidence intervals that clnicians are left uncertain as to whether the treatment effect is trivial or huge. Clearly, many if not most small trials reside at this level of evidence, too small to rule in or rule out efficacy.

The advent of meta-analysis (the quantitative synthesis of relevant, high-quality study results) has a major impact here, for it can show that two or more high-quality, homogeneous but small (and therefore Level II) trials really provide Level I evidence of treatment efficacy. Stated another way, when the results of Level II studies are aggregated, the lower limit of the confidence interval around the pooled estimate may then become greater than the minimally important benefit, rendering the aggregate of several Level II studies now Level I evidence.

The most compelling rationale for meta-analysis is its ability to generate more precise estimates (reflected in narrower confidence intervals) of the true treatment effect, such as a relative risk reduction, than can be provided by any individual trial. A key element in interpreting this confidence interval is its relation to the ''minimally important benefit'' which, if met or exceeded, will lead clinicians to use the treatment. If the entire confidence interval surpasses this minimally important benefit, the inference that the treatment is effective is very strong. For example, if the lower limit of a 90% confidence interval of a relative risk reduction exceeded a minimally important benefit, this means that there is 95% chance that the true treatment effect is greater than the minimally important benefit.

If, on the other hand, the confidence interval brackets the minimally important benefit, the strength of the inference that treatment should be administered in such patients is much weaker. Finally, when sample sizes are very small or events very rare, even though the point estimate of benefit may favor active treatment, the lower limit of the confidence interval may suggest not only the possibility that the treatment is harmful, but also that the degree of harm is important. Under these circumstances, the strength of inference in a positive treatment recommendation is very weak.

Thus, the advent of meta-analysis permits us to sharpen this classification further by generating a ''pooled'' estimate of the treatment's efficacy across all the high-quality, relevant trials, especially when these trials are small in size. Meta-analyses also reveal any inconsistencies in the estimates of efficacy between trials (''heterogeneity''), highlighting those that require further scrutiny before an overall treatment policy can be generated.

In the most recent conference, high-quality overviews were incorporated into the determination of Levels of Evidence. If no high-quality overview was available, the Levels were determined as previously. If, however, a rigorous overview was available, it becomes the basis for determining the Level of Evidence. A rigorous overview, in which the quality of the original studies is high and there is no unexplained heterogeneity in trial results, could raise the designation of the Level of Evidence.

For example, if the lower limit of the confidence interval for a relative risk reduction (the estimate that was least favorable to active treatment, but still consistent with the trial resutls) *exceeded* the minimally important benefit that would trigger its clinical use, the treatment effect was judged both large and important. Therefore, the treatment was rated at Level I+ (regardless of whether the individual trials were Level I or Level II) if the result was homogeneous over a collection of high-quality trials. This rating was lowered to I− if a rigorous overview documented heterogeneity in the trial results.

If the lower limit of the confidence interval for a relative risk reduction *fell below* the minimally important benefit that would trigger its clinical use (but the point estimate of its effect was at or above the minimally important benefit), the effect of treatment might be trivial. It was rated at Level II+ (regardless of whether the individual trials were Level I or Level II) if the result was homogeneous over a collection of high-quality trials. As before, this rating was lowered to II− if a rigorous overview documented heterogeneity.

SUMMARY

In summary, then, we can learn three useful things from small clinical trials. First, we can learn when to challenge conventional but untested therapeutic wisdom. Second, because the patient number in any trial is the number of events, rather than the number of study patients, some small trials are so definitively positive that they are sufficient to identify the best therapy. And third, small trials, even when individually inconclusive, can serve as the basis for convincingly conclusive overviews and meta-analyses that carry, and deserve, greater credibility than a single large trial of similar size to their sum.

REFERENCES

1. National Institutes of Health Consensus Development Conferences. 1977–1978. **1:** 1–43.
2. Coronary Drug Project Research Group. 1980. Influence of adherence treatment and response of cholesterol on mortality in the Coronary Drug Project. N. Engl. J. Med. **303:** 1038–1041.
3. ASHER, W. L. & H. W. HARPER. 1973. Effect of human chorionic gonadotropin on weight loss, hunger, and feeling of well-being. Am. J. Clin. Nutr. **26:** 211–218.
4. HOGARTY, G. E. & G. E. GOLDBERG. 1973. Drug and sociotherapy in the aftercare of schizophrenic patients. Arch. Gen. Psychiatry **28:** 54–64.
5. FULLER, R., H. ROTH & S. LONG. 1983. Compliance with disulfiram treatment of alcoholism. J. Chronic Dis. **36:** 161–170.
6. PIZZO, P. A., K. J. ROBICHAUD, B. K. EDWARDS, C. SCHUMAKER, B. S. KRAMER, & A. JOHNSON. 1983. Oral antibiotic prophylaxis in patients with cancer: A double blind randomized placebo-controlled trial. J. Pediatr. **102:** 125–133.
7. HORWITZ, R. I., C. M. VISCOLI, L. BERKMAN *et al.* 1990. Treatment adherence and risk of death after myocardial infarction. Lancet **336:** 542–545.
8. SACKETT, D. L., R. B. HAYNES, G. H. GUYATT & P. TUGWELL. 1991. Clinical Epidemiology: A Basic Science for Clinical Medicine, 2nd ed:36, 39. Little, Brown. Boston, MA.
9. COBB, L. A., G. I. THOMAS, D. H. DILLARD, K. A. MERENDINO & R. A. BRUCE. 1959. An evaluation of internal-mammary-artery ligation by a double-blind technique. N. Engl. J. Med. **260:** 1115–1118.
10. BARSAMIAN, E. M. 1977. The rise and fall of internal mammary artery ligation in the treatment of angina pectoris and the lessons learned. *In* Costs, Risks and Benefits

of Surgery. J. P. Bunker, B. A. Barnes & F. Mosteller, Eds.: 212–220. Oxford University Press, New York.

11. FISH, R. G., T. P. CRYMES & M. G. LOVELL. 1958. Internal-mammary-artery ligation for angina pectoris. Its failure to produce relief. N. Engl. J. Med. **259:** 418.

12. DIMOND, E. G., C. F. KITTLE & J. E. CROCKETT. 1958. Evaluation of internal mammary artery ligation and sham operation for angina pectoris. Circulation. **18:** 712.

13. Veterans Administration Cooperative Study Group on Antihypertensive Agents. 1967. I. Results in patients with diastolic blood pressures averaging 115 through 129 mm Hg. JAMA **202:** 1028–1034.

14. COOK, D. J., G. H. GUYATT, A. LAUPACIS & D. L. SACKETT. 1992. Rules of evidence and clinical recommendations on the use of antithrombotic agents. Chest **102**(Suppl): 305S–311S.

15. GUYATT, G. H., L. B. BERMAN, M. TOWNSEND *et al.* 1987. A measure of quality of life for clinical trials in lung disease. Thorax **42:** 773–778.

DISCUSSION

RICHARD DOLL (*Cancer Research Fund, Oxford, U.K.*): I'd like to add my personal experience to that of Drs. Sackett and Cook. The smallest conclusive control trial that I know of was one on 12 patients treated with beta blockers when they were first introduced for use in angina. But the design of this trial was one which is perfect statistically, but is so seldom actually practical in ordinary medical practice, namely a crossover trial in which each patient had each treatment twice so that you were able to compare the variations within patients as well as between patients. And that trial on 12 patients gave a *p* value of 0.001.

DAVID SACKETT (*McMaster University Clinic, Ontario, Canada*): We have a service where we can carry out randomized trials on individual patients. The issue here is one in which one randomizes the sequence with which patients receive active drug or placebo. The purpose, of course, is not to determine efficacy as clinical policy, but an issue of quality of care of the individual patient. As it happens, a number of these patients have had a disorder called fibrositis and have negotiated with the clinicians to try to achieve identical treatment outcomes in terms of removing sleep disturbances and aches and pains. As it worked out, the first such group of patients all had quite positive effects in these N of 1 trials and, of course, in these kinds of terms it's possible just with simple sign tests to get positive overall results with about six patients.

UNIDENTIFIED SPEAKER: Dr. Sackett, essentially you spoke about the retrospective evaluation of the benefits of small trials, and you found quite a number that have proven of great benefit. But the question is, in embarking on research, since we don't know what the results are going to be, when should we do small trials? What situations lend themselves to a purposefully designed small trial?

SACKETT: The short answer is that we don't do them—because of concerns about ethics. If one is randomizing patients to alternative treatments where there is a possibility of toxic side effects, that trial would have to be begun with reasonable assurance that useful answers are going to be derived. Otherwise you've subjected patients to, at the least, an invasion of privacy, and, at the worst, side effects and toxicity, without a guarantee of a rational objective answer at the conclusion of the trial. So we would not engage in randomized trials in which we did not feel we'd identified high-risk high-response groups.

TOM CHALMERS (*New England Medical Center, Boston, Mass.*): I'd like to add two points to this presentation. With regard to the fact that patients who are compliant and take their pills live longer than those who don't, there is one notable exception—the case of the University Group Diabetes Program. When those assigned at random to the active drug were dichotomized into compliant and noncompliant patients, the latter lived longer than the former, a reversal of the usual. That point has been forgotten by a lot of people.

SACKETT: And, of course, the same thing occurred in encainide and flecainide.

CHALMERS: I was going to ask whether that had been found in the other long-term study and in the arrhythmic drug study. The second point I want to make is that it's nice to be able to recognize one's mistakes publically. When you contemplate a randomized control trial but don't have enough patients to satisfy a type 1 and type 2 error of reasonable importance, I used to advocate abandoning the trial. But the last part of your presentation, Dr. Sackett, shows the absolute fallacy of that concept in that one should not pay any attention to the number of patients available but should go ahead and do a small trial in the anticipation that provided we solve the publication bias problem, which will be discussed later, eventually the small trials can be combined and the type 2 error reduced.

SACKETT: But again, there is the ethical dilemma of the individual's doing a trial that she knows to be too small.

Doing Good Before There's Harm

WILLIAM L. ROPER

Centers for Disease Control and Prevention
Mailstop D14
1600 Clifton Road, NE
Atlanta, Georgia 30333

STEPHEN B. THACKER[a]

National Center for Environmental Health
Centers for Disease Control and Prevention
Mailstop F29
4770 Bufard Highway, NE
Atlanta, Georgia 30341-3724

INTRODUCTION

In his foregoing chapter,[1] Dr. William Silverman clearly articulates the theme of this book, "Doing More Good Than Harm," and Dr. Mosteller gives a stimulating presentation on the theme of evaluating interventions.[2] Together, these two themes are reflected strongly in the activities at the Centers for Disease Control and Prevention (CDC)—formerly, the Centers for Disease Control—that we call "prevention effectiveness."

In this paper, we define prevention effectiveness, describe the CDC's activities and plans for the future, and illustrate these activities with two case studies, one of measles and the other of breast cancer. Finally, we discuss the importance of prevention in health care reform and how prevention-effectiveness methods should be used in any reform programs.

The authors of the articles in this book make it clear that the "gold standard" for evaluating clinical prevention activities is the clinical randomized controlled trial (RCT). Meta-analysis consolidates information from many RCTs to give us a broader view of a particular intervention or clinical problem. Some researchers, however, emphasize the importance of observational data in many clinical situations. In public health, we rarely have the luxury of doing RCTs, yet we must still develop sound public health policy on the basis of available information. Consequently, we have had to develop expertise in assessing the effectiveness of programs and intervention methods. As a result, we have an excellent record in conducting studies of effectiveness and cost in fields such as immunization as well as in using tools such as decision analysis and meta-analysis to formulate policy.

Nevertheless, more has been demanded from prevention activities than from clinical medicine.[3] A surgical procedure may need only to be safe; a medical procedure may need only to be effective. Prevention activities, on the other hand, must often be cost-effective or even cost-saving. This situation, in fact, reflects the reality that, despite rhetoric to the contrary, prevention has a role secondary to clinical care. This reality is underscored by the fact that less than three percent of the federal dollar is spent on prevention activities.[4]

---

[a] To whom correspondence should be addressed.

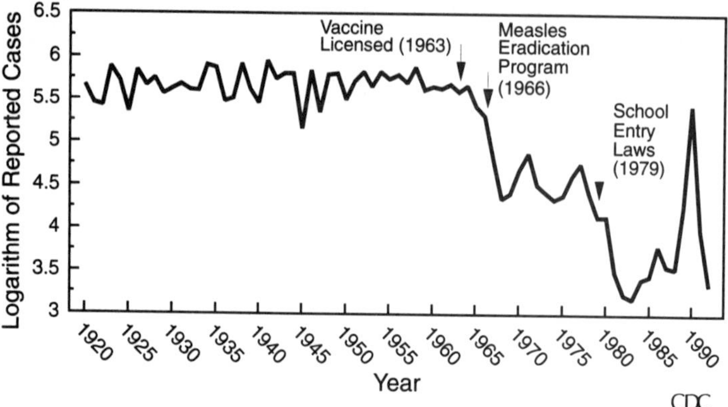

FIGURE 1. Reported cases of measles in the United States: 1920–1992 (1992 provisional). SOURCE: National Notafiable Diseases Surveillance System.

In the past three years, the CDC has focused on three priority areas. The first of these is strengthening the nation's public health system, the second is making prevention a practical reality, and the third is improving the health of children. Assessing prevention effectiveness is an important part of making prevention real for every American. The assessment of prevention effectiveness is an ongoing process that uses both quantitative and qualitative analyses to measure the impact that prevention policies, programs, and practices have on public health.[5] Thorough analysis extends beyond assessment of effectiveness, safety, and cost: it involves examining the societal consequences of disease and injury prevention activities and includes medical, legal, and ethical considerations. An underlying principle is that a procedure, drug, or practice can be analyzed for measured value, such as benefits versus cost and efficacy versus risk. I will illustrate these methods with two case studies. The first concerns measles vaccination, a tool for primary prevention. The second describes the use of mammography screening for secondary prevention of breast cancer.

MEASLES CASE STUDY

Before the measles vaccine was licensed in 1963, childhood measles infection was universal. In the United States,[6] thousands of deaths due to measles were recorded annually, reaching a peak of more than 10,000 deaths in 1923. In 1966, a campaign was launched to eradicate measles in the United States, and the next quarter century saw a dramatic decline in the incidence of measles. The average annual number of reported cases decreased from more than 500,000 prior to 1966 to only 1,497 in 1983 (FIG. 1).

Several analyses of the benefits and costs of measles immunization programs have been done. Studies of the benefit:cost ratios of vaccination against measles with a single antigen vaccine showed ratios ranging upward from 5 : 1, depending on the techniques and assumptions used.[7-9] These results contributed strongly to the acceptance and formulation in 1979 of a new national policy of measles elimination. A 1985 analysis of a combination measles-mumps-rubella vaccine showed a benefit : cost ratio of 14 : 1.[10] This finding highlighted the advantages of combined vaccines in any immunization program. Looked at another way, these data showed that the cost per case of any of the three diseases prevented was $16.85.

In recent years, however, a series of developments has undermined the assumptions and estimates used in previous analyses of programs to vaccinate children against measles. Sporadic outbreaks among schoolchildren in 1989 led to a reassessment of the national vaccine strategy. Because 5 percent of children are not protected by the initial dose of measles vaccine, a second dose is now recommended to protect this small proportion of children.[11]

The national measles epidemic in 1989 and 1990 shows that even a cost-effective primary prevention technique, such as measles vaccination, is not without flaws. Public health surveillance data show that measles cases rose from 1,500 in 1983 to 18,000 in 1989 and nearly 28,000 in 1990. The epidemic affected primarily unvaccinated preschool children in high-risk areas. More than 97 percent of U.S. children are vaccinated against measles before they enter school. The proportion of poor inner-city preschoolers who are vaccinated is substantially lower, which suggests a failure of the vaccine-delivery system. In some areas, the rate of measles vaccination for 2-year-old children may be as low as 50 percent.

Concerns about the possible adverse effects of vaccines, the limited access of some people to health care, and the practice of exempting some children from vaccination on religious grounds have all contributed to imperfect vaccine delivery in the United States. However, because the public health community focused on finding the causes for failures in vaccine delivery and then on instituting large-scale programs to overcome the delivery problems, the number of cases dropped to fewer than 10,000 in 1991 and to 2,200 in 1992.

Measles vaccine is an example of an effective technology that has had a dramatic impact on disease, but that has still fallen short of its anticipated effect. A series of pilot demonstration projects have been launched to assess alternative proposals to extend this prevention technique to all children at the recommended age of 12 to 15 months. In addition, the effectiveness of the two-dose vaccine strategy merits assessment.

BREAST CANCER CASE STUDY

In 1991, in the United States, 175,000 women contracted breast cancer, and nearly 45,000 of them will die from the disease.[12] A woman's lifetime risk of contracting breast cancer is nearly 10 percent.[13] The evidence from epidemiologic studies is strong that mammographic screening for women older than 50 years of age can reduce mortality from breast cancer, with reductions ranging from 20 to 70 percent. Current guidelines for mammography screening differ because they are based on different assessments of the effectiveness, safety, and cost of such screening. Ongoing studies in Sweden, the United Kingdom, and Canada should clarify the best ages and intervals for breast cancer screening.

Currently, we are failing to deliver breast cancer screening successfully to populations at risk. In 1987, 38 percent of women 40 years or older reported having had at least one mammogram; only 15 percent had a mammogram in the year preceding the interview.[14] The proportion of women who had ever had a mammogram increased with age among women 40 to 54 years, peaking at 45 percent for the 50- to 54-year-old age group. By age 70 or older, however, fewer than 30 percent of women reported having had a mammogram in the previous year. The women least likely to be screened for breast cancer are those who are poor or less educated.

The average cost of a mammogram in the United States is just over $100, ranging from $25 to $250.[15] Concerns about aggregate costs have been a barrier to establishing national policy recommendations about breast cancer screening, to convincing doctors and insurers that mammography is cost-effective, and to providing access for persons without health insurance. In addition, the technology for breast cancer screening is economically inefficient. By 1990, about 10,000 mammography units had been installed throughout the United States, whereas fewer than 3,000 would be needed in a moderately efficient health care delivery system.[16]

The cost-effectiveness of screening can vary according to the delivery strategies chosen and the risk of groups of women targeted. Analysts have estimated that if all women 50 years or older were screened annually by a physical breast examination alone, more than 4,000 lives would be saved, and the cost of saving an additional year of life would be $10,000 to $15,000.[13] If mammography were combined with a physical examination, more lives could be saved, but the cost of an additional year of life would be as high as $105,000. If annual screening by a physical breast examination and mammography were extended to all women 40 years or older, the cost of an additional year of life could be as high as $165,000.

In summary, although the efficacy of mammographic screening for individual women is evident, the effectiveness of screening programs for women as a group must be increased and the cost of such programs decreased. To accomplish these goals, screening should be standardized, implemented systematically, and delivered more efficiently and effectively. Future assessment of the effectiveness of breast cancer screening should include economic analyses of mammography programs, diagnostic testing, follow-up treatment, and management. Assessors must consider changes in the average age at which breast cancer is diagnosed and changes in mortality rates. Certainly, variations in breast cancer rates within racial, ethnic, and socioeconomic groups must also be assessed.

PREVENTION EFFECTIVENESS AT CDC

Policymakers should learn to use the results of prevention-effectiveness assessments to help them answer questions about a program's effectiveness, safety, and cost. To develop tools for answering such questions, we at the CDC have undertaken several activities. We first set up an advisory committee with representatives from all the major organizational units in the agency and began a strategic planning process. We also set up a Prevention Effectiveness Activity in the Epidemiology Program Office, one of our cost-cutting organizational units at the CDC. Through this activity and through the efforts of a technical work group that reports to the advisory committee, we have begun several activities that focus on training, methods development, and technical assistance.

To train the senior staff in the tools of prevention effectiveness, we identified experts in the appropriate methods to work with the CDC in developing and implementing training courses. In addition, a special course was developed for our Epidemic Intelligence Service officers, young men and women who are a vital part of the CDC's ongoing efforts in epidemiology and public health and who will be the future leaders of CDC programs. We are expanding the availability of the training to all CDC staff members as well as to colleagues in state health departments. In addition, we have developed case studies in prevention effectiveness for training purposes, and we have developed computer software for meta-analysis.

To develop methods, we established a prevention effectiveness technical work group with representatives from all parts of the CDC. We are developing a workshop to teach prevention methods to epidemiologists in state health departments and to help them identify state needs in the area of prevention. We have also published a series of articles on prevention effectiveness in the *Morbidity and Mortality Weekly Report* (*MMWR*), the CDC's major organ of communication to the world. The first of these was a special supplement that outlined information on the tools of prevention effectiveness.[17] Subsequently, the *MMWR* has regularly published articles written by the staff of a variety of CDC programs, focusing on the results of prevention-effectiveness research.

Finally, in the area of research, we are working with several large health maintenance organizations that have exceptional records in research in order to determine how well we can use their patient populations to assess interventions of public health importance.

Ultimately, I expect programs throughout CDC to integrate these assessment tools into routine evaluations of all program activities, whether these programs are conducted at the CDC or in state and local health departments.

CONCLUSIONS

As the CDC's new name emphasizes, we see prevention as central to the good health of individuals and our country. As we look forward, we must ask ourselves: What can we do to lessen the degree of uncertainty in a changing world and to make prevention a practical reality?

I think that the answer to this question lies in five areas. First, we must apply systematic strategies when assessing the effectiveness of prevention. Traditional scientific methods can make these assessments more concrete and measurable. Basic cause-and-effect relationships need to be established clearly to confirm that a particular change in behavior actually leads to a better health outcome. This step in the process is often overlooked or assumed. Information gaps need to be identified, and research needs to be conducted to fill those gaps. Economic analyses need to become routine.

Second, to maximize the usefulness of analyses, we must assess prevention effectiveness, using consistent methods for determining outcomes and economic impact. It is important for us to have comparable data when choosing which prevention strategy to recommend. Therefore, standard guidelines for selecting methods and measuring outcomes are critical in prevention-effectiveness studies.

Third, research priorities must be set with prevention in mind. Prevention-effectiveness studies help us recognize what we know and can act upon. Such studies also help us recognize what we do *not* know and, therefore, where specific research is needed. Using data from prevention-effectiveness studies, we can target our research efforts to critical questions, and we can increase our cost-efficiency by directing our resources to the areas with the greatest potential for reducing morbidity and mortality.

Fourth, the results of prevention-effectiveness studies should be used to design prevention programs. It is important to develop intervention programs that will reach people effectively and promote the best health outcomes. With effectiveness information available, we can make intelligent choices about public health activities. We can implement programs knowing with confidence that the programs we choose will make the positive health changes we want.

Fifth, effectiveness data must be used more often during policymaking. When Congress is in session, few days go by without a member of Congress calling the CDC for information on the effectiveness of a program under consideration in Washington. The reality is that a greater emphasis on accountability has put not only Congress, but business, academia, and community organizations under increasing pressure to provide quantifiable data that show the effectiveness of programs.

Finally, in the new Administration and the new Congress, health reform is an issue of primary importance. We believe that prevention must be a critical element in the new health system. Without strong active efforts at this time, much ground could be lost to the long-term detriment of the public's health. We need to clearly and forcefully make the case for prevention in a reformed system, both for community-level public health services and clinical prevention services. This goal can best be achieved by using the results of prevention-effectiveness studies.

We believe that the tools of prevention effectiveness will help us to understand better how effective our prevention activities are and to articulate better for others the real impact and importance of such efforts. At the CDC, we feel that all our programs should be based on the best available science. In public health, the scientific evidence produced by assessing prevention effectiveness will help us provide the best possible programs.

REFERENCES

1. SILVERMAN, W. A. 1993. Doing more good than harm. Ann. N.Y. Acad. Sci. This volume.
2. MOSTELLER, F. 1993. Some evaluation needs. Ann. N.Y. Acad. Sci. This volume.
3. FOEGE, W. H. 1983. Budgetary medical ethics. J. Public Health Policy **4:** 149–151.
4. BROWN, R. E., A. ELIXHAUSER, J. COREA, B. R. LUCE & S. SHEINGOLD. 1991. National expenditures for health promotion and disease prevention activities in the United States. Batelle: Medical Technology Assessment and Policy Research Center. Washington, DC.
5. THACKER, S. B., J. P. KOPLAN, W. R. TAYLOR, *et al.* 1993. Assessing the effectiveness and cost of prevention activities in health: The challenge to use data to drive program decisions. Public Health Rep. In press.
6. SENCER, D. J., H. B. DULL & A. D. LANGMUIR. 1967. Epidemiologic basis for eradication of measles in 1967. Public Health Rep. **82:** 253–256.
7. WITTE, J. J. & N. W. AXNICK. 1975. The benefits from 10 years of measles immunization in the United States. Public Health Rep. **90:** 205–207.
8. ALBRITTON, R. B. 1978. Cost-benefits of measles eradication: Effects of federal interventions. Policy Analysis **4:** 1–22.
9. KOPLAN, J. P. & C. C. WHITE. 1985. An update on the benefits and costs of measles and rubella immunization. *In* Immunizing against mental disorders: Progress in the conquest of measles and rubella. E. M. Greenberg, C. Lewis & S. Goldston, Eds. Oxford University Press. New York.
10. WHITE, C. C., J. P. KOPLAN & W. A. ORENSTEIN. 1985. Benefits, risks, and costs of immunization for measles, mumps, and rubella. Am. J. Public Health **75:** 739–744.

11. Centers for Disease Control. December 29, 1989. Measles prevention: Recommendations of the Immunization Practices Advisory Committee (ACIP). MMWR **38**(S-9): 1–18.
12. 1991. Cancer facts and figures—1991. American Cancer Society. Atlanta, GA.
13. EDDY, D. M. Screening for breast cancer. 1989. Ann. Intern. Med. **111:** 389–399.
14. DAWSON, D. A. & G. B. THOMPSON. 1989. Breast cancer risk factors and screening: United States, 1987. Vital Health Stat. **10:** 172.
15. DODD, G. D. 1987. The major issues in screening mammography: The history and present status of radiographic screening for breast cancer. Cancer **60:** 1669–1702.
16. BROWN, M. L., L. G. KESSLER & F. G. RUETER. 1990. Is the supply of mammography machines outstripping need and demand? An economic analysis. Ann. Intern. Med. **113:** 547–552.
17. TEUTSCH, S. M. 1992. A framework for assessing the effectiveness of disease and injury prevention. MMWR **41**(RR-3): 1–12.

DISCUSSION

MICHELE ORZA (*U.S. General Accounting Office, Washington, D.C.*): Dr. Roper brings a very different and important perspective to this issue. A lot of the fussing that we've been doing about outcomes research versus randomized trials versus observational studies is all taking place within a fairly small sphere and sometimes it seems as if we're going to come down to the question of comparing the prevention with the intervention. As William Silverman asked earlier: If the outcome that we desire is reduced infant mortality, are we going to get that through better prenatal care or through what he referred to as fetal salvage? Do we have the tools to make those kind of comparisons and to make that kind of judgement?

WILLIAM ROPER (*Centers for Disease Control and Prevention, Atlanta, Ga.*): I guess I would have to say no, we don't have those tools to any great extent, but we need to be setting up the kinds of studies that will permit those choices to be made more rationally. We are, of course, as a society making those decisions now—we're just not making them overtly or explicitly and we're certainly not making them very wisely.

ALAN MORRIS (*LDS Hospital, Salt Lake City, Utah*): I was very pleased to hear your emphasis, Dr. Roper, on the evaluation of the prevention techniques you're going to use. The tools you're developing might be very effectively used by the Agency for Health Care Policy and Research to evaluate the impact of the guidelines that will be generated to control care and perhaps ultimately to determine payment in the American system. Is there any chance that you might collaborate with them to see how information can be shared between the two agencies with regard to impact evaluation?

ROPER: It's an interesting proposal.

RICHARD PETO (*Clinical Trial Service Unit, Radcliffe Infirmary, Oxford, U.K.*): I can't believe that anybody in this country is serious about prevention when 3 billion dollars a year is being spent on advertising and smoking cigarettes. How can we be talking about prevention in such a context? It makes nonsense of everything. And yet the CDC has done more than corresponding agencies in almost any other country to get smoking taken seriously. But, still, as a society, the United States spends vastly more on promoting cigarettes then it spends on any sort of prevention despite the fact that cigarette smoking contributes to 40%

of all deaths in middle-aged males and in a rapidly increasing proportion of middle-aged women as well. Can you get President Clinton to actually put a 2-dollar tax on a pack of cigarettes, as was mentioned in the *New York Times* yesterday?

ROPER: I think it's going to happen simply because the government needs the money. And I hope the tax will be 4 dollars a pack. I think we're going to see a whopping increase in the tax and a corresponding decrease in the numbers of young people who take up smoking. The habit is price-sensitive—our studies have shown that.

On the Proper Use of Clinical Trials

HENRY GREENBERG

Division of Cardiology
St. Luke's/Roosevelt Hospital of
Columbia University
College of Physicians & Surgeons
428 West 59th Street
New York, New York 10019

The clinical trial, and its gigantic progeny, the meta-analysis, are powerful and effective tools with which we can measure the efficacy of therapy. The impact of drugs, therapeutic interventions, and even psychosocial manipulations on carefully defined patient groups can be precisely assessed. With care and reason these results can be extrapolated to larger groups with wide clinical relevance.

This process, part of what is known as "outcomes analysis," will be an integral component of the design of health care finance planning in the United States. In cardiology, the field I know best, prior and potential impact have been, and continue to be, extraordinary. Interventions as disparate as drug therapy following myocardial infarction, the timing of thrombolysis, angioplasty, and exercise stress tests, and even coronary artery bypass surgery have all been studied in carefully designed and carried-out controlled clinical trials. The translation of the results of clinical trials to improved patient treatment is an ongoing, sustaining fact of professional life for all of us.

But there are some pitfalls that must be avoided, and as cost-containment clouds an ever larger portion of the medical care horizon, the potential for both short- and long-term errors is high. The results of clinical trials, after appropriate replication and verification, can be applied to the clinical practice of medicine in either of two ways, which for want of better terms I will call "guidelines" and "outlines."

In the present dispensation we tend to use trial results as guidelines. The results of trials are taken as recommendations that emerged from group data and are to be applied to individual patients with the filtering we know as clinical judgment. Powerful, and usually replicated, data are incorporated into practice quite quickly. Beta blockers became widely used following myocardial infarction after the Norwegian Timalol Study[1] and the Beta Blocker Heart Attack Trial (BHAT)[2] were published. The use of antiarrhythmic drugs plummeted after the data of the Cardiac Arrhythmia Suppression Trial (CAST)[3] were made available, without even waiting for replication. After a shaky start due to study design problems, aspirin gained an enormous foothold when its beneficial long-term effects post infarction were recognized.[4] But we find the results of well-done studies relatively ignored if the results are only weakly positive and the alternatives not appealing. The use of aspirin for primary prevention of myocardial infarction was quickly adopted after the Physician's Health Survey[5] published its report, whereas the nearly simultaneous British physicians study,[6] with its negative results, was essentially ignored in this country.[7] It is possible that the low event rate in the British study precluded a positive result from emerging, thus negating the impact of the study.[7]

An "outline" approach to the interpretation of clinical trials would be far more literal. The result of a trial or a meta-analysis would be converted to a set of rules for managing clinical problems, for determining eligibility for drugs or procedures, or for defining length of hospital stay. The individual patient would be subject to the results of the analysis of the group data in the trial. Defined therapeutic algorithms would govern this managed care approach to therapeutics. While it may be argued that this approach differs from a "guidelines" approach only in the rigidity with which the clinical template is applied, the difference in reality is much greater. The difference is subtle, profound, and comes into focus only when a longer view is contemplated.

The obvious difference is that group data results would forge a rigid therapeutic cocoon for an individual patient. If the patient did not fit the template in terms of a numerical assessment of left ventricular function (ejection fraction), minutes elapsed since the onset of chest pain, or the duration of symptom-free activity on a treadmill test, the patient would be excluded from consideration for a more aggressive—and more importantly—a more expensive plan of management. Clinically germane variables either not accounted for in the trial or not even available at the time it was done, are unable to sway the pendulum to the clinician's choice. Short-term results of this rigidity may exclude only a small or modest number of patients from receiving treatment, itself usually of modest significance since most clinical trials deal with clinical choices that are not overwhelmingly clear cut. Thus the traditional sorts of outcomes analysis will most likely show little influence on national, regional, or even insurance unit morbidity or mortality.

There may even be a short-term improvement in the clinical outcome following the managed care application of therapeutic algorithms. Those physicians who do not keep abreast of the literature, those who order excessive tests out of uncertainty, fear of litigation, or greed, and those who practice medicine outside their range of expertise will all be brought up to a minimal standard of competence. This improvement represents the "quality" that managed care supporters claim, with some justification, will emerge from the systematic application of defined algorithms. The long-term effects of the "outline" approach can be devastating, however, reaching far beyond minor blips in the clinical outcome data. The translation of clinical management to recipe-like formulas will reduce and finally eliminate a role for clinical judgment. In cardiology, clinical trials have defined—or soon will—therapeutic algorithms for most major disease categories. If this help, this organized, well-compiled wisdom of the ages becomes dogma rather than lesson, the role of clinical judgment will be fatally curtailed. As Anthony described Cleopatra, so clinicians understand complex diseases, "Age cannot wither her nor custom stale her infinite variety."

With "cookbook cardiology" in place there may not be an increase in morbidity and mortality for some time. The current downward slope in mortality may even accelerate initially as those practitioners who do not follow the "guidelines" of evolving trials are drawn into the "outline" of their results. But in time there will be a reduced clinical capacity to deal with new problems, to anticipate new directions for clinical investigation, to push for greater command over the new reaches of heart disease. The capacity for excellence will be lost. There are many threats to the conservation of the capacity for excellence in medicine and the misapplication of the results of clinical trials is only one of them. As the designers of the trials, we have a special responsibility to perpetuate their strengths and not incorporate their weaknesses.

REFERENCES

1. THE NORWEGIAN MULTICENTER STUDY GROUP. 1981. Timalol-induced reduction in mortality and reinfarction in patients surviving acute myocardial infarction. N. Engl. J. Med. **304:** 801–807.
2. B-BLOCKER HEART ATTACK RESEARCH GROUP. 1982. A randomized trial of propanolol in patients with acute myocardial infarction I. Mortality results. JAMA **247:** 1707–1714.
3. CARDIAC ARRHYTHMIA SUPRESSION TRIAL. 1989. Preliminary report: Effect of encainide and flecainide on mortality in a randomized trial of arrhythmia suppression after myocardial infarction. N. Engl. J. Med. **321:** 406–412.
4. ISIS-2 (SECOND INTERNATIONAL STUDY OF INFARCT SURVIVAL) COLLABORATIVE GROUP. 1988. Randomized trial of intravenous streptokinase, or aspirin, both, or neither among 17,187 cases of suspected myocardial infarction. Lancet **2:** 349–360.
5. THE STEERING COMMITTEE OF THE PHYSICIANS' HEALTH STUDY RESEARCH GROUP. 1989. Preliminary report: Findings from the aspirin component of the ongoing Physicians' Health Study. N. Engl. J. Med. **321:**129–135.
6. PETO, R., R. GRAY, R. COLLINS, *et al.* 1988. Randomized trial of prophylactic daily aspirin in British male doctors. Br. Med. J. **296:** 313–316.
7. LAMAS, G., M. A. PFEFFER, P. HAMM, J. WERTHEIMER, J-L. ROULEAU & E. BRAUNWALD. 1992. Do the results of clinical trials of cardiovascular drugs influence medical practice? N. Engl. J. Med. **327:** 241–247.

Regional Organization
for Outcomes Research

GERALD T. O'CONNOR, STEPHEN K. PLUME, AND
JOHN E. WENNBERG

Center for the Evaluative Clinical Sciences
Dartmouth-Hitchcock Medical Center
Lebanon, New Hampshire 03756

BARRIERS TO IMPROVEMENTS IN MEDICAL AND SURGICAL CARE

The U.S. health care system is appropriately the target of calls for substantial reform. In addition to the problems of access to care, and inflation of medical care costs, there are flaws in the traditional role of the physician as a decision-making agent of the patient and important problems based on the inadequacy of clinical science. Flaws in clinical science may adversely affect physicians' judgment and the lack of an infrastructure severely limit the ability of physicians to improve the quality of their work. In addition, the actual effectiveness of interventions may differ substantially between institutions or individual clinicians. These flaws in the current health care system have important effects on the goal of medical and surgical interventions to "do more good than harm."

Methods for achieving improvement in medical and surgical outcomes are often discussed, but actual improvements are rarely achieved. A number of factors contribute to the failure of medical quality improvement. Among these factors are the following:

1. *The insular nature of clinical medicine makes benchmarking difficult or impossible.* Much of medical and surgical care involves the clinician and patient alone. The theories of care and the processes of care are hidden from view. A consequence of this structure is that it is difficult for clinicians to compare their theories of care and their approach to problems with each other. Since care delivered by other clinicians is rarely observed, benchmarking, a commonly used technique for industrial quality improvement is virtually unknown in clinical medicine.

2. *The inadequacy in the detail of information on current clinical practice prevents knowledge of the fine structure of care and makes studies linking practices to outcomes difficult.* In many settings, health care is, within loosely defined limits, based on the individual style of the clinician as modified for the setting and the individual patients. This individualized care is rarely described in a manner that would make it available to other clinicians nor in enough detail to scrutinize it or to derive general principles from it. Guidelines, which attempt to prevent only unintended variation, are often spurned by clinicians as "cookbook medicine."

For some clinical problems there is *no* regular method of assessing the outcomes of medical or surgical care, as in, for example, the routine care of hypertension, bronchitis, or chronic obstructive pulmonary diseases; for other problems, like coronary artery bypass grafting, rates of adverse events such as in-hospital mortality are regularly collected either by the hospital, the government, or a regulatory agency such as the Joint Commission on Accrediting Healthcare Organizations.

These rates provide a performance metric of variable quality, but do not provide insight on the root causes of adverse outcomes. Understanding of the etiology of adverse outcomes requires a deep understanding of the fine structure of the situation, that is, both an understanding of the clinical details of the care and a knowledge of the cause-specific mortality rate (or other appropriate outcome).

3. *The lack of a reliable and trusted data-gathering infrastructure and of technical expertise limits attempts by individual clinicians and hospitals to improve the quality of medical and surgical care.* As we discuss the changes now occurring in the U.S. health care system and the seeming rush toward managed competition, it is important to recall that most clinical care is provided by independent practitioners or groups of practitioners. The fee-for-service system creates a competitive environment in many areas, while in other areas of the country virtual monopolies exist. Neither financial competition nor monopoly compels individual clinicians to organize themselves to compare the processes or outcomes of the care that they provide. As a consequence, the individual clinician rarely knows with certainty the quality of care that he or she is providing.

Evaluation of clinical care requires the design and analysis of observational studies. This kind of epidemiology is often difficult. Differences in outcomes can be the result of chance, bias, or confounding. Multivariate statistical techniques are routinely required. Collaborations between clinicians and epidemiologists may occur by chance, but are by no means routine. The combination of skills and resources required to assess outcomes of clinical care are rarely available.

4. *Many adverse outcomes are quite rare. Even the thoughtful analysis of the experience of an individual institution may be inadequate to draw strong inference on the etiology of adverse outcomes.* Consider a cardiothoracic surgeon performing 100 coronary artery bypass grafts per year. Four of these patients die in the hospital: One dies of hemorrhage in the recovery room, one dies of sepsis after mediastinitis, another dies of low-output heart failure after a postoperative myocardial infarction, and the last is found dead in bed on postoperative day 7. In each of these cases, some analysis of the situation is possible, but no comparison with the outcomes of other surgeons is available. These four deaths cannot by themselves be the basis for informed and beneficial changes in procedures of care. No one can derive from this experience the risk factors for mediastinitis or the preferred manner for myocardial protection or for screening for coagulopathies. There are too many questions and too few data. Yet, if data were available from thousands of patients, and if processes of care were known, patterns might emerge that could be studied to improve the quality of care.

5. *Failed theory and the punitive nature of many "quality improvement" efforts create fear and limit the acceptability of these efforts to clinicians and hospitals.* Two aspects of failed theory merit mention.

First, we know from Deming's work that it is absolutely essential to quality improvement that we drive out fear.[1] The postulate that we can improve the outcomes of medical or surgical care by frightening physicians to higher levels of performance is absurd. The rank ordering of clinical outcomes and the publication of that information creates only denial and attempt to manipulate the system through the choice of patients or other means. No clinician prefers that their patients experience adverse outcomes. Most clinicians are trying as hard as they can to provide good care.

Second, the improvement of the quality of medical or surgical care is not largely a "bad apples" problem. Although there is substantial variability in the outcomes of care, the vast majority of adverse outcomes are not related to negligence or incompetence, but rather to variability in the processes of care and failures in the system of delivering the care. Some of these defects result from the skills or judgment of the clinician, some result from failed clinical theory and incomplete knowledge, and some result from confusion and failures of the many systems of care within our institutions. Inspection focuses its attention on the "tails" of the statistical distribution, distracting us from appreciating that the most important opportunities for quality improvement will result from changing the mean rate of adverse outcomes. The important differences between monitoring performance and depending upon inspection to assure quality are not well understood.

REGIONAL ORGANIZATION FOR OUTCOMES RESEARCH

We report on a regional voluntary consortium founded in 1987 to provide information about the management of cardiovascular disease in Maine, New Hampshire, and Vermont. This consortium, called the Northern New England Cardiovascular Disease Study Group (NNECVDSG), is an inter-institutional model for the improvement of medical and surgical care. The members include all cardiothoracic surgeons, interventional cardiologists, scientists, and administrators from the participating institutions. The NNECVDSG maintains registries for all patients receiving coronary artery bypass grafting (CABG), percutaneous transluminal coronary angioplasty (PTCA), and heart valve replacement surgery. During the last six years, data on approximately 20,000 procedures were collected and analyzed. The group meets three times per year to review data reports and to plan studies. An executive committee composed of two representatives from each institution and the data center director constitutes the administrative structure for the group.

The NNECVDSG has investigated: institutional differences in in-hospital mortality rates associated with coronary artery bypass grafting (CABG)[2]; development and validation of a clinical prediction rule incorporating predictors of in-hospital mortality associated with CABG[3]; management of unstable angina pectoris[4]; subjective probability estimation by clinicians[5]; reasons for excess mortality among women undergoing CABG surgery[6]; the trend toward increasing predicted risk among CABG patients[7]; use of a pericardial flap and its effect on the incidence of mediastinitis and sternal dehiscence[8]; use of techniques for continuous quality improvement in cardiac surgery[9]; and studies of small-area variation in the performance of myocardial revascularization procedures. Other work in progress includes the study of regional outcomes associated with PTCA, and development of a multivariate prediction rule to estimate the risk of in-hospital mortality and nonfatal adverse effects associated with PTCA.

During 1987–1989, a study of patient case mix and predictors of in-hospital mortality associated with CABG was conducted. Data about patient demographic and historical information, cardiac catheterization results, priority at surgery, intensity of therapy, and co-morbidity and status at hospital discharge were collected by five clinical centers. The overall crude in-hospital mortality rate for isolated CABG, based on 3,055 patients, between July 1, 1987 and April 15, 1989, was 4.3%. Patient, clinical, and laboratory data were combined and logistic regression analysis was used to predict the risk of in-hospital mortality. The clinical prediction rule was developed on a training set of data and then validated on a test set. The logistic regression model of in-hospital mortality incorporated the following variables: age, sex, left ventricular end diastolic pressure, ejection fraction score, priority of surgery (elective, ugent, or emergent), the presence of co-morbid disease, history of prior coronary artery bypass grafting, and body surface area. This regression model significantly ($\chi^2[8 \text{ df}] = 57.7, p < 0.0001$) predicted the occurrence of in-hospital mortality. The area under the receiver operating characteristic curve was 0.74 (perfect = 1.0) and the clinical prediction rule was robust when used on a test set of data (area = 0.76). The correlation between observed and expected numbers of deaths was 0.99.

Considerable variability between medical centers ($3.1–6.3\%, p = 0.021$) and between surgeons ($1.9–9.2\%, p = 0.025$) was observed, and persisted after adjustment for potentially confounding variables. We concluded that the multivariate clinical prediction rule, based on risk factors identified in this study, significantly predicted the likelihood of in-hospital mortality in this patient population. Furthermore, the observed differences in in-hospital mortality rates among institution and surgeons are not solely attributable to differences in case mix, as described by these variables, and may reflect differences in patient care which have yet to be identified.

Another current project is to develop a scoring system to allow reliable calculation of cause-specific mortality rates associated with CABG and PTCA. The NNECVDSG is currently conducting a case-control study comparing processes of clinical care among 406 patients who died and 812 survivors of CABG surgery.

The overall approach that has evolved is to:

(1) Create an infrastructure that allows the collection and sharing of data;
(2) Develop an agreed upon performance metric;
(3) Study variability in outcomes and report these results to the clinicians and institutions;
(4) Develop methods of assessing cause-specific outcomes;
(5) Link clinical processes to cause-specific outcomes; and
(6) Continuously monitor processes and outcomes

One measure of the success of the NNECVDSG is the level of participation of its members. Since 1987, enthusiasm for the process has grown. Regional meetings now regularly attract more than 50 participants, and institutions and individual clinicians support the data collection efforts.

LIMITATIONS OF THE PROPOSED MODEL

Structural Limitations of the Proposed Model

The model of quality improvement that we have described has several important limitations. In most areas of the U.S., there is no existing infrastructure for such an endeavor. Region-wide relationships between clinicians do not exist, nor does the required technical expertise or financial support. In addition, devising an appropriate and relevant performance metric will be a challenge for some medical and surgical specialties. These problems are real, but not insurmountable. Coalitions can be forged, technical help can be found, and the expenses are rather modest (less than 0.1% of the cost of care). Recent work on acurately assessing functional health status may provide an important and clinically relevant performance metric for certain conditions.

Managed Competition Has a Currently Unknown Effect on Quality Improvement Efforts

The trend toward managed competition may have substantial effects on attempts toward regional organization for quality improvement. Aggregation of medical and surgical care into the functional units required for managed competition may provide an important infrastructure that would aid the development of quality improvement groups. A principle of managed competition is that hospitals, or aggregates of hospitals, will compete for market share based on both price and quality. Quality of care may assume a new priority when it is regularly assessed. However, cooperation and the sharing of information may be very difficult when hospitals compete head-to-head in this new financial environment. Scientific progress requires the free flow of information; "trade secrets" are not often shared. An example of the inhibiting effects of competition on scientific discourse may be found in molecular biology before and after the development of biotechnology enterprises. The actual effects of managed competition on the quality of medical and surgical care are as yet unknown.[10]

Current Models of Regional Organization Do Not Deal With the Problem of Supplier-Induced Demand

Another substantial limitation of the proposed approach is inherent in the structure of fee-for-service medicine. Networks for improving quality involve working to free the doctor-patient relationship from the burden of supplier-induced demand. The Deming strategy of quality management assumes the sovereignty of the consumer in choosing among alternative products. In medical markets, the consumer must be given sovereignty through reform of the doctor-patient relationship to disentangle the preferences of the doctor from those of the patient.

The struggle for quality in medicine requires attention to the quality of the decision process in choosing treatments and diagnostic tests as well as the quality with which they are produced. Networks of quality have not dealt effectively with the problem of supplier-induced demand. The incentives of fee-for-service medicine pose a great barrier to the prospects for the shared-decision model. Strategies for quality management in medicine must be enlarged to include recognition of the requirement to free medical decisions from supplier-induced demand.

Financial and Structural Instability of Existing Examples of Regional Organization

Lastly, a limitation of this approach is its inherent instability. No policy is yet in place to support networks of quality. Hospitals do not financially support these efforts. Nor, thus far, do third-party payers. Regional quality improvement efforts in health care are, for the most part, undersupported and dependent on the whims of granting agencies. Such funding may be adequate for trying new ideas, but will not suffice for durably maintaining the infrastructure and providing the technical expertise required.

Lack of Societal and Governmental Tolerance for Variability in Outcomes

There is no doubt that "real" inter-institutional and inter-clinician differences exist in the outcomes of medical and surgical care. Considering the insular nature of clinical practice and the inadequacies of clinical science, it would be astounding if this were not so. Yet, although variations in performance and outcome undoubtedly occur in all fields of endeavor, societal and governmental tolerance to variations in the outcomes of medical and surgical care is quite low. Furthermore, in the past, organized medicine has not dealt effectively with even extreme examples of poor performance among its ranks. In the name of consumerism, publication of clinical outcomes has met the societal need to "do something". There is a substantial challenge to medicine to organize itself to improve the quality of care. In these differences in outcomes are the clues to the improvement of processes of care. In our view, it is only through a continuing effort to understand how and why outcomes differ that medical and surgical care can be improved, public confidence can be regained, and control of the process of quality improvement can be retained by the profession.

CONCLUSION

The combination of the inherent professionalism of health care workers with increasing demands from health policy makers and consumers mandates attention to the study of the outcomes of medical and surgical treatment. Patients require accurate, quantitative estimates of the risk of treatments to make fully informed decisions. Physicians require valid estimates of the expected number of deaths or other relevant outcomes so that they can constantly reassess their own performance and that of their institutions. Quality improvement requires a detailed study of the etiology as a vital step toward useful examination of the multiple processes that constitute excellent or less than excellent care of patients. Yet there are barriers to progress: crude mortality rates are distrusted as performance metrics for physicians or institutions; quantitative risk estimates given to patients may often be inaccurate or not attempted at all; quality assurance is usually based on the discussion of a few sentinel adverse events and only rarely on an adequate epidemiologic understanding of the situation; only rarely are relevant, contemporaneous data available to guide decisions. All of these are symptoms of the underlying fact that medicine has not yet built an infrastructure for quality improvement. Furthermore, we do not sufficiently understand the fine structure of the problems to be able to act definitively for the benefit of patients, society, or the profession.

The Northern New England Cardiovascular Disease Study Group is an attempt to create an infrastructure for health care improvement. We have emphasized a regional approach for building population-based systems of care based on professional responsibility for managing discrete subsystems of the regional health care system. We believe that this approach has both theoretical and practical advantages. This consortium is a multi-institutional, regional model for continuous improvement of medical and surgical care, one which may have applications in other settings.

SUMMARY

Methods for achieving improvement in medical and surgical outcomes are often discussed, but rarely achieved. We report on a regional voluntary consortium founded in 1987 to provide information about the management of cardiovascular disease in northern New England. Members include all cardiothoracic surgeons and interventional cardiologists in the region, as well as administrators and scientists associated with the five institutions that provide advanced cardiac services in this region. The group maintains registries for coronary artery bypass grafting, coronary angioplasty, and heart valve surgery and has investigated institutional differences in mortality rates; the development and use of clinical prediction rules; the reasons for excess mortality among women undergoing bypass graft surgery; and time trends in the use of myocardial revascularization. This consortium is an inter-institutional model for the continuous improvement of medical and surgical care.

REFERENCES

1. DEMING, W. E. 1986. Out of the Crisis. MIT-CAES. Cambridge, Mass.
2. O'CONNOR, G. T., S. K. PLUME, E. M. OLMSTEAD, *et al.* 1991. A regional prospective study of in-hospital mortality associated with coronary artery bypass grafting. JAMA **266**(6): 803–809.
3. O'CONNOR, G. T., S. K. PLUME, E. M. OLMSTEAD, *et al.* 1992. Multivariate prediction of in-hospital mortality associated with coronary artery bypass grafting. Circulation **85**(6): 2110–2118.
4. WASSON, J. H., G. T. O'CONNOR, D. J. JAMES & E. M. OLMSTEAD. 1992. A physician-completed patient registry system: Pilot results for unstable angina in the elderly. J. Gen. Intern. Med. **7**: 298–303.
5. O'CONNOR, G. T., S. K. PLUME, J. R. BECK, C. A. S. MARRIN, W. NUGENT & E. M. OLMSTEAD. 1988. What are my chances? It depends on whom you ask. The choice of a prosthetic heart valve. Medical Decision Making **8**: 341.
6. O'CONNOR, G. T., E. M. OLMSTEAD, L. H. COFFIN, C. T. MALONEY, J. R. MORTON, S. K. PLUME, D. MALENKA & M. J. DIEHL. 1991. Gender and in-hospital mortality associated with coronary artery bypass grafting (CABG). Circulation **83**: 723.
7. DISCH, D. L., G. T. O'CONNOR, J. D. BIRKMEYER, D. G. LEVY, E. M. OLMSTEAD & S. K. PLUME. 1992. Trend toward increasing predicted mortality among patients undergoing coronary artery bypass grafting. Clin. Res. **40**(2): 347.
8. NUGENT, W. C., E. L. MAISLEN, G. T. O'CONNOR, C. A. S. MARRIN & S. K. PLUME. 1988. Pericardial flap prevents sternal wound complications. Arch. Surg. **123**: 636–639.
9. KASPER, J. F., S. K. PLUME & G. T. O'CONNOR. 1992. A methodology for QI in the coronary artery bypass grafting procedure involving comparative process analysis. Quality Rev. Bull. **18**(4): 129–133.
10. KRONICK, R., D. C. GOODMAN, J. WENNBERG & E. WAGNER. 1993. The marketplace in health care reform. The demographic limitations of managed competition. N. Engl. J. Med. **328**: 148–152.

DISCUSSION

ALAN MORRIS (*LDS Hospital, Salt Lake City, Utah*): I found an interesting juxtaposition between this very interesting paper and Dr. Greenberg's concern about being constrained by guidelines and being prevented as a physician from doing what we as physicians want to do, and that is to use our independent judgment for the treatment of individual patients. There seems to be an incompatibility here if harm has in fact followed from individual judgmental decision making;

then it seems that the concern about being constrained by guidelines, assuming the guidelines are based upon good information, is one which we should put aside.

I believe that your attention to the detail of process is on the right track, and I would recommend that we go even further. For example, it has been demonstrated by Dr. Sackett's group and by others dealing with protocols that control the management of anticoagulant therapy, that Boswell's dictum that man more often needs to be reminded than instructed is well applied in the clinical environment. Reminders alone are extremely important for helping physicians prevent the overlooking of important elements of therapy and diagnosis. An extension of this truism might figure in the form of guidelines that would be applicable in available digital systems to help physicians with decision support tools that would remind them of important elements in care that need to be considered.

This brings us to the issue of information overload. The clinical environment is extremely complex and as few as four to seven variables can overload human decision-making abilities. The clinical environment easily presents hundreds of such variables to the physician, and so the concept of providing support tools by means of guidelines will be very helpful.

DR. GERALD O'CONNOR (*Dartmouth-Hitchcock Medical Center, Lebanon, New Hampshire*): Currently we are conducting a case-control study of 406 cardiac deaths that have occurred between 1987 and 1992. This case-control study is a study comparing a wide range of patient and treatment variables between survivors and non-survivors of CABG, matched on site, age, sex, and priority at surgery. We're looking at 170 variables that were defined by a clinical group to look at processes of care in heart surgery. In comparing these 406 deaths with 812 non-deaths from the same institutions we are looking at differences in process and trying to relate them to cause-specific mortality. At that point both data and process will be tied together and the use of total quality management techniques will be used to develop process flow diagrams.

Outcomes Research, PORTs, and Health Care Reform

JOHN E. WENNBERG,[a] MICHAEL J. BARRY,[b]
FLOYD J. FOWLER,[c] AND ALBERT MULLEY[b]

[a]*Center for the Evaluative Clinical Sciences*
Dartmouth Medical School
Hanover, New Hampshire 03755-3863

[b]*Medical Practices Evaluation Center*
Massachusetts General Hospital
Boston, Massachusetts 02119

[c]*Center for Survey Research*
University of Massachusetts at Boston
Boston, Massachusetts 02125-3393

On behalf of my colleagues, I am very pleased to have been asked to contribute to this celebration of Iain Chalmers and Richard Peto. These men, whose brilliant careers amply demonstrate the wisdom of an organized investment in randomized clinical trials and the synthesis of results through meta-analysis, also provide an essential example of the type of science and form of scientist that Archie Cochrane sought to promote. The influence of Cochrane and the model of the evaluative scientist he inspired have shaped many of those who are contributing to this volume.

The Patient Outcomes Research Team or PORT strategy is a novel approach for organizing an interdisciplinary attack on Archie Cochrane's problem of efficiency and effectiveness. Nested within the Agency for Health Care Policy and Research's Medical Treatment Effectiveness (MEDTEP) program, these modestly expensive programs (circa $1 million per year) were designed to provide a mechanism for policymakers to assure the systematic evaluation of all relevant treatment theories, not just those that are the subject of formal regulatory evaluation or are of particular interest to investigators. Priorities have been set to attack "big ticket" conditions such as benign prostatic hyperplasia (BPH) or early-stage prostate cancer. PORTs thus were conceived to occupy a policy niche between research that is part of formal regulation (such as Food and Drug Administration–mandated clinical trials of new drugs) and investigator-initiated studies in which the subject matter and priorities are specified by the investigator. My principal task is to give a brief report on the work of the Prostate Disease PORT (of which I have been the Principal Investigator), emphasizing the role we have attempted to forge for PORTs in the spectrum of responsibility for evaluation.

A BRIEF BACKGROUND OF THE PROSTATE DISEASE PORT

The Prostate Disease PORT began well before the enabling legislation that brought the Agency for Health Care Policy and Research into being. In the mid-

1980s, a group of researchers from Dartmouth, the Massachusetts General Hospital, and the University of Massachusetts began meeting with practicing urologists in the state of Maine to learn the reasons for the extraordinary variations in rates of prostate surgery throughout the different hospital districts in that state. In some communities, we estimated that the cumulative incidence of prostate surgery for benign prostatic hyperplasia (BPH) approached 50% by age 85, while in others, often barely 20 miles away, the chance was less than 15%. In retrospect, the differences in practice style behind the variations can be traced to two problems:

(1) Lack of clarity (and certainly consensus) among urologists on the main reason (theory) for undertaking surgery; and
(2) Adherence to a model for clinical decision making (the rational agency or delegated decision model) that left the choice of treatment more or less to the physician.

In the early years, our research agenda concentrated on he first of these problems. We spent time with our urological colleagues to learn the nature of their disagreement. Some physicians believed that the natural course of untreated BPH was for most men a relentless one, leading to the need for surgery to prevent serious, irreversible kidney disease or bladder decompensation. They recommended early surgery, even when symptoms were mild, in order to obviate the need for operations when patients were older and sicker. Others believed that the natural course was not so malignant and that for most men the reasons for operating were to reduce symptoms and improve the quality of life.

EVALUATING THEORY TO LEARN WHAT WORKS

We then undertook a series of studies to clarify the theoretical basis for undertaking surgery, looking first at the preventive theory: Does early intervention improve life expectancy? Drs. Michael Barry and Albert Mulley built an actuarial model predicting life expectancy for those men undergoing surgery and for those choosing what we called "watchful waiting"—expectant treatment that delays surgery until BPH complications or intolerable symptoms appear. While no randomized clinical trial had been reported to provide the probability estimates for the critical events in the model, we found a few cohort studies in the literature that provided estimates of the crossover rates from watchful waiting to surgery; we also used large claims databases to learn about the failure rates among men operated upon (deaths associated with operations and probability for subsequent re-operations). The model revealed that for all age groups, early surgery failed to provide a life expectancy gain: The rate of progression of untreated BPH to irreversible end-stage renal disease or life-threatening infection was not sufficient to warrant early intervention with the rationale of improving the chances for survival.

We then turned to the quality-of-life theory to find that the published literature was even less helpful. Never mind that no randomized clinical trials existed. We couldn't find a cohort study or even a case series report that adequately addressed the subjective responses of patients to surgery. The case for the efficiency of prostate surgery in improving symptoms was built on anecdote and the analogy that since prostatectomy demonstrably improved urinary flow, it must also improve symptoms and quality of life. To solve this missing data problem, we undertook our own study.

The first task was to learn what mattered to patients and to develop an instrument that captured the events.

Dr. Floyd J. Fowler undertook unstructured interviews with patients (using a focus group format), some of whom were contemplating surgery, some of whom were confirmed watchful waiters, and others who had surgery with both good and bad outcomes. From these conversations, Dr. Fowler amassed a list of all the outcomes that mattered to patients and then set out to build and validate a questionnaire to quantify symptoms, complications, and quality of life states as well as to measure the subjective impact that the BPH condition had on the individual patient—how much he was bothered by his symptoms and what his expectations were from treatment.

When the measurement tool was ready, we and our urologist colleagues in Maine undertook a cohort study of consecutive patients who underwent prostatectomy. All in all, some 400 patients were interviewed at the time of operation and their outcomes measured three, six, and twelve months after surgery. Just as our urologist colleagues had predicted, the benefits of surgery in reducing symptoms was a "slam bang" effect: about 76% of severely symptomatic men reported only mild or virtually no symptoms after surgery. This outcome is much better than that obtained by watchful waiting, where the best that can be expected is some slight improvement.

But the news was not uniformly good. Seventeen percent of those interviewed after surgery reported they still had moderately severe symptoms, and 7% said they were no better off than before. Moreover, well over half reported difficulty with sexual function (retrograde ejaculation), 5% of previously potent men reported no erections, and 4% reported problems with dribbling of urine which they had not had before the operation.

THE IMPORTANCE OF PATIENT PREFERENCE

In our study of patients we also learned that men were not all the same in the way they reviewed the impact of BPH upon their lives. Some men, even those with severe symptoms, told us that they were not very much bothered by them. Moreover, as we learned from the interviews conducted prior to surgery, they differed in their concerns about the risk of impotence and incontinence. The more our studies took us into the subjectivity of the patient experience, the more variegate and nonuniform the typology of preference appeared to be. Nothing in the objectivity of the patient—his clinical history, his physical findings, his laboratory scores, his urine flow, even his symptom level—strongly predicted the degree of BPH botheredness or the aversion to the risks of surgery. To learn what the individual patient wants—to make the normatively correct treatment choice from the perspective of the individual—the patient must be asked to participate in a decision process that disentangles the patient's preferences from those of others, in particular, the physician.

We had arrived at this conclusion as early as 1987. We then began experimenting with ways to inform patients about their options. Al Mulley, who had explored the concept of interactive videos for other projects, suggested that this medium might be useful for explaining complicated decision problems to patients. The medium proved very useful for explaining the structure of the BPH problem: The reality that patients do have a choice was made evident by showing the testimonies of two physician-patients, each severely symptomatic; one who chose surgery, the other watchful waiting. The possible outcomes were made vicariously accessible by filming patients who had good outcomes, as well as those who had experienced the principal complications of surgery and watchful waiting. The computer, which is part of the technology, made it possible to store the probability estimates for the risks and benefits on a subgroup-specific basis. We thus could provide the estimates for the relevant outcomes acording to the patient's age, clinical status, and symptom score.

We have learned from studying patient reactions to the interactive videodisc program for BPH that most patients, including those with less than high school education, want considerable information and feel this experience is valuable in making a treatment decision. More important, the choices they make seem to reflect their preferences: Degree of bother and fear of impotence were the most important predictors of choice of treatment—more important than symptom level. Risk aversion seems to be emerging as another major factor in patient decision making; despite its superior effect on reducing symptoms (the "main effect" outcome), only one in five men whose symptom score ranked as severe chose surgery in a cohort study of videodisc viewers. Indeed, the change in pattern of choice provoked by the interactive videodisc has significantly reduced the per capita rate of surgery in two prepaid group practices.

THE SHARED DECISION-MAKING MODEL

The emergence of patient preferences as central to rational decision making has deeply influenced our thinking. When the outcomes of a particular treatment are multiple and when more than one treatment option exists, an optimal treatment choice for individuals depends on the evaluations they give to the risks and benefits associated with the outcomes that matter to them. The evaluation will differ from one individual to another. Some men, as we found in the BPH situation, valued the present state of their sexuality more than the prospect of reducing their urinary tract symptoms; when given the chance, they chose watchful waiting on the basis of their wish to avoid the risk of impotence and/or retrograde ejaculation. Others find the opportunity to reduce their symptoms a compelling one and choose surgery.

Learning how to create the opportunity for patient preferences to guide clinical choice has become a central focus of our PORT team effort. In shared decision making, it is the role of the physician to convey information about diagnostic or treatment options in a way that patients understand that they truly do have choices and those choices depend upon their own goals. Yet the tradition of Western medicine is steeped in the notion that physicians should act as agents for patients and that it is rational to delegate decision making to physicians. Achieving the shared decision-making model is predicated on the ability of the physician to give up the old model, to share power and to give up the disequilibrium that now exists between the supply of resources and "demand" as expressed in terms of utilization.

While the critical requisites for adopting shared decision making involve economic and other social structures well beyond the scope of our PORT project, our research has lead to several "spin-off" projects concerned with the psychological and ethical issues related to shared decision making. The interactive videodisc is proving useful as a tool for studying the doctor–patient relationship, for evaluating preferences and for measuring and studying other subjective impacts of medical care on patients.

THE PREFERENCE TRIAL CONCEPT

We have also been pursuing lines of thought about the conduct of clinical trials. The classic randomized clinical trial (RCT) is clearly the most efficient way for estimating the relative risk or risk difference associated with a single end-point such as death from breast cancer for Treatment A compared to Treatment B. For relative risks in the range of 1.2–1.5, as Richard Peto maintains, this design may be the only reasonable way to avoid the confounding associated with unmeasured initial differences among treatment cohorts. But when the relevant outcomes are multiple and patient preferences are essential to the construction of rational choice, then "patient preference" itself represents an array of important dependent variables that must be taken into account.

To make this concept less abstract, consider the example of BPH. Through our focus groups we learned about the outcomes that matter to patients. Patients want to know about the chances for these outcomes as they occur in everyday clinical practice (where patients should be free to choose their treatments according to their own evaluations). Thus, the required probability estimates for educating patients are those that apply under circumstances of active choice. Clearly, active choice is confounded with the placebo effect, the poorly understood phenomena in which the expectations patients have for benefit become realized in their subjectivity. But when, as in the case of BPH, symptom reduction and improvement in the quality of life are the "main effects" of treatment and the proper decision involves the evaluation of risk aversion and degree of botheredness, then these topics cannot be ignored; they must be made the object of investigation.

Our PORT has become interested in compare the advantages and limitations of the RCT and what we have come to call the preference clinical trial (PCT). Under either design, patients are offered (standardized) information about what is known and not known about the benefits and risks of conventional and experimental treatments and the patient populations followed-up according to their choice of treatment. The sole difference is that in the RCT design, patients are asked to accept randomization (and sometimes can only receive an "experimental" treatment if they accept randomization). In the PCT design, patients choose among all treatments.

Elsewhere, I have proposed a head-to-head comparison of the RCT and the PCT. Under this proposal, patients are randomly assigned to the PCT or the C-RCT design. In the example proposed, patients see an interactive videodisc describing what is known and not known about the outcomes of watchful waiting, surgery, and a "new" drug for BPH, Pfizer's Prazosin (Minipress®), a selective alpha-1 receptor drug which reached the market under a NDA as an antihypertensive agent, but which is now being used by clinicians to treat BPH. FIGURE 1 gives one way I have proposed of designing the trial.

Such a trial would explore a number of interesting problems. Would more patients elect the drug under active choice than under randomization? (Our hypothesis is *yes*: Risk aversion would drive patients to avoid the chance of randomization to surgery.) Would the probabilities for symptom reduction and other outcome estimates obtained under the RCT be the same as those under the PCT? (Our hypothesis is *no*: Expectations associated with active choice should result in better outcomes for all treatments.) A series of RCT-PCT comparisons seem critical to the development of outcomes research methodology, to an understanding of the various dimensions of confounding, including the bias that emerges when clinical investigation fails to investigate the interdependency of therapeutic effects with preferences, placebo, and compliance.

THE PORT-AUA CONNECTION

The story of the BPH-PORT would not be complete without a brief review of the history of its relationship with the AUA—the American Urological Association. In late 1988, as news of the BPH interactive videodisc strategy traveled, the leadership of the American Urological Association learned of our work and arranged to come to Hanover to review what we were doing. This early contact lead to several subsequent meetings, including one in the spring of 1989, when we presented to the AUA the results of a study that raised the possibility that transurethral prostatectomy (TURP) might carry with it an elevated risk of death in the years after surgery compared to the risk with open prostatectomy. The evidence rested in large claims databases in several countries. When survival studies were performed comparing the outcomes of transurethral prostatectomy with those of open prostatectomy, a relative risk of death of between 1.2 and 1.4 over a five-year period after surgery was evident from databases covering experiences in the United States,

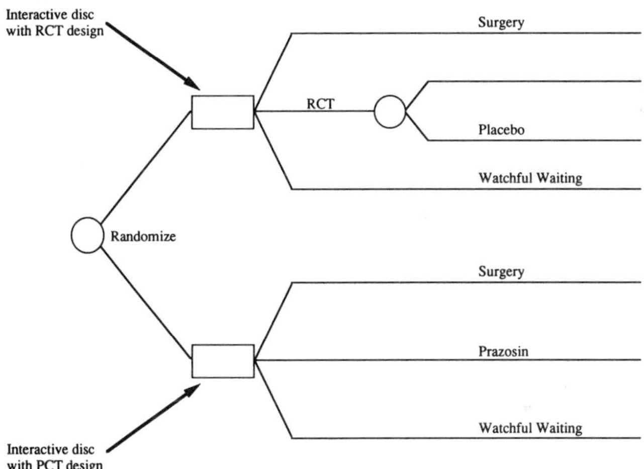

FIGURE 1 Proposed trial of a trial: Preference clinical trial (PCT) design versus randomized (RCT) design.

Canada, the United Kingdom, and Denmark. In a further study of the Canadian experience in which hospital records were abstracted to obtain data to adjust for severity of disease, the effect persisted. A small randomized clinical trial comparing the open to the transurethral procedure was consistent with the database observations. Our concern that TURPs might be causally associated with higher death rates lead us to propose that the AUA and the PORT sponsor a randomized clinical trial to test this hypothesis.

The response of the AUA was extraordinary: Within three months, under the leadership of its president, Paul Peters, its then treasurer and secretary, and Logan Holtgrewe and Abe Cockett (now president and president-elect), the AUA committed itself to undertake a clinical trial to test the painful proposition that the most common procedure used in American urology—which had been adopted into clinical practice without benefit of randomized clinical trials—was somehow causing an elevation in death rates.

The AUA-PORT collaboration lead to a comprehensive strategy for evaluation that would make Archie Cochrane proud. The AUA committed itself to see that in the future new BPH treatment technologies were adequately evaluated. To do this, the PORT and AUA would plan a technology assessment network—a network of investigators that would examine, in sequence, all new promising technologies before they became widely diffused into practice, comparing them to current treatment strategies in a series of randomized trials.

The importance of the AUA's technology assessment network is underscored by the veritable explosion of new ideas and new technologies that have emerged over the life of our PORT. When we began our studies, surgery and watchful waiting were the only serious treatment options, but by 1993 the situation was much more complex and other methods of treatment had been developed, including the following:

Balloon dilation: Reasoning from analogy, clinicians proposed that balloon angioplasty technology be adopted to treat BPH. Balloon dilation became a BPH treatment—a strategy in which the offending prostate tissue causing urination problems is stretched out of the way by inflating a balloon that is inserted as part of a catheter.

Alpha blockers: I mentioned above that drugs approved by the FDA for treatment of hypertension have been adoptd for use in BPH since physicians noted that patients who are taking this drug for their blood pressure seem to gain some relief from their urinary symptoms.

Finasteride: A major drug company undertook an elegant research project to come up with a drug that inhibits production of the hormone that contributes to growth of the prostate, thereby reducing prostate size.

Hyperthermia and thermal therapy: The NIH's investment in biomedical technology produced a machine capable of heating organs selectively. Although designed with the intention of treating cancer, curious researchers tried it out on the prostate, where it may help with symptoms.

Stents and coils: Other physicians have developed devices which, when inserted into the urethra, shore up the offending prostate tissue, rather like a mine tunnel is shored up with timbers to prevent cave-ins.

TUIP: Surgeons have invented (or, rather, actually rediscovered) a new way of doing surgery in which an incision is made into the offending prostate tissue, but the prostate tissue is not extensively removed as is the case in conventional prostatectomy.

Laser surgery: Yet another application in the fast-growing field of lasers in medicine: in some medical centers, prostate tissue is now being ablated using one of a number of laser devices.

The concept shared between the PORT and the AUA was that each of these technologies would be reviewed and prioritized for study to ascertain, in everyday practice on sequential patients, the probabilities for all of the outcomes that mattered to patients. The comparison groups would include TURP, open prostatectomy (for men with larger prostates), and watchful waiting. Each patient would be offered a randomized clinical trial, but everyone would be followed up, including those who refused the randomization. The objective was to learn as much as possible about each of the subgroups that are offered treatment, even when they did not accept randomization. (We were particularly interested in seeing if the TURP mortality effect would disappear when good baseline co-morbidity data could be collected prospectively and documentd through randomization).

The AUA-PORT collaboration has had another important outcome: the standardization of measurement tools used for assessing patient-centered outcomes.

The AUA Symptom Index questionnaire is now being widely adopted for the evaluation of BPH treatments. We are now following a similar approach for measuring BPH-specific health status. The standardization of instruments is a critically important step in the evolution of outcomes research. The PORT–specialty society collaboration provides a means for accomplishing this end.

The commitment of the AUA to the technology assessment network included their underwriting of a pilot study which has demonstrated the feasibility of the approach. More than $1 million of the AUA's own funds have been spent on this project. But the story does not have a happy ending. The necessary federal support for the full-scale network has not been forthcoming. Four years later, with funds and patience exhausted, the pilot study is about to be terminated, even though it successfully demonstrated the feasibility of the network.

The consequences of the failure of the Agency for Health Care Policy and Research to muster support for the AUA-PORT technology assessment network does not bode well for the future of the Medical Treatment Effectiveness Program. The nonexperimental tasks of our PORT have by and large been completed, and the future value of our work in BPH will depend increasingly on the conduct of clinical trials. More significant, however, is the lost opportunity. The AUA has distinguished itself in the tradition of Cochrane by stepping forward to embrace the ethic of evaluation as an emblem of professional responsibility. Its leadership has made a valiant and expensive effort to set the example of a knowledge-based standard of practice. So much the pity that its efforts fall on deaf ears.

LIFE AFTER PORT AND HEALTH CARE REFORM

The PORT experiment is hanging in policy limbo, having run its course to the point where the tasks and functions that need to be done can be reasonably well specified, but the resources and the policy are not yet in place to assure their orderly accomplishment. Archie Cochrane was not the first, nor will the leadership of the AUA be the last, to experience the frustration of seeing what appears to be so sane an idea—that we should learn what works in medicine—fall between the cracks of indifference. But the energy keeps coming back. No matter how prepared we seem to be to accept ignorance, the counter-argument that ethical medicine must be science-based always waits in the wings. I am sure it will emerge again and soon, and that the need for policy-initiated research that assures the orderly evaluation of all treatment options will be widely recognized.

The lessons from the PORTs seem worth recording, for surely there will be more vigorous sons and daughters of PORTs. We need policy-directed research that captures the full richness of the innovative processes. Much innovation is inaccessible to regulation, arising (as so well-illustrated by the recent explosion of BPH treatments) in the problem-solving context of everyday practice. To assure orderly evaluation, much of policy-initiated research like the PORT program should be organized on an interdisciplinary and condition-specific basis. The priorities should be set by the government on the basis of a simple notion that those conditions should be studied first that: (1) affect the most people, (2) cost the most, (3) share the fact that preferences of patient are an important component of rational choice, but (4) have treatment patterns that vary in the typical way suggestive of supplier-induced demand. I have listed some examples in TABLE 1.

TABLE 1. Common Conditions and Their Current Treatment Options for Which Outcomes Research and Shared Decision Making Can Lead to the Rationalization of Patient Demand

Condition	Major Treatment Controversies
Noncancerous condition of the uterus	Surgery (by type) vs. hormone treatment vs. drugs vs. watchful waiting
Angina pectoris	Bypass surgery vs. angioplasty vs. drugs
Gallstones	Surgery vs. stone-crushing vs. medical management vs. watchful waiting
Peripheral vascular disease	Bypass surgery vs. angioplasty vs. medical management
Cataracts	Lens extraction (by type) vs. watchful waiting
Arthritis of hip and knee	Surgery (by type) vs. medical management
Prostatism (BPH-benign prostatic hyperplasia)	Surgery (by type) vs. balloon dilation vs. drugs vs. microwave diathermy vs. watchful waiting
Herniated disc	Surgery (by type) vs. various medical management strategies
Atherosclerosis of carotid artery with threat of stroke	Carotid endarterectomy vs. aspirin

The tasks for evaluation should also be clearly specified. The orderly advance of the science of clinical medicine depends on the routine and iterative accomplishment of certain tasks. While our research agenda in prostate disease has taken many twists and turns, we have been guided by an underlying set of principles to assure that:

(1) all of the outcomes that matter to patients are routinely identified;
(2) measurement tools are developed and maintained that capture the outcomes from the patient perspective;
(3) the probabilities that these outcomes will occur, given the treatment used and conditioned on patients' comorbidities and severity of illness, are estimated as accurately as possible;
(4) the importance of patient preference for optimal treatment choices is constantly evaluated;
(5) new ideas and technologies, whatever their source, are identified as early as possible and brought into an evaluative network; and
(6) information is made available to patients, health care providers, policymakers, and the public in ways that empower shared decision making and improve policy decisions.

But these tasks cannot be accomplished without the appropriate level of funding. Much of the difficulty we have encountered in getting the AUA-PORT technology assessment network established is the intense competition over priorities and funds in the Agency of Health Care Policy and Research, which has a total budget for effectiveness research of less than $44 million in fiscal year 1993. Less than 5% of approved grants are now being funded.

Iain Chalmers and Richard Peto know well the frustrations of attempting to build systems capable of learning from experience. But the need for these has never been greater. Biomedical technology has fired the medical imagination; an unprecedented cascade of novelty inundates the everyday practice of medicine, but we learn very little from change. Federal research policy, which generously supports the biomedical sciences while neglecting the evaluative sciences, is largely responsible for the present predicament. It is a credit to the work of the British evaluative scientists that it should be the British National Health Service that was the first to recognize the level of funding required to establish and support the evaluative sciences. A program is under way there to spend up to 1.5% of the NHS budget on outcomes research and the building of networks among providers for improving the quality of health care. This percentage far exceeds the 0.5% proportion of the Medicare budget I once proposed as a source of funding for the evaluative sciences.

The value of health care is ultimately a question both of what works and what patients want. Health care reform that ignores the depth of our uncertainty about the outcomes of care and the needs and wants of patients repackages the status quo. It is time to get right the scope and scale of this nation's investment in the evaluative sciences.

REFERENCES

1. BARRY, M. J., A. G. MULLEY, F. J. FOWLER & J. E. WENNBERG. 1988. Watchful waiting vs. immediate transurethral resection for symptomatic prostatism. JAMA **259**(20): 3010–3017.
2. WENNBERG, J., N. ROOS, L. SOLA, A. SCHORI & R. JAFFE. 1987. Use of claims data systems to evaluate health care outcomes: Mortality and re-operation following prostatectomy. JAMA **257**(7): 933–936.
3. FOWLER, F. J., J. E. WENNBERG, R. P. TIMOTHY, et al. 1988. Symptom status and quality of life following prostatectomy. JAMA **259**(20): 3018–3022.
4. WENNBERG, J. 1992. A challenge to HMOs. HMO Practice **6**(2): 5–17.
5. BARRY, M. J. et al. 1993. Patient reactions to a program designed to facilitate patient participation in treatment decisions for benign prostatic hyperplasia. Submitted for publication.
6. WENNBERG, J. E. 1992. Innovation and the policies of limits in a changing health care economy. *In Medical Innovations at the Crossroads*, Vol. 3: *Modern Methods of Clinical Investigation*. A. C. Gelijns, Ed.:9–33. National Academy Press. Washington, DC.
7. FLOOD, A. B., D. LORENCE, J. DING, K. MCPHERSON & N. BLACK. 1993. The role of expectations in assessing outcomes during post-operative recovery. Med. Care. In press.
8. WENNBERG, J. E. 1990. What is outcomes research? *In Medical Innovations at the Crossroads*, Vol. 1: *Modern Methods of Clinical Investigation*. A. C. Gelijns, Ed.: 33–46. National Academy Press. Washington, DC.
9. ROOS, N. P., J. E. WENNBERG, D. J. MALENKA, E. S. FISHER, K. MCPHERSON, T. F. ANDERSON, M. M. COHEN & E. RAMSEY. 1989. Mortality and reoperation after open transurethral resection of the prostate for benign prostatic hyperplasia. N. Engl. J. Med. **320**: 1120–1124.
10. ANDERSEN, T. F., H. BRONNUM-HANSEN, T. SEJR & C. ROEPSTORFF. 1990. Elevated mortality following transurethral resection of the prostate for benign hypertrophy. Med. Care **28**(10): 870–881.
11. D. J. MALENKA, N. ROOS, E. S. FISHER, D. MCLERRAN, F. S. WHALEY, M. J. BARRY, R. BRUSKEWITZ & J. E. WENNBERG. 1990. Further study of the increased mortality following transurethral prostatectomy: A chart-based analysis. J. Urol. **144**: 224–228.
12. MEYHOFF, H. 1987. Transurethral versus transvesical prostatectomy. Scand. J. Urol. Nephrol. Suppl. **102**: 2–26.

13. BARRY, M. J., F. J. FOWLER, M. P. O'LEARY, R. C. BRUSKEWITZ, H. L. HOLTGREWE,
     W. K. MEBUST & A. T. K. COCKETT. The Measurement Committee of the AUA.
     1992. The American Urological Association Symptom Index for benign prostatic
     hyperplasia. J. Urol. **148:** 1549–1557.
14. GRAY, B. H. 1992. The legislative battle over health services research. Health Affairs
     11(4): 38–66.

Use of Claims Data to Monitor Patients over Time: Acute Myocardial Infarction as a Case Study[a]

BARBARA J. McNEIL

Department of Health Care Policy
Harvard Medical School
25 Shattuck Street
Boston, Massachusetts 02115

INTRODUCTION

Since the initiation of the outcomes movement there has been considerable interest in the use of administrative data for the assessment of health outcomes. While early forays into this area suggested the possibility that many diseases or techniques could be evaluated with claims data, recent experiences indicate that current systems in place in the United States allow only limited use of such data for purposes of evaluation or monitoring and are inadequate for judging the appropriateness of the care of individual patients. This paper will be based on experiences from the Patient Outcomes Research Team (PORT) selected to evaluate processes of care and outcomes of care for patients with an acute myocardial infarction (AMI). As a case study, the paper will indicate the conditions under which the AMI PORT was able to use claims data successfully. Our experiences and those of others are largely based on the use of Medicare claims data, particularly inpatient data, and most of our conclusions are based on these data. Supplemental data sources exist for specific applications in selected populations, however, and will be discussed briefly.

DATA SOURCES FOR PATIENTS

Two data sources provided us with particularly useful information for the monitoring of patients. Medicare provided one source and a private billing company the other. Almost all older (≥ 65 years) Americans are currently covered by Medicare. For these individuals Medicare maintains databases that include detailed information on their demographic and enrollment status as well as their utilization of medical care in a variety of settings.

For example, the Health Insurance Skeletonized Eligibility Write-off (HISKEW) file contains administrative information on all patients who are enrolled in Medicare including age; gender and race; residence; reason for and length of entitlement under Medicare Part A and Part B; enrollment in an Health Maintenance Organization (HMO); and occurrence and time of death. The Medicare

[a] This work was supported in part by Grant HS-06341 from the Agency for Health Care Policy and Research.

Provider Analysis and Review (MEDPAR) file contains information on the care of all enrollees who are hospitalized, including reason for admission and other diagnoses (5) and procedures (3) done in the hospitalization.[1] The Part B Medicare Annual Data (BMAD) file contains information on physician care of 5% of the Medicare population whether hospitalized or not. Until recently this was the only file that provided information on routine ambulatory encounters. Beginning with 1991, however, Medicare has significantly augmented its databases. The National Claims History (NCH) File has replaced the MEDPAR, BMAD, and other utilization files and documents on procedure use in inpatient, outpatient, skilled nursing facility, and home health agencies for 100% of the Medicare population. Because encounters with the medical profession by Medicare patients utilize unique identifiers known as the patients' Health Care Insurance Claim (HIC) numbers (as well as individual hospital numbers), it is possible using the NCH and its predecessors to track patients across hospitals and providers and over time.

Shared Medical Systems (SMS) Corporation is a nationwide supplier of health care information and billing systems to hospitals, physician groups, and multi-entity integrated health care providers. Hospitals that contract with SMS agree to provide data on all patients (i.e., over and under 65 years of age). The database is constructed using an on-line real-time "order entry" system whereby data on use of drugs and other services are automatically entered into the SMS database at the time the drugs or services are ordered. Like the Medicare database, the SMS database contains full diagnostic and procedural profiles as well as information on gender, age, race, and primary payer status (Medicare, Medicaid, or private insurance). Unlike Medicare databases, however, SMS files also include data on in-hospital use of medications. Because the database is constructed for patients in SMS hospitals, it is not possible to link patients across hospitals that are not part of the SMS network. With the use of Social Security numbers and other identifying data, it is possible, however, to link patients to the National Death Index and thus to obtain information on their survival status post discharge.

DESIDERATA FOR USE OF CLAIMS DATA FOR MONITORING

Several kinds of information must be available before administrative data can be used for evaluation or monitoring such as information about the patient (e.g., disease severity, co-morbidity, types of outcomes); processes of care provided to the patient; and his/her status over time. For each of these factors, information about coding practices (accuracy, completeness, and timeliness) is also essential. A few words about each of these will indicate why patients with an AMI are particularly good for study with claims data.

1. *Patient Characteristics.* In order to evaluate the impact of treatment on outcomes either initially or during a follow-up period, it is necessary to have an unbiased sample of patients for study. In prospective clinical work this is usually accomplished by use of randomization procedures. In retrospective observational studies, this is obviously not possible, and it is necessary to ensure that chance, bias, or confounding are not the cause of the observed effects. Their effects will be minimized if, in the case of claims data, the following conditions hold.

First, all patients are identified. In the case of AMI, with the exception of patients who have a sudden death out of hospital, patients with a known AMI are universally hospitalized in this country, and hence the Medicare data capture the fact, duration, and many details of the hospitalization. *Second,* the disease code is unambiguous. In the case of AMI a specific code exists (410.), and although the code initially applied to individuals with a new as well as a previous AMI, these states have subsequently been differentiated into two (410.x1 for the initial episode of care for a newly diagnosed MI and 410.x2 for a subsequent episode of care). Moreover, unlike other diseases or conditions (cataract extraction or hip fracture or replacement, for example), there is no need to specify laterality of disease. *Third,* the disease code is complete. Because payments for Medicare patients in the United States are based on the principal reason for hospitalization, in the case of AMI patients, this code will always exist. Were the disease being studied incidental to the reason for admission, it would be reliably coded only if its presence changed DRG assignment. *Fourth,* if there is interest in linking the effects of processes of care with outcomes (e.g., the effect of cardiac catheterization after an AMI on long-term survival), the data must allow creation of "natural experiments" and the ability to analyze the data in an unbiased fashion; techniques like hierarchical modeling or instrumental variables are useful for this purpose because they allow the investigator to control for *unobservable* differences in patients having alternative treatments. McClellan and Newhouse have used geographical distance as the basis for a "natural experiment." By comparing patients "close" to facilities providing catheterization and hence who are more likely to undergo catheterization with patients "far" from catheterization facilities and hence who are less likely to undergo catheterization, they were able to assess the impact of *marginal* catheterization use on survival four years later.[2]

And finally, depending upon the scope of the analysis, use of claims data for evaluation requires the ability to eliminate in an unbiased fashion patients who might be systematically different from the population of general interest or patients for whom complete data are not available. Patients in the former group might be those who are eligible for Medicare by virtue of having end stage renal disease or premature disability instead of by age (i.e., 65 years of age or older). Patients in the latter group would be Medicare beneficiaries who belong to an HMO and for whom Medicare does not reliably receive complete information. Coding practices allow for consideration or elimination of both of these groups of patients.

When these conditions apply, it is possible to obtain general descriptive data on outcomes for the whole cohort or for cohorts selected on the basis of age, gender, or race. Data on other subgroups are generally not possible to obtain because of difficulties in adequately controlling for disease severity and/or co-morbidity even when codes for these states appear to exist on the claims record.

2. *Processes of Care.* Tracking processes of care with the Medicare data also has limitations. Although the NCH administrative files include room for many (10) procedure codes, hospitals have an incentive to code only those procedures that influence payment through changes in DRG assignment, so only major procedures are believed to be accurately identified. In the case of AMI patients several such procedures exist: cardiac catheterization, coronary artery bypass surgery (CABG) and percutaneous transluminal angioplasty (PTCA). On the other hand, for this disease and others, drug therapy is an equally important component of care, but drugs are not identifiable from Medicare claims data. An important example involves thrombolytic therapy (e.g., tissue plasminogen activator [t-PA], streptokinase, urokinase), considered the most important advance in the care of AMI patients in the past decade. The SMS database allowed us to study trends in the use of these drugs in more than 65,000 patients seen in 88 hospitals over a five-year period.

3. *Follow-up Information.* Follow-up information generally involves assessment of outcomes, and for retrospective observational studies, only selected out-

comes are reliably captured from administrative data. They include mortality (available from the HISKEW file), reinfarction, and readmissions (available from the utilization files). As noted above, patient-specific data can be obtained across years and medical facilities by linking files on the basis of patient HICs. However, whether or not a readmission is *related* to the previous admission cannot be easily determined from claims data and such a determination must instead be obtained through a series of inferences. Several investigators at Harvard Medical School are attempting to use the Medicare data set to create algorithms that identify "related adverse readmission rates" for AMI patients.

TABLE 1. Characteristics of Medicare Patients with AMI and General Medicare Population with AMI[a]

	AMI Cohort (n = 218,427)	Random Sample of Medicare Population without AMI (n = 1,158,579)
Age (years, mean ± SD)	76.0 ± 7.3	73.1 ± 5.8
<65	0	0
65–69	48,605 (22%)	391,205 (34%)
70–74	52,351 (24%)	327,299 (28%)
75–79	48,897 (22%)	241,271 (21%)
80–84	37,472 (17%)	156,365 (14%)
85 & over	31,102 (14%)	42,439 (4%)
Gender		
Male	109,168 (50%)	470,510 (41%)
Female	109,259 (50%)	688,069 (59%)
Race		
White	198,368 (91%)	1,023,306 (88%)
Black	11,946 (5%)	85,611 (7%)
Other	8,113 (4%)	49,662 (4%)

[a] Reprinted in part with permission from JAMA **268:** 2533 (1992).

USE OF MEDICARE CLAIMS DATA TO STUDY PATIENTS WITH AN AMI: CHARACTERISTICS OF THE PATIENT POPULATION

Claims data allow identification of cohorts of patients that differ either by their year of entry into the study or by the presence or absence of disease. For the AMI study both types of groups were used.[b] The AMI patients themselves came from several different cohorts, the first (reported in detail in this paper) involved patients with an AMI in 1987 but not in 1986,[b] and who were followed for a period of 24 months. The second involved control groups free of that diagnosis in the year in question. These two groups were compared in several ways, as described in TABLE 1 and below. In the 1987 cohort the average ages for the patients and

[b] The exclusion criterion was introduced in this study to attempt to minimize differences in disease severity in the population. By excluding patients with two AMIs in a one-year period, we believed we were limiting our analysis to less severely ill patients for whom treatment strategies would be more comparable.

the control group were 76 and 73 years, respectively. The most commonly occurring co-morbidities in the AMI group (not shown here) included congestive heart failure, chronic ischemic heart disease, minor and major arrhythmias, uncomplicated hypertension, uncomplicated diabetes, and chronic pulmonary disease. Because significant co-morbidities are usually coded in the discharge abstract form, it is possible to use these data to control analyses for co-morbidity, using either a Charlson type index[3,4] or an index developed from the data set itself.[5] In either case, obviously, the adjustment will not be as good as that obtained with more detailed data on co-morbidity and disease severity obtained from the medical record itself. The conclusions drawn from all analyses reported below did not change with adjustments for co-morbidity.

Medicare patients with an AMI have remarkably similar characteristics from year to year.[6] For example, the mean age for patients changed little from 76 in 1987 to 76.3 years in 1990. Moreover, the distributions by age, gender and race were virtually identical. These similarities facilitate cross-cohort comparisons.

PROCESSES OF CARE AFTER AN AMI

For the 1987 cohort, approximately 23% of the Medicare population had an inpatient cardiac catheterization within 90 days of the index admission; 43% of those 65–69 years, 32% of those 70–74, 19% of those 75–79, and under 10% for those over 80 had the procedure.[6-8] These rates varied by geographic location, ranging, for example, from 15% in New York to 26% in Texas. Over time, the catheterization rate has increased; in 1990 33% of all AMI patients underwent cardiac catheterization. But the geographic diversity has been maintained; there is still an 11 percentage point difference between Texas and New York in the 1990 cohort of Medicare AMI patients (i.e., 33% and 22%, respectively).

Approximately half of these Medicare patients went on to a subsequent CABG or PTCA in 1987; the rates of these procedures varied markedly by age (TABLE 2).[1] Over time, new cohorts showed that, as with cardiac catheterizaton, use of revascularization procedures increased over time, but the relative use of CABG versus PTCA has declined. In fact, the usage of CABG had essentially flattened by 1990, whereas that for PTCA had nearly doubled, relative to usage rates in 1988.[6]

Improved drug therapy is believed to be a major accomplishment of the 1980s and '90s with regard to patients with an AMI. The SMS data set indicated that patients of all ages appear to be receiving thrombolytic therapy less frequently than would have been expected, that they are also receiving beta-blockers less frequently than recommended, and that they are receiving calcium channel blockers more often than recommended. Over time, the trends in usage for all three drugs appear to be going in the direction suggestions by guideline panels.[9]

OUTCOMES FOR MEDICARE BENEFICIARIES AFTER AN AMI: THE 1987 COHORT

Survival is the most important endpoint after an AMI, and results from more than 218,000 Medicare patients tracked by claims data show results considerably worse than those conventionally reported from clinical trials data.[1] These differences are undoubtedly due to differences in the ages of patients in clinical trials (generally younger) or differences in their overall health (generally healthier).

TABLE 2. Cardiac Procedure Use within 90 Days after an AMI[a]

	N	Cardiac Catheterization		CABG		PTCA	
		90-Day Rate[b]	Adjusted[c] Relative Risk	90-Day Rate[b]	Adjusted[c] Relative Risk	90-Day Rate[b]	Adjusted[c] Relative Risk
Overall	218,427	23%		8%		5%	
Age (yr)							
65–69	48,605	43%	1.00	14%	1.00	10%	1.00
70–74	52,351	32%	0.76	11%	0.78	7%	0.71
75–79	48,897	19%	0.47	7%	0.48	4%	0.42
80–84	37,472	8%	0.21	2%	0.19	2%	0.19
85+	31,102	2%	0.06	1%	0.04	1%	0.07
Gender							
Male	109,168	28%	1.00	10%	1.00	6%	1.00
Female	109,259	18%	0.82	6%	0.71	4%	0.87
Race							
White	198,368	23%	1.00	8%	1.00	6%	1.00
Black	11,946	18%	0.72	4%	0.50	3%	0.52
Other	8,113	26%	0.99	9%	0.98	6%	1.03

[a] Reprinted with permission from JAMA **268:** 2533 (1992).
[b] Rates of procedures used are for all patients in the AMI cohort.
[c] Comparisons by age are adjusted for gender and race, comparisons by gender are adjusted by age and race, comparisons by race are adjusted for age and gender. The reference groups were: for age—65–69; for gender—male; for race—white. All differences in relative risk by age, gender, and race are significant at $p < 0.0001$, based on the Mantel-Haenszel Chi-square statistic.

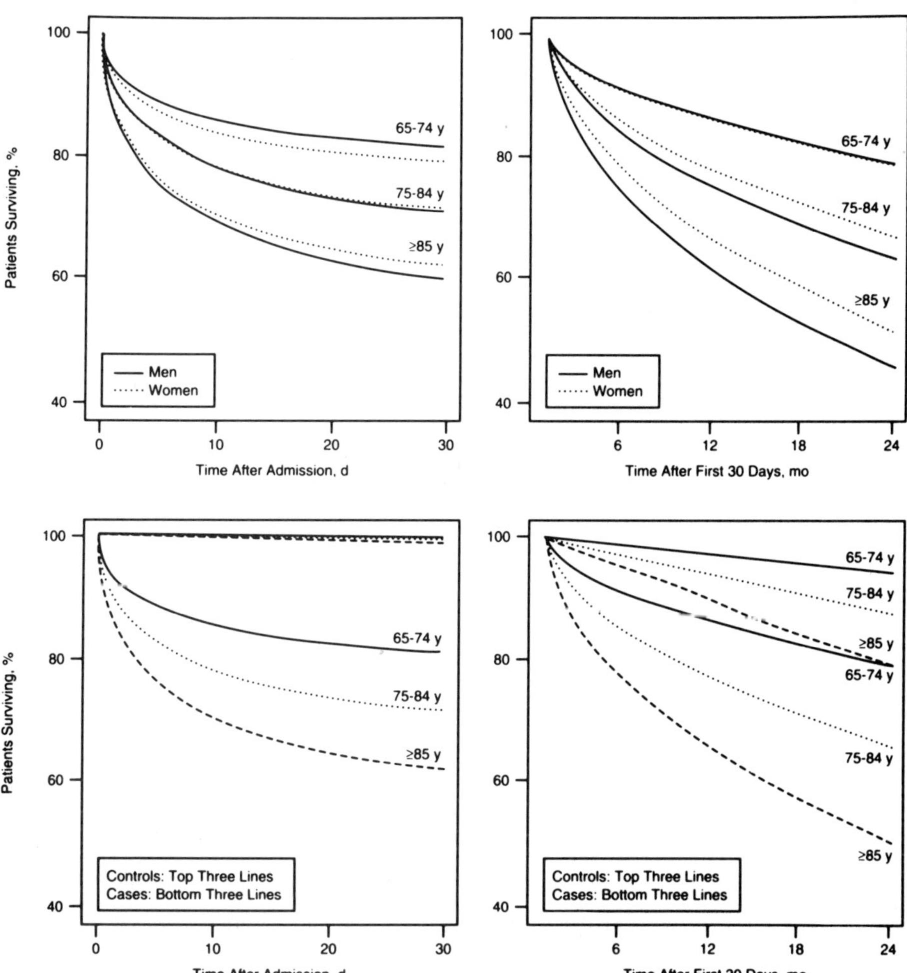

FIGURE 1. Gender- and age-specific survival during the two years after an AMI for the 1987 AMI cohort and the Medicare control population. The ordinate represents the cumulative proportion of patients surviving over time. (*Upper left panel*): Differences in survival between men and women during the first 30 days after their index AMI. Men are represented by the solid curves in each age group and women by the dotted lines. (*Upper right panel*): Differences in survival between men and women for those surviving the first 30 days. Men are represented by the *solid curves* in each age group and women by the *dotted lines*. (*Lower left panel*): Survival of AMI cohort by age compared to control population for first 30 days. The control patients are represented by the overlying lines at the top near 1.0. The AMI cohort groups are represented as follows: 65–74 years (*solid line*), 75–84 years (*dotted line*), and over 85 years (*dashed line*). (*Lower right panel*): Survival of AMI cohort by age groups compared to control population for those surviving the first 30 days. The controls are represented by the top three lines and the AMI patients by the lower three lines. Reprinted with permission from JAMA **268:** 2535 (1992).

FIGURE 1 shows, for example, gender- and age-specific survival during this two-year period for these individuals 65 years of age or older. Mortality rates for AMI patients were high; they also varied by age and less so by gender and race (FIG. 1, top). These rates were significantly higher than those of the control group, so much so, for example, that the mortality rate for individuals 65–74 years who survived the first 30 days after an AMI was approximatley equal at 2 years to that for individuals over 85 years without an AMI (FIG. 1, bottom).

Reinfarction is another relevant endpoint for patients after an AMI (TABLE 3). Overall, 7.3% of the AMI cohort was readmitted in the first year with a diagnosis of a second AMI. The risk of reinfarction increased slightly with age, was higher for women than for men, and was similar across all races. Forty-four percent of the cohort had either reinfarction or death within the first year after their index AMI.

TABLE 3. Rates of Reinfarction[a] or Death within the First Year after AMI

	Reinfarction		Reinfarction or Death	
	Rate	Adjusted RR[b] (95% CI)	Rate	Adjusted RR[b] (95% CI)
Overall	7.3%		44.1%	
Age (yr)				
65–69	6.7%	1.00	30.8%	1.00
70–74	6.9%	1.02 (0.98, 1.07)	37.7%	1.22 (1.20, 1.24)
75–79	7.7%	1.14 (1.09, 1.19)	45.7%	1.48 (1.46, 1.50)
80–84	8.2%	1.20 (1.14, 1.26)	53.1%	1.72 (1.69, 1.75)
85+	6.9%	1.01 (0.95, 1.06)	62.3%	2.01 (1.98, 2.04)
Sex				
Male	7.1%	1.00	42.4%	1.00
Female	7.5%	1.05 (1.01, 1.08)	45.8%	0.99 (0.98, 1.00)
Race				
White	7.3%	1.00	44.3%	1.00
Black	7.3%	0.98 (0.92, 1.05)	42.4%	0.97 (0.95, 0.99)
Other	7.5%	1.03 (0.95, 1.11)	42.3%	1.00 (0.98, 1.03)

[a] These data were calculated using the definition of reinfarction that maximizes sensitivity (see Ref. 1).

[b] Adjusted for age, gender, and race. The reference groups were: for age—65–69; for gender—male; for race—white.

Quality of life is also likely to be an important outcome after an AMI, particularly if revascularization surgery or angioplasty is done in the follow-up period. Such data are not available, however, from claims data and must be obtained directly either from the patients themselves or, less likely, from medical records. Claims data do serve an important pupose in this regard, however, by providing identification of a random sample of patients with an AMI stratified in whatever way desired (e.g., by geographic location, age). As part of the AMI PORT such a study is being done. Among the random sample selected, approximately 80% of those alive at 18 months have participated in a phone interview to assess quality of life.

OUTCOMES FOR MORE RECENT COHORTS

New cohorts of patients with AMIs in 1988 (but not 1987), 1989 (but not 1988), and 1990 (but not 1989) have been created and preliminary analyses concluded.

The results show some improvement in survival (approximately 4 percentage points) from the 1987 cohort. This is particularly true for younger patients. Survival advantages persist for at least two years.[6]

The average level of improvement in survival appears to be greater than would have been expected on the basis of thrombolytic therapy alone (posited to lead to about a 20% advantage in survival, based on pooled analyses of different studies[10]). During this same time interval there also appears to be an increase in the incidence of hemorrhagic strokes at a rate considerably larger than what would be expected from use of thrombolytic therapy alone[11,12]; it is possible that the use of additional drug therapies (e.g., heparin) could be responsible for this increase.

CONCLUSIONS

The experience of the AMI PORT indicates that claims data can be extremely useful for measuring processes of care as well as outcomes of care for cohorts differing in age, race, gender, or year of AMI. The experience is driven by some unique characteristics of patients with AMI, and it is unlikely that our experience with AMI will be able to be generalized to many other diseases.

REFERENCES

1. UDVARHELYI, I. S., C. GATSONIS, A. M. EPSTEIN, C. L. PASHOS, J. P. NEWHOUSE & B. J. McNEIL. 1992. Acute myocardial infarcton in the medicare population. JAMA **268:** 2530–2536.
2. McCLELLAN, M. & J. P. NEWHOUSE. 1993. Medical treatment intensity and patient outcomes: The care of acute myocardial infarction in the elderly. Econometrica. Submitted for publication.
3. CHARLSON, M. E., P. POMPEI, K. L. ALES & C. R. MacKENZIE. 1987. A new method of classifying prognostic comorbidity in longitudinal studies: Development and validation. J. Chronic Dis. **40:** 373–383.
4. DEYO, R., D. CHERKIN & M. CIOL. 1992. Adapting a clinical comorbidity index for use with ICD-9-CM administrative data bases. J. Clin. Epidemiol. **45:** 613–619.
5. NORMAND, S. L., B. J. McNEIL, J. P. NEWHOUSE & A. M. EPSTEIN. 1993. Development and validation of a comorbidity index for patients with an acute myocardial infarction. Submitted for publication.
6. PASHOS, C. L., C. GATSONIS, A. M. EPSTEIN, J. P. NEWHOUSE & B. J. McNEIL. 1993. Temporal changes in the care and outcomes of elderly patients with acute myocardial infarction, 1987 to 1990. JAMA **270:** in press.
7. GATSONIS, C., S. L. NORMAND, C. LIU & C. MORRIS. 1993. Geographic variation of procedure utilization: a hierarchical approach. Med. Care **31:** 4554–4559.
8. GATSONIS, C., A. M. EPSTEIN, S. L. NORMAND, J. P. NEWHOUSE & B. J. McNEIL. 1993. Geographical variations in the use of cardiac catheterization after an AMI. Submitted for publication.
9. PASHOS, C. L., S. L. NORMAND, J. B. GARFINKLE, J. P. NEWHOUSE, A. M. EPSTEIN, & B. J. McNEIL. 1993. Trends in the use of drug therapies in patients with acute myocardial infarction: 1988–1992. Submitted for publication.
10. GRINES, C. L. & A. N. DeMARIA. 1990. Optimal utilization of thrombolytic therapy for acute myocardial infarction: Concepts and controversies. J. Am. Coll. Cardiol. **16:** 223–231.
11. KRUMHOLZ, H. M., R. C. PASTERNAK, M. C. WEINSTEIN, G. C. FRIESINGER, P. M. RIDKER, A. N. A. TOSTESON & L. GOLDMAN. 1992. Cost effectiveness of thrombolytic therapy with streptokinase in elderly patients with suspected acute myocardial infarction. N. Engl. J. Med. **327:** 7–13.

12. O'CONNOR, C. M., R. M. CALIFF, E. W. MASSEY, *et al.* 1991. Stroke and acute myocardial infarction in the thrombolytic era: Clinical correlates and long term prognosis. J. Am. Coll. Cardiol. **16:** 533–540.

DISCUSSION

RICHARD PETO (*Radcliffe Infirmary, Clinical Trial Service Unit, Oxford, U.K.*): I found the fact that the number of people who weren't using treatments of demonstrated value a bit depressing, given how strong the evidence of benefit is. But the one thing that you weren't claiming, Dr. McNeil, is that one can actually find out what works and what doesn't work from analysis of such data. In your list of four points that claim wasn't made. Would you agree that you can't actually use such data for making reliable inferences about what does or doesn't work in terms of saving lives when we know from other sources that certain things do work? Your data are useful in drawing attention to the fact that doctors aren't using such treatments, but whether by instrumental variables or any other way, you can't work out whether specific treatments save lives or not from analysis of such data. Do you agree?

BARBARA MCNEIL (*Harvard Medical School, Boston, Mass.*): That is a very good question. I tried to be quite specific in my paper about the four areas where I thought these data were most useful. I also tried to say that there may be some potential, given the variability that we see, to use instrumental variables or hierarchical modeling to relate process of care to outcomes of care. That's a newer effort which has not been widely used or evaluated and so we need to defer judgement on it until we've had a chance to have more peer review. My economics colleagues and many clinicians who have seen these data seem to think that this kind of instrument—this division on the basis of geography—is a reasonable one that allows us to hold the case mix constant and that should provide us with some glimmer of evidence to link process with outcome. I don't think that it will make you happy and it may not work in the long run, but I think it's a reasonable thing to try at this point.

PETO: But you *are* looking for small differences and therefore your method can't give reliable information. You're suggesting comparing people who lived in the inner city near one of these more technologically sophisticated facilities with people who don't and then determining whether or not the outcome is rather similar. You talk about differences in outcome, but you are going to see differences in *patients*. There are going to be small differences in the types of patients who get referred from the inner cities from those being treated further away, and you can't adjust for those biases.

MCNEIL: You're probably right . . .

PETO: Then you can't produce serious evidence about whether things work or not.

MCNEIL: I think that perhaps your initial question was probably not the right one to be asking me. My paper was designed to indicate what claims data were useful for and I thought I was quite clear about that. Again, I'm not proposing this particular approach as an alternative to a randomized clinical trial.

PETO: I do agree with the value of such an inquiry for the purposes that you stated.

ALAN H. MORRIS (*LDS Hospital, Salt Lake City, Utah*): Dr. McNeil, you pointed to myocardial infarction as a particularly instructive disease to study because the diagnosis was rather specific, so I assume that you recognize that the quality of the data for drawing other diagnostic conclusions might be questionable. For example, it is pretty challenging to try to ferret out information in a patient with profound pulmonary failure after trauma who has thromboembolic disease and gets an infection and multiple organ failure. Could you comment further on the quality of the data for drawing inferences about the use of drugs in these cases? The issue of quality in this database, which is financially directed and thus fraught with uncertainty, is an important one.

McNEIL: That's an excellent question to which, regrettably, I can't give a precise answer. We have no drug database except for Medicaid patients, who have drug coverage benefits. So if we want to look at drug usage we have to find some way to do it. For this particular database we took comfort in the fact that it recorded thrombolytic therapy because such therapy, at least in the early stages when it was largely tissue plasminogen activator, resulted in an average charge of $3,000 in these SMS hospitals. Now it seems unlikely for a hospital not to bill a $3,000 item. In these particular hospitals a drug would not be filled by the pharmacist without this order entry. That suggested to us that there may be situations in which these drugs were ordered, but not given, and no credit was given to reflect that, leading to a possible overestimate of its use. Unfortunately, considerations of confidentiality prevented our getting a random chart review.

JONATHAN LOMAS (*McMaster University, Ontario, Canada*): I'd like to make an observation contrasting one of your results, Dr. McNeil, with Peto's earlier results with regard to thrombolysis. This disparity points to a need for methodologic rigor in assessing clinical evidence. One potential explanation for the fairly sizeable difference in the apparent rate of thrombolytic therapy in the U.K. versus that in your study is that self-reporting from physicians is fairly extensive in the U.K. in contrast with more chart-ordered or claims data reports in the U.S. So the size of the difference between nearly 70%, as Richard Peto reports for the use of streptokinase in the U.K., versus the figure of less than 40% in your survey may turn out in the real world to be no different. It's merely a reporting error, and given what we know from McPhie's studies on preventive practices and our own studies and almost any other study that contrasts these hard outcomes versus the physicians' self report, a major "halo effect" seems to be indicated, especially when clinical trials are reported. Physicians sometimes report what they think they *should* be doing, rather than what they are actually doing. Again, this calls for greater methodologic rigor.

McNEIL: That point is very good. In a similar study from Duke University that asked physicians in the U.S. what percentage of their patients received thrombolytic therapy the number was higher than what we observed in the SMS data, but considerably lower than that reported by Richard Peto.

Using Scientific Information to
Improve Quality of Health Care

ROBERT H. BROOK

Health Sciences Program
RAND Corporation
Santa Monica, California 90406-2138

Departments of Medicine and Health Services
UCLA Center for Health Sciences
Los Angeles, California

In writing a paper on using scientific information to improve quality of health care, it is possible for me to take two perspectives—both that of a health services researcher who has contributed to the subject and that of a practicing internist who must use scientific information and expert judgment to provide, on a day-to-day basis, actual care to patients. The former perspective is more scholarly and politically appropriate for this symposium, while the latter is more pragmatic, less theoretical and may serve to more crisply define some of the issues in this field. It is for this set of reasons that this paper will examine efficacy, effectiveness, and quality from the point of view of a practicing physician.

A practicing physician is called upon to make decisions each day. He cannot fall back on the response often attributed to academicians, which is to do a study. Like the academician, the practicing physician wants to make the right decision—that is, he wants to maximize the patient's own set of health outcomes (in economic terms he wants to act as the perfect agent for the patient)—but unfortunately the practicing physician has less than adequate data on which to make a decision. If he is lucky he has some information on the efficacy of medical care—that is, the benefit of medical care performed under *ideal circumstances.*

Data on *efficacy* will answer the question: is drug A better than drug B or is procedure A better than procedure B when both are prescribed or performed by the best physicians and under ideal circumstances?[1] Sometimes information from a randomized trial or, better yet, a scientifically valid meta-analysis of randomized trials is available. However, the patients included in the randomized trials or the analysis of randomized trials may not reflect the physician's current patient. His patient might have been excluded from the trial because of the presence of co-morbidities or other factors such as advanced age or other health conditions. More importantly, the therapies studied, although having the same name as those currently available to the physician, may not actually be the same. For instance, most of the information about coronary artery bypass surgery comes from randomized controlled clinical trials, but those trials were conducted more than a decade ago, and although coronary artery bypass surgery is still called by the same name, it is a very different procedure today from the one evaluated a decade or more ago. Among the differences are the way the heart is stopped in surgery, the way obstructive lesions are bypassed, and other aspects of pre- and postoperative care. Likewise, medical therapy for coronary artery disease, although still called medical therapy, has also changed radically in the last decade. Yet, it is extremely unlikely that scientists will repeat the controlled clinical trials that demonstrated the efficacy of "old" coronary artery bypass surgery versus the "old" medical therapy. Thus, new medical therapies for coronary artery disease will never be tested rigorously against the new surgical techniques. The practicing physician will need to rely on expert judgment or indirect evidence.

Even more important than the fact that the studies may be out of date or not generalizable is the concern that the outcomes achieved by the surgical and medical arms of a randomized trial when both are performed under ideal conditions may not reflect the outcomes achievable in a patient who often must go to the average doctor, not the best one. Again, the *effectiveness* of care, that is, the outcomes of care when performed under conditions available in the community, may be very different from that obtained under ideal circumstances. This difference may be due to differences in quality. Thus, a randomized trial or a meta-analysis based on randomized trials may not provide the right information for a practicing physician to make the best decision on the patient's behalf.

These comments do not imply that my practicing physician is anti-science but, rather, that information from randomized trials about clinical efficacy is a necessary, but not sufficient basis on which to make a decision regarding a treatment plan for a particular patient. Information produced by randomized trials should not be revered or regarded as having been brought down on tablets from Mount Sinai. Such information will not change the practice of medicine forever, but rather has an extraordinarily limited half-life and, because of the difference between efficacy and effectiveness, can be misleading if not applied carefully by the practicing physician.

Three specific examples may make this point clearer. Consider a 70-year-old man who had had a transient ischemia attack and on carotid angiography is shown to have a 70 percent obstruction of the carotid artery. An elegant randomized trial published in the *New England Journal of Medicine* demonstrated that carotid endarterectomy for this patient is efficacious, that is, it produces a better outcome than is achievable by state-of-the-art medical therapy.[3] However, the complication rate (5%) obtained by surgeons who were allowed to participate in this trial may not reflect that achieved by the average U.S. surgeon who does the procedure. In particular, the best community-based data suggest that a complication rate from this operation of 10 to 12% may be more representative.[4] This figure is far different from the 5% rate reported in the randomized trial. Moreover, an average U.S. surgeon performs only one to two carotid endarterectomies per year.[5]

Now what should our practicing internist do who has taken the time to read the *New England Journal of Medicine*? (And this in itself makes him unusual.) Should he ignore the results reported in the *New England Journal*? Should he hope that the surgeon he knows is as good as those used in the trial? Should he bet on the fact that his managed-care patient, who belongs to an accountable health care plan, will only receive medical care of average rather than high quality? Should he treat the patient by saying to him, "you decide"? I submit that the data published in the *New England Journal of Medicine* may harm more people than it helps in the absence of a system to identify which surgeons and their hospital teams have complication rates that are sufficiently low to justify performing this procedure. Without a commitment to making information available on outcomes by physician and hospital, efficacy data produced by randomized trials may be elegant, but may also be misleading. If we are going to invest money in performing expensive randomized trials, should we also insist that valid information on performance at the physician and hospital level must also be released so that the trial results can be properly used?[6]

Let us now consider a woman with stage 1 cancer of the cervix. As in the above example, two therapeutic courses of action are available: surgery or radiation therapy. Unlike the above example, however, the cure rate of both procedures is about equal. But the complication rate of surgery under ideal circumstances is greater than (worse) that from radiation therapy. However, a study of the effectiveness of radiation therapy demonstrated that in the average hospital, radiation therapy was so poorly applied that its complication rate exceeded that of surgery by two- to three-fold.[7] As in the previous example, on the basis of efficacy data, I would have urged my patient to have had radiation therapy, but I would recommend surgery on the basis of the effectiveness data. Again, since the average physician has no information about the quality of care of either his surgical colleagues or his radiation therapy colleagues, what should he do? Should he follow the efficacy data or the effectiveness data?

The third example relates to a man who calls his physician in the middle of the night and complains of crushing chest pain. The physician's classical response in the United States probably is to hang up the phone and call 911. An ambulance would take the patient to the nearest hospital, where he or she would be admitted to the coronary care unit and a myocardial infarction ruled in or out. But what evidence has the physician used in making this decision? And is this decision the correct one? There has been only one study of home versus hospital care for patients with possible symptoms of an acute myocardial infarction. It was performed in the United Kingdom many years ago and showed no benefit of coronary care units.[8] However, coronary care units have substantially improved since the time that randomized trial was performed, and most researchers in the United States would consider it unethical to repeat such a randomized trial today. The U.K. study was also criticized on methods grounds. On the other hand, effectiveness of care for patients with a heart attack varies markedly by hospital. In a nationally representative sample of more than 300 U.S. hospitals, we showed that the worst 25% of U.S. hospitals had a 30-day post-hospital admission mortality rate that was about 30% higher than that of the other 75% of hospitals. This amounted to about six additional deaths per 100 patients who were admitted to the hospital with a myocardial infarction. Analyses that have led to these conclusions carefully adjust at a clinical level for differences by hospital in the patients' sickness at admission.[9]

Considering these data about both effectiveness and efficacy, what should my confused doctor do? If he had data about hospital quality, knew which of the hospitals in the immediate vicinity of the patient's home was the worst one, and also knew that this worst hospital was also the closest one, then instead of calling 911 he might have gotten dressed and driven to the patient's house. He would have put his patient in his car and taken him not to the nearest hospital but to the best hospital. This course of action would certainly expose the patient to a longer period of time without any medical care and the excess risk of death associated with this longer time without treatment. However, the excess risk may, and probably would, have been offset by the better quality of care rendered to the patient in the better hospital. Of course, the best solution of all would be for the ambulance driver to know which was the best hospital and to take that patient to that facility and bypass the nearest one.

I have presented these rather simplistic clinical examples to illustrate the following points:

1. No matter how much clinical research is performed, physicians will need to make most of their decisions in the absence of complete data.
2. The results of randomized trials when they are available may not be as useful as we hope. In many cases the therapy that has been evaluated in

the clinical trial, although the same in name as the therapy now being used, may be so fundamentally different as to make the results from the randomized trials misleading. For example, the angioplasty catheter used today is very different from the one used five years ago.[10] Coronary artery bypass surgery is a different operation than that available five years ago. Yet, we still talk about angioplasty and coronary artery bypass surgery as if they have not changed.[11] In addition, the quality with which each arm of the randomized trial can be carried out in the community may overwhelm any differences between alternative therapies that are demonstrated in the trial itself. Data on the quality of community practice by hospital and physician are essential for making proper use of data from randomized trials.

3. Data on efficacy that are produced by designs other than a randomized controlled clinical trial will always be viewed as nondefinitive. People will always worry about whether there were adequate adjustments to control for selection effects that resulted in good-risk patients selecting one therapy versus another.

4. We must therefore design new methods that synthesize knowledge and expert judgment. These methods will never be perfect, but will help physicians make better decisions regarding what they should do when they are faced with decision-making in the absence of definitive knowledge, wisdom, or data on efficacy, effectiveness, and quality.[12,13] It is my contention that this circumstance will exist forever in medicine whether we like it or not and no matter how much we invest in learning more about what works and doesn't work. If anything, the current explosion of medical technologies will make the situation worse and in the future it is likely there will be less data from randomized trials about what works or not in relationship to the new battery of tools than what we currently have from our existing tools.

Because of these four beliefs, assertions, or truths (depending on your viewpoint), the rest of this paper will describe a method that uses specific information and judgments to provide guidelines to physicians that can be used to improve the appropriateness of medical care. By appropriateness we mean that the benefits of a medical service exceed its risks by a sufficiently wide margin that the service should be rendered. In developing a method for assessing appropriateness, we applied five criteria.

First, we wanted to assure the timeliness of guidelines and thus set a six-month to one-year time frame for the full process of guideline development. Second, we wanted to assure that the guidelines incorporated the best information that was available in the medical literature on effectiveness, efficacy, use, cost, and complications. Third, we determined that the available literature was not adequate by itself for reaching conclusions about the appropriateness of the use of procedures. In particular, when we reviewed the entire world's literature in 1981[14] we found 18 randomized trials for coronary artery bypass surgery, 19 for coronary angiography, 11 for cholecystectomy, 18 for colonoscopy, 10 for upper GI endoscopy, and 1 for carotid endarterectomy. The literature analysis would need to be coupled with some sort of a group judgment process. Fourth, we wanted the guidelines to represent a medical rather than a cost viewpoint, a decision that was more than philosophical, for if we were to include cost considerations we would have had to decide *whose* cost we would consider. Should the guidelines reflect what a person with a large amount of disposable income should do? Or should the guidelines reflect what society should do if it were wealthy? Or should the guidelines reflect what a society should do when it does not even have enough money to provide food to its population? So, by eliminating the cost element, we were able to produce appropriateness standards or guidelines that were independent of such decisions. Finally, we wanted the guidelines to have a multispecialty perspective and not be based on or reflect the opinion of a single specialty. This last criterion is important in terms of the makeup of the group judgment process and the decision that the leader of it be a physician with expertise in epidemiology, statistics, or research design, but not in the content of the guideline.

We began our efforts at establishing guidelines by studying procedures that were either expensive or dangerous, rather than by considering conditions or diseases. We chose this path because it was easier to set guidelines for procedures than for conditions. The literature on procedures is more focused than that for conditions. In addition, a large amount of the expense in the health care system, as well as its benefit, is related to whether or not a procedure should be performed, and thus studying procedures appeared to be a good way to begin.

In order to select our procedures, we began by determining from national data how often the procedures were performed and then used clinical judgment to determine their likelihood of being associated with great benefit or great risk. We identified the following procedures for examination: coronary angiography,[15] coronary artery bypass surgery,[11] coronary angioplasty,[10] carotid endarterectomy,[16] colonoscopy,[17] upper GI endoscopy,[18] cholecystectomy,[19] cataract surgery,[20] hysterectomy,[21] back manipulation,[22] and abdominal aortic aneurysm resection.[23] After selecting the procedure for study, we did a review of the literature. Because of the criteria stated above, we required that the literature review be finished in six months. It was conducted by a physician with training in statistics, epidemiology, and/or health services research. All relevant articles were identified from a MEDLINE search under the subheadings of efficacy, use, complications, cost, and indications for the use of the procedure. We examined reference lists from leading textbooks in the field as well as from the articles we identified and categorized the literature into randomized controlled trials, prospective non-randomized trials with a cohort design, prospective non-randomized trials with a registry design, retrospective cohort studies, cross-sectional studies, surveys, editorials, and reviews. We eliminated articles that did not appear in English and we also eliminated articles that were based on a single case.

On the basis of this literature analysis, we produced outcome evidence tables which summarized, for a group of clinically homogeneous patients, information about complications, effectiveness, and efficacy. For instance, we tried to differentiate the effect of coronary angioplasty in patients with stable angina, or in the post myocardial infarction patient, or in patients with one set of stress test results versus another. We did not do a formal meta-analysis of the literature and in some cases we were even uncomfortable in averaging the results in the outcome evidence tables because that calculation could possibly be misleading.

As information about the strength of evidence regarding effectiveness and efficacy is being gathered, the same physician who is performing that task begins the development of a preliminary list of clinical scenarios or indications for which the procedure may or may not be done. The literature is used to suggest the critical variables in these scenarios and how many of them might be needed to put a patient in one category. These scenarios may categorize patients in terms of their symptoms, past medical history, and the results of previous diagnostic tests. The indication list is designed to be detailed, comprehensive, and manageable. The indications should be detailed enough so that patients presenting with a particular indication are reasonably homogeneous in the sense that performing the procedure is equally appropriate or inappropriate for all patients in that group.

In addition, the list should include all indications for performing the procedure that might occur in clinical practice and it should be short enough so that all indications can be rated by the panelists within a reasonable length of time (1–2 days).

We have had as few as 49 indications for cholecystectomy to as many as 3,000 or more for colonoscopy. A typical indication might be as follows: coronary angiography is indicated in an asymptomatic patient in a high-risk occupation (pilot) if there is no evidence of the performance of an exercise EKG or exercise thallium or MUGA test. This one indication contains the following terms: asymptomatic, high-risk occupation, exercise EKG, exercise thallium, and exercise MUGA. Most of the indications contain about this number of clinical variables and every term in each indication must be precisely defined.

After the list of indications or clinical scenarios is drafted and after the literature review is performed, we send it to specialists who review both the structure of the indications and the literature review and answer the following questions: Is the literature review biased in any way? Are major studies overlooked? Is the indication structure sufficiently detailed to achieve the objective of dividing patients into clinically homogeneous groups? Using this process we have been able to produce a literature review with outcome evidence tables for nine procedures and an indication structure that was considered complete and unbiased. It is interesting, however, that different issues are raised in each literature review, such as the question: how dependent are estimates of complication rates on the performance at a small set of institutions? In addition, results for patients who were referred from long geographic distances may be biased. These patients may experience better outcomes than patients whose profiles appear to be absolutely similar, but who reside in the community in which the procedure is performed.

At the same time that the literature review and indication structure are being completed, a panel of experts is selected whose job it will be to also review the literature review and the indication structure, and in addition to rate the indications on a scale of 1–9, where 9 indicates that the procedure is appropriate (i.e., the health benefits of performing the procedure greatly exceed its risks) and 1 indicates the opposite.

In deciding how to structure the group judgment process, we examined a variety of options, and for many reasons (some of which are listed below) agreed on the following format. First, we wanted to ensure that every member had an equal say in the final decision and that the opinion of the group was explicitly recorded. We thus thought that a modified Delphi process met this need, in which individuals would provide their appropriateness rating for each indication at home alone, then convene as a group to discuss their ratings, and then re-rate all of the clinical indications.[24] The group meeting was felt to be necessary to ensure that sufficient attention was paid to the task to perform it accurately. It could be the case that some ratings would be wrong simply because the physician expert was interrupted while doing this work. We believed that we needed a defined process such as this because committees made up of physicians often result in a single physician's dominating the entire meeting and it is unclear at the end of the meeting whether the judgment arrived at reflects the opinion of one or two physicians or of all the physicians in the room.

We selected nine physicians because, when a moderator and a facilitator are added, the group reaches 11, and we did not believe that the group could function if it were larger. We determined that a multispecialty group was needed. A typical group to consider coronary artery bypass surgery might consist of one family physician, two internists, three cardiologists, two cardiac surgeons, and one radiologist. A panel to consider the use of cholecystectomy and endoscopy might consist of one family physician, two internists, three gastroenterologists, two general surgeons, and a radiologist. We know that an all-doer panel (a panel of physicians who actually perform the procedure) produces higher ratings than a mixed panel, but we are not yet sure which panel produces the most valid ratings.[25] We attained nominations for the panels by asking specialty societies to nominate at least five persons for each of the panel slots and we then examined the *curriculum vitae* of each nominee to select a panel with diversity in terms of geography and practice style. We have had a great deal of professional interest in this process. In a recent experience of five panels, of 190 panelists nominated, 90 percent responded with a *curriculum vitae*, and of the 45 whom we asked to participate, only four declined, all because of a conflict on the date of the panel meeting.

Although the panelists are nominated by specialty and subspecialty societies, they are told that their participation on the panel does not represent endorsement by the society, but seeks to determine their individual judgments concerning the circumstances under which a procedure should or should not be used. Before we convened the panel, we sent the panelists the preliminary list of indications and the literature review and determined whether they also believed that the literature review was unbiased and that the indications structure was a good starting place. We then asked each of the panelists to rate the indications. The ratings were returned to the RAND Corporation, where they were summarized and the panel convened for a face-to-face meeting where all indications were discussed and re-rated. We can do both rounds of ratings in about five days of panelists' time, which includes usually a two-day meeting.

The instructions given to the panelists in doing the ratings are as follows: They are asked to consider the use of the procedure for the specified clinical scenario (i.e., indication), and then to determine its appropriateness (using the previous definition) if the patient undergoes that procedure at the hands of the average physician or at the average hospital. After the ratings of the first round are obtained, they are analyzed. If the panel's median rating is 7, 8, or 9, the indication is considered appropriate. If the median is 4, 5, or 6, the indication is considered to be equivocal, and 1, 2, or 3 is considered to be inappropriate. Agreement and disagreement are also defined.

The panel meeting consists of a series of exchanges among the panel leader (that is, the physician who did the literature review and developed the indication structure) and the rest of the panel. The meeting tends to focus on rating trends. Each physician at the meeting knows his rating and knows the ratings of all other panelists, but not which panelist produced what rating. The group leader knows how each individual panelist rated an indication as well as whether the indication was rated with agreement or disagreement or was considered to be appropriate, inappropriate, or uncertain. The discussion focuses on those ratings for which there is disagreement or where there may be some misunderstanding. The process of resolving disagreement is to first suggest that the indication needs to be clarified. This can be done by clarifying definitions or by dividing indications so that they reflect more clinically homogeneous groups. If disagreement persists, we try to understand the evidence on which the disagreement is based. The panel process does not result in or force consensus. Once positions are stated and defended with the literature we move on.

Recently we have added a third set of ratings to this process—rating the indications for necessity. A procedure is considered necessary to the extent that all four of the following criteria are met: (1) The procedure is appropriate; (2) it would be improper not to provide the service; (3) there is a reasonable chance that the procedure will benefit the patient; and (4) the benefit to the patient is not small. A procedure could be appropriate but not necessary if it had a low likelihood of benefit but few risks or if it produced a minor but almost certain benefit. The necessity ratings so far have been completed at home. The results are tabulated as described for the appropriateness analysis.

If this literature review and group judgment process is carried out correctly, it produces within about a nine-month to one-year time window, a reasonably complete analysis of the literature; a structure of all possible appropriate and inappropriate uses of a procedure (i.e., a set of indications); ratings for each of these indications; and a standard text of definitions that would allow one to assess either prospectively or retrospectively whether a procedure was necessary, appropriate but not necessary, equivocal, or inappropriate.

There are, of course, many research questions that could and should be asked about this method. It represents a model T that needs to be improved. This method does, however, provide a means by which ratings for the 100 or so procedures that make up most of what we do in medicine could be developed within a time frame of about three years. The success of such an effort would increase if there were cooperation from research groups around the world.

We have demonstrated that the indication structure and literature review can be transported from one country to another country with very little modification and the indications can be re-rated by experts from that second country. The ratings may differ, but the structure of the indications and the literature analysis provides a template to make the process go faster. For instance, we have used coronary angiography, coronary artery bypass surgery, and angioplasty literature reviews and indications structures developed in the United States to serve as a template for rating these procedures in the U.K.,[26] the Netherlands, Canada, and Sweden. A U.S. cholecystectomy literature review and indication structure has been used in the U.K. and in Israel.[27] Switzerland is using some indications without even asking their physicians to re-rate them.

The method produces an explicit track record of what was done and each physician is accountable for his action, and it quickly identifies those indications for which the physician community believes we do not know whether the risks and benefits favor performing or not performing the procedure. Such indications, if they are frequently used to justify performing a procedure, would be perfect ones to use as the basis for randomized controlled clinical trials. One of the byproducts of this method could be information that would help determine what randomized trials should be performed on which clinical populations. Similarly, indications for which there is major disagreement might also be ones for which randomized trial data would be useful. Finally, we avoided producing a vague document that nobody can use by trying to become more rather than less precise and by not worrying if indeed consensus was not reached. Thus, we did not seek the lowest common denominator but, rather, tried to come up with well-defined patient groups for which all participants could give an explicit opinion.

We have applied our ratings to many procedures in the United States and abroad and have demonstrated that as many as one-third of procedures may be performed for less than appropriate reasons.[28] Thus, this method, if valid, identifies a large percentage of medical care that could be eliminated without sacrificing a person's health. Appropriateness has also been shown to vary by country,[29] hospital,[30] and procedure.[28]

However, the method and its conclusions have also come under a great deal of fire from many fronts, and we recognize that the method represents but a beginning step. A number of critical questions concerning this method need to be addressed, the most important, of course, being its validity. For instance, if we follow the indications for a given procedure in one region of the country and follow usual practice in another region of the country, what happens to health expenditures as well as to health for people with those conditions who might benefit from or be harmed by the procedure? On a more methodologic note, would a meta-analysis, when feasible, improve the validity and reliability of the ratings? Should the ratings process itself be changed to reflect probabilities and utilities? If utilities are estimated for different outcomes, whose utilities—the physicians' or the patients'—should be used? Should decision analysis be used to aid the group's deliberation? Should different criteria be used to select the physician experts? Should cost be introduced into the model explicitly? How reliable are the ratings? All of these questions need to be addressed, but in general most of them would require the expenditure of greater resources and require more time to complete the development of ratings for a procedure. The question is whether they are worth the additional time and financial cost. This should be a matter of scientific investigation. Of course, the ratings, the indications, the structure, and the literature review need to be updated as knowledge changes. Finally, the question of quality addressed by the case examples at the beginning of this paper should also be addressed by this method. Should ratings be adjusted for circumstances in which the procedure is done by a superior performer versus an average performer versus an inferior one?

Where then are we? I believe that the method described above complements nicely the investigations of efficacy that are now being done throughout the world. It provides a convenient, feasible way of synthesizing information so that it can be used by physicians when faced with a real decision for a real patient. It has been used both in research studies and prospectively to help physicians make better decisions. The guidelines we have produced are in the public domain and are available for use by patients as well as physicians. They could help patients to increase their power to reach an informed decision when they visit their physicians.

I am sure that in the future better methods will be devised to translate scientific knowledge into tools to help physicians, but current methods are sufficiently sensitive to identify a large proportion of procedures that are not needed. Perhaps we are in a situation very similar to where we were in laboratory medicine 30 years ago. In the past, techniques for measuring serum sodium or potassium were rather crude compared to those of the modern laboratory. Yet, the measures were sensitive enough to identify most illnesses and they helped physicians to make better treatment decisions. In like manner, while methods to translate effectiveness and efficacy data into practice guidelines also need to be improved, they still appear to be sufficiently valid and reliable to be used now. Work should proceed on developing such guidelines for the 100 or so common procedures carried out in medicine today. In addition, work on improving the methods by which the guidelines are developed should also proceed rapidly.

REFERENCES

1. BROOK, R. H. & K. N. LOHR. 1985. Efficacy, effectiveness, variations, and quality: Boundary-crossing research. Med. Care **23**: 710–722.
2. LEAPE, L. L., L. H. HILBORNE, J. P. KAHAN, *et al.* 1991. Coronary Artery Bypass Graft: A Literature Review and Ratings of Appropriateness and Necessity. JRA-02-CWF/HF. RAND Corporation, Santa Monica, CA.
3. BARNETT, H. J. M., D. W. TAYLOR, R. B. HAYNES, *et al.* 1991. Beneficial effect of carotid endarterectomy in symptomatic patients with high-grade carotid stenosis. N. Engl. J. Med. **325**(7):445–453.

4. WINSLOW, C. M., D. H. SOLOMON, M. R. CHASSIN, *et al.* 1988. The appropriateness of performing coronary endarterectomy. N. Engl. J. Med. **318**(12): 721–727.
5. LEAPE, L., R. E. PARK, D. H. SOLOMON, *et al.* 1989. Relation between surgeons' practice volumes and geographic variation in the rate of carotid endarterectomy. N. Engl. J. Med. **321**: 653–657.
6. BROOK, R. H. 1992. Improving practice: The clinician's role. Br. J. Surg. **79**: 606–607.
7. HANKS, G. E., D. F. HERRING & S. KRAMER. 1983. Care outcome studies: Results of the national practice in cancer of the cervix. Cancer **51**: 959–967.
8. MATHER, H. G., N. G. PEARSON, *et al.* 1971. Acute myocardial infarction: Home and hospital treatment. Br. Med. J. **3**: 334–338.
9. KAHN, K. L., E. B. KEELER, M. J. SHERWOOD, *et al.* 1990. Comparing outcomes of care pre- and post-implementation of the DRG-based prospective payment system. JAMA **264**: 1984–1988.
10. HILBORNE, L. H., L. L. LEAPE, J. P. KAHAN *et al.* 1991. Percutaneous Transluminal Coronary Angioplasty: A Literature Review and Ratings of Appropriateness and Necessity. JRA-01-CWF/HF. RAND Corporation. Santa Monica, CA.
11. LEAPE, L. L., L. H. HILBORNE, J. P. KAHAN *et al.* 1991. Coronary Artery Bypass Graft: A Literature Review and Ratings of Appropriateness and Necessity. JRA-02-CWF/HF. RAND Corporation. Santa Monica, CA.
12. BROOK, R. H., M. R. CHASSIN, A. FINK, *et al.* 1986. A method for the detailed assessment of the appropriateness of medical technologies. Int. J. Technol. Assess. Health Care **2**(1): 53–63.
13. KOSECOFF, J., A. FINK, R. H. BROOK, *et al.* 1987. The appropriateness of using a medical procedure: Is information in the medical record valid? Med. Care **25**(3): 196–201.
14. FINK, A., R. H. BROOK, J. KOSECOFF, *et al.* 1987. Sufficiency of the clinical literature for learning about the appropriate uses of six medical and surgical procedures. West. J. Med. **147**(5): 609–615.
15. BERNSTEIN, S. J., M. LAOURI, L. H. HILBORNE, *et al.* 1992. Coronary Angiography: A Literature Review and Ratings of Appropriateness and Necessity. JRA-03-CWF/HF. RAND Corporation. Santa Monica, CA.
16. MATCHAR, D. B., L. B. GOLDSTEIN, D. C. MCCRORY, *et al.* 1992. Carotid Endarterectomy: A Literature Review and Ratings of Appropriateness and Necessity. JRA-05-CWF/HF. RAND Corporation. Santa Monica, CA.
17. FINK, A., C. P. ROTH, R. H. BROOK, *et al.* 1986. Indications for Selected Medical and Surgical Procedures—A Literature Review and Ratings of Appropriateness: Colonoscopy. R-3204/5-CWF/HF/HCFA/PMT/RWJ. RAND Corporation. Santa Monica, CA.
18. KAHN, K. L., C. P. ROTH, J. KOSECOFF, *et al.* 1986. Indications for Selected Medical and Surgical Procedures—A Literature Review and Ratings of Appropriateness: Diagnostic Upper Gastrointestinal Endoscopy. R-3204/4-CWF/HF/HCFA/PMT/RWJ. RAND Corporation, Santa Monica, CA.
19. SOLOMON, D. H., R. H. BROOK, A. FINK, *et al.* 1986. Indications for Selected Medical and Surgical Procedures—A Literature Review and Ratings of Appropriateness; Cholecystectomy. R-3204/3-CWF/HF/HCFA/PMT/RWJ. RAND Corporation. Santa Monica, CA.
20. LEE, P. P., J. TOBACMAN, L. H. HILBORNE, *et al.* Cataract Surgery: A Review of the Literature Regarding Efficacy and Risks. JRA-06/CWF/HF. RAND Corporation, Santa Monica, CA. In press.
21. BERNSTEIN, S. J., E. A. MCGLYNN & C. J. KAMBERG. 1992. Hysterectomy: A Literature Review and Ratings of Appropriateness. JR-04. RAND Corporation, Santa Monica, CA.
22. SHEKELLE, P. G., A. H. ADAMS, M. R. CHASSIN, *et al.* 1991. The Appropriateness of Spinal Manipulation of Low-Back Pain: Indications and Ratings by a Multidisciplinary Expert Panel. R-4025/2-CCR/FCER. RAND Corporation, Santa Monica, CA.
23. BALLARD, D. B., J. A. ETCHASON, L. H. HILBORNE, *et al.* 1992. Abdominal Aortic Aneurysm Surgery: A Literature Review and Ratings of Appropriateness and Necessity. JRA-04-CWF/HF. RAND Corporation, Santa Monica, CA.

24. FINK, A., J. KOSECOFF, M. R. CHASSIN, *et al.* 1984. Consensus methods: Characteristics and guidelines for use. Am. J. Public Health **74:** 979–983.
25. LEAPE, L. L., R. E. PARK, J. P. KAHAN, *et al.* 1992. Group judgments of appropriateness: The effect of panel composition. Quality Assurance in Health Care **4**(2): 151–159.
26. BERNSTEIN, S. J., J. KOSECOFF, D. GRAY, *et al.* 1993. The appropriateness of the use of cardiovascular procedures: British versus U.S. perspectives. Int. J. Technol. Assess. Health Care **9**(1): 3–10.
27. FRASER, G. M., D. PILPEL, S. HOLLIS, *et al.* 1993. Indications for cholecystectomy: The results of a consensus panel approach. Quality Assurance in Health Care **5**(1): 75–80.
28. BROOK, R. H., C. J. KAMBERG, A. MAYER-OAKES *et al.* 1990. Appropriateness of acute medical care for the elderly: An analysis of the literature. Health Policy **14**(3): 177–280.
29. GRAY, D., J. R. HAMPTON, S. J. BERNSTEIN, *et al.* 1990. Clinical practice: Audit of coronary angiography and bypass surgery. Lancet **335:** 1317–1320.
30. WINSLOW, C. M., J. KOSECOFF, R. H. BROOK, *et al.* 1988. The appropriateness of performing coronary artery bypass surgery. JAMA **260**(4): 505–509.

DISCUSSION

HENRY GREENBERG (*St. Luke's-Roosevelt Hospital, New York, N.Y.*): I'd like to open Dr. Brook's rather challenging talk with a quick story suggested by the first patient he mentioned, the man who needed an endarterectomy for a carotid stenosis. I recently asked a neurology consultant to recommend a surgeon for a patient who unequivocally needed an endarterectomy. The neurologist advised me to use another hospital here in New York saying that they had done so many inappropriate operations there during the past decade that they had become really good at it!

ROBERT BROOK (*Rand Corporation, Santa Monica, Calif.*): By the way we have demonstrated that the doctors that do a greater number of inappropriate operations on persons who are less sick have better mortality statistics; we actually have data to substantiate that anecdote.

GREENBERG: Clinical judgment got me there also.

DAVID L. SACKETT (*McMaster University Clinic, Hamilton, Ontario, Canada*): While we're talking about the first patient, if you look at the randomized trials, both in North America and in Europe, you can identify the centers where you could send such patients.

First I'd like to note that Bob Brook and his colleagues are extraordinarily generous in sending out their reports. They make extremely interesting and instructive reading and represent a major contribution. In terms of how to improve things I'd like to note that the information provided about complication rates in different locations is extraordinarily important. But I think you should pay more attention to levels of evidence and be more formal about it. Adopt the sorts of procedures that, for example, characterize the Canadian task force on the periodic health examination or the American College of Chest Physicians, where strong statements are permitted but are coupled with information about whether conclusions are based upon randomized trials, big trials, little trials, meta-analysis, concurrent or historical controls, or clinical judgment. Otherwise you risk perpetuating the bleeding, cupping, purging, and puking, so to speak, of the 1890s.

BROOK: Let me interrupt to ask whether you think that in the next round of doing these that we ought to double or triple the price of the analysis in the literature review.

SACKETT: Yes, you should do it right. The American College of Chest Physicians has a group of researchers who work at this and do quite a bit of work every four years. This has had some interesting spinoffs, not the least of which has been that when the College put out grade C recommendations about atrial fibrillation, members of that same group were involved in carrying out three of the five randomized trials that converted the recommendation from a grade C to a grade A.

Secondly, I'd like to make a plea from those of us who carry out randomized trials that before you make a judgment you look around to see whether any randomized trials are currently under way. We think that your report on carotid endarterectomy probably had a major chilling effect on our efforts in North America and in Europe to carry out randomized trials of this procedure. Because you made a pronouncement about efficacy at the same time that we were trying to randomize patients to determine efficacy clinicians were negatively influenced as to whether or not they were willing to enter patients into such a randomized trial. Your report had a chilling effect on recruitment. I would thus ask the trialists to hold off in circumstances in which a preliminary publication would make it more difficult for us to find the truth.

KENT JOHNSON (*Federal Drug Administration, Bethesda, Md.*): I sympathize with your attempts to disentangle these questions about indications and procedures, but maybe the whole process is much more complicated than you assume and your methods impose an artificial simplification on them. My impression of the Delphi approach, for instance, is that it forces a false consensus. The situation may be much more complicated, but not totally chaotic.

BROOK: We don't try to force consensus with our process—we try to report differences. The meeting is spent trying to go back to the literature, look at the randomized trial data and the data that we publish in our outcomes evidence tables to make sure that the panel is at least reflecting what's in the literature. I think we have done what David Sackett has suggested by analyzing the recommendations against randomized trial data. There is absolutely no question that indications that are supported by randomized trials are always rated as appropriate. There's an interesting difference in philosophy between physicians in the Trent region of the U.K. versus those in the U.S. Most of the U.K. physicians that we worked with demand a lot of evidence before they are willing to make a strong recommendation for doing a procedure, while those in the United States seem to regard evidence drawn from animal and other basic or laboratory studies as sufficient for making clinical recommendations.

Patient Outcomes Research Teams: Examples from a Study on Knee Replacement

DEBORAH A. FREUND,[a] BARRY P. KATZ,[b] AND
CHRISTOPHER M. CALLAHAN[c]

[a]Bowen Research Center
School of Public and Environmental Affairs
IUPUI, and
Department of Family Medicine
Long Hospital
Indianapolis, Indiana 46202-5102

[b]Indiana University School of Medicine
Division of Biostatistics
Riley Research Wing
702 Barnhill Drive
Indianapolis, Indiana 46202

[c]Regenstrief Institute
1001 West 10th Street
Indianapolis, Indiana 46202

BACKGROUND

The 1960s were a decade full of important health legislation. Along with the regional medical program and comprehensive health planning, this decade saw the ushering in of Medicaid and Medicare. As well intentioned as the original legislators were, what they could not have foreseen was that the next three decades would be filled with legislation meant, in great part, to undo the cost problems created by the introduction of Medicare and Medicaid. If the 1960s was the decade of Medicare and Medicaid, then the 1970s should be called the regulatory decade, the 1980s the competitive decade, and the 1990s the outcomes decade. The purpose of this paper is to describe the genesis of the outcomes movement and one of the major research programs it comprised—the Patient Outcomes Research Teams (PORTs). By means of examples from a PORT on knee arthritis, we discuss some of both the potential highlights and methodologic difficulties associated with the conduct of outcomes research.

What has become known as outcomes research had its genesis in two streams of inquiry—small area variations and guideline development. The first, small area variations (SAV) analysis, was pioneered in the early 1970s by Jack Wennberg, an epidemiologist at Dartmouth Medical School. Small area variation studies were born from the observation that two small areas—towns, counties—that appeared demographically similar often had different procedure rates. For example, in their classic work, Wennberg and Gittelsohn found more then a three-fold variation in the tonsillectomy rate from one town to another in New England that could not be explained by differences in demographics, insurance, or health status.[1] After the multiple replication of similar results across a variety of procedures, investigators turned their interest toward understanding (1) the underlying causes of such variation and (2) implications of the variation for health status and clinical practice. Of interest for the development of PORTs were several findings. First, Wennberg has reported that physicians often have different underlying philosophies about when to operate on patients and what to do. In his now famous research on prostatectomy, Wennberg finds that some physicians view a transurethral resection of the prostate as an opportunity to forestall the underlying disease and, hence, they recommend surgery sooner than do those who believe in its relief of symptoms; thus, prostatectomy rates across communities may differ because some physicians recommend waiting while others recommend surgery. Though infrequently studied in the past, another compelling suggestion of SAV research is that patient preferences toward risk may explain some of the variation in procedure rates; some patients choose surgery more readily than others. Similarly, other authors suggest that the prevalence of hospital beds in a community is the culprit. For example, Perrin *et al.*[2] find a three-fold difference in the risk of hospitalization for children in Rochester, New York, New Haven, Connecticut and Boston, Massachusetts. The rates were highest in Boston and lowest in Rochester. These communities were selected for study because the health care delivery system in each community is dominated by one or more medical schools but differs in the number of hospital beds per capita, again with Boston the highest and Rochester the lowest.

Regardless of whether the underlying reason for variation is due to physician practice style, patient preferences, or other variables that have been suggested such as bed supply or access to care, there remains the question of what consequences such variation has for patient and population health as well as for how medicine "should" be practiced. Wennberg and Noralou Roos and colleagues extended some of the earlier prostatectomy research to address the difference in outcomes, as measured by mortality and reoperation, of men who had their prostates removed via transurethral prostatectomy (TURP), popular in North America, versus open resection, relatively more common in Europe and elsewhere.[3] Using claims data and other sources from three countries—England, Denmark, and Canada (the Province of Manitoba)—their findings were startling. Reoperation rates and death rates were higher in males undergoing TURP rather than open prostatectomy. Even though many analysts believe that the study did not adequately control for patients' underlying health status, implying that sicker men were more likely to get TURP, these findings opened up an entire new field exploring the effectiveness, costs, risks, and benefits of different approaches to managing clinical problems in the community. Several words are worth emphasizing. *Effectiveness* is different than *efficacy* and refers to outcomes that obtain under nonexperimental conditions when new technologies and clinical strategies are disseminated beyond teaching centers to the community. Medical studies are often confined to rarified settings, which makes it impossible to address the question of whether the long-term outcomes are equivalent, better, or worse than those that result in the community.

Unlike SAV, where the aim is to understand variation in outcomes or procedure rates, guideline development was born from the belief that appropriate and inappropriate care could be defined and measured; thus, variation is due to the large amount of inappropriate care. Robert Brook and colleagues at the Rand Corporation and the University of California at Los Angeles have developed a process for assessing appropriateness that has the following distinct steps[4]:

(1) A procedure is selected for scientific evaluation and scrutiny;

(2) An extensive literature review is conducted, aided by techniques such as meta-analysis, in order to identify indications for the use of the procedure(s) and attendant risks, benefits, and effectiveness;

(3) A specific list of indications is developed based on the literature and with input from expert physicians in the relevant discipline. Disease severity and co-morbidity are taken into consideration in developing the list;

(4) After the list of indications is completed, an expert panel of nine nationally regarded physicians is appointed to review the results of the literature review and indications list;

(5) The expert panel ranks the indications on the basis of their experience, giving a score of 1 for inappropriate and 9 for the most appropriate indications;

(6) Results of the ratings of the panel are collated and discussed at a face-to-face meeting. At the end of this meeting, panelists re-rate the indications;

(7) Retabulations of the results yield a set of medical guidelines with the following scores: 1–3 inappropriate, 4–6 equivocal, and 7–9 appropriate.[5]

This method has been applied multiple times since its development to conditions including, but not limited to, carotid endarterectomy and coronary artery bypass graft surgery.[4]

Even though they were both developed over a 10- to 20-year period, SAV and appropriateness research gained particular stature during the late 1980s during a time characterized by extreme frustration over continued double-digit increases in health care costs. Diagnosis-related groups had helped, but only marginally, and neither competition in its earlier forms nor the regulatory programs the competitive philosophy replaced (such as certificate of need) had proven any better. Looking for yet another strategy with promise, the U.S. Senators Durenberger (D-Minnesota) and Mitchell (D-Maine) and Congressman Willis Gradison (R-Ohio) turned to outcomes research. At the urging of Dr. Wennberg, a close friend of Mitchell's, and the Association for Health Services Research, a bill was introduced and passed in late 1988 creating the Agency for Health Care Policy and Research (AHCPR). In actuality, as early as 1986, Durenberger had pushed passage of a bill creating the Patient Outcome Assessment Research Program; however, an adequate appropriation never followed. The AHCPR replaced the existing National Center for Health Services Research and elevated it within the Public Health Service's organizational chart to the level of the National Institutes of Health. The mission of the AHCPR was to coordinate and fund outcomes research placing an emphasis on some of the costliest and most frequent procedures reimbursed by Medicare. The AHCPR was placed in the Public Health Service rather than in the Health Care Financing Administration (HCFA) after a fight because of the belief that improving patient care rather than cutting costs through reimbursement should be its major focus.

PATIENT OUTCOME RESEARCH TEAMS

Not surprisingly, guideline development and outcomes research became the main concerns of the AHCPR. The legislation creating the AHCPR mandated the staff to develop guidelines for at least 20 different problems during the first three years and three problems in the first 9 months. This group within the AHCPR called the Forum, which is charged with guideline development, embraced, with some modifications, the RAND method. The main outcome research thrust was the PORT initiative. Since the original request for application (RFA) was published in the last quarter of 1988, 14 PORTs have been funded. The RFA suggested that research essentially follow many of the steps that had been so successful for Wennberg, as well as a few of the RAND Methods. As a result, the majority of PORTs include the following components: (1) meta-analysis of clinical controversies and indications; (2) analysis of claims data from a variety of sources to investigate small area variations and a limited number of outcomes such as death, cost, complications, and readmission; (3) surveys of patients and physicians to measure other outcomes not estimable from claims such as pain, function, and quality of life; (4) decision analytic models to develop practice guidelines; (5) activities to disseminate the findings or practice guidelines to physicians and/or patients; (6) a study of the impact of the dissemination activities on clinical practice patterns. Currently, more than 14 PORTs are ongoing: for cataracts, prostate disease, low back pain, coronary artery disease, total knee replacement, total hip replacement, diabetes, stroke, ischemic heart disease, community-acquired pneumonia, low birthweight, schizophrenia, gallbladder disease, and pediatric gastroenteritis. Each of the PORTs are large multidisciplinary enterprises involving people from a range of disciplines including medicine, biostatistics, and economics and representing a variety of expertise in such fields as meta-analysis, claims analysis, survey research, and often from multiple organizations within the U.S. and abroad.

THE PORT AT INDIANA UNIVERSITY

The focus of the PORT at Indiana University is on determining the best ways of treating patients with severe arthritis of the knee, with particular emphasis on the role of total knee replacement (TKR) and osteotomy. A glimpse of the questions being investigated by this PORT as well as the issues that have arisen in the analyses should give the reader an appreciation of the promise and challenges of conducting outcomes research. In particular, we discuss the areas of creating analysis files using claims and conducting surveys of patients and physicians, and we focus on our experience in conducting meta-analysis and using claims to estimate mortality and analyze variation in procedure rates and length of stay (LOS).

META-ANALYSIS FOR TOTAL KNEE REPLACEMENT

Most meta-analyses concerned with medical interventions have focused on systematic review and pooling of clinical trials relevant to the intervention of interest. In general, the extant literature relevant to TKR is composed of retrospective or prospective cohort studies reporting the experience of individual surgeons or institutions (often well-known teaching hospitals). Only a small minority of available studies are clinical trials that randomize patients to competing treatments, and typically these studies are investigations of postoperative care as opposed to the knee replacement procedure itself. For this reason, we have attempted to confine our meta-analysis to issues of prognosis after knee replacement. Our goal is to delineate more precise estimates of expected rates of success as defined by patient outcomes of pain, function, and range of motion. We also wish to more precisely estimate rates of mortality, infection, thromboembolism, and revision based on available reports in the literature. Each of these outcomes may vary as a function of type of prosthesis, and perhaps also by differences in surgical technique, postoperative care, and patient characteristics.

Even though we have limited our meta-analysis to issues of prognosis, we have encountered three major problems in the systematic literature review. First, the patient populations in individual studies are often poorly described, which makes it difficult to determine to whom the results apply. The majority of the studies report that the primary indication for surgery was pain, but authors rarely specify how individual patients were referred to the surgeon, how a particular prosthesis was chosen, how many patients were evaluated but deemed ineligible, or how many had co-morbid illnesses, previous knee procedures, or concomitant therapies. Second, knee replacement is a moving technology. Many of the prostheses reported in the literature are no longer in use, yet the outcomes from these studies cannot be ignored because they help to define how far the procedure has advanced. Hundreds of different prosthetic types have been tested, and surgeons have hundreds of minor surgical technique and postoperative care options that may affect patient outcomes. Therefore, two centers reporting on the same prosthesis may have different results because of variation in surgical technique or postoperative care and these differences may not be apparent from the published methods. Third, there are more than 30 knee-specific rating scales that have been developed for assessing TKR. An individual investigator may choose from among these scales or use an outcome measure that assesses a single construct such as pain. Even among studies employing the same rating scale, there is variation in the method of applying the scale and in aggregating the results. This variation in outcome measures makes it exceedingly difficult to compare outcomes across studies. We expect to present a summary from the literature of patient outcomes based on broad categories of prosthetic types, but we are less optimistic that we will have sufficiently detailed data to allow explanation of outcomes variation due to patient characteristics, surgical technique or postoperative care.

USING CLAIMS DATA IN OUTCOMES RESEARCH

Arthritis of the knee is primarily, though not exclusively, a problem of elders who have osteoarthritis (OA) and/or rheumatoid arthritis (RA). Younger individuals may be at risk because of injuries (post-traumatic arthritis) or because of the early onset of either OA or RA. For this reason, for investigating outcomes such as mortality, complications, readmission, cost, and length of stay, it was important to acquire claims data on all age groups. Thus, the total knee replacement PORT team includes claims from U.S. Medicare, which provides a 100% sample of U.S. elders over 65, Blue Cross/Blue Shield of Western Pennsylvania (WPA), which provides a sample of patients under 65 years of age, and the Ontario Health Insurance Plan which provides a 100% sample of all individuals residing in this province. The Canadian data are desirable because of the PORT's additional goal of understanding Canadian and U.S. differences. Using claims data which are collected as a basis of payment and not for research purposes on outcomes is tricky and requires a laborious list of tasks. Even so, there are many rewards including the cost of acquiring data, the representativeness of samples, and the large number of patient observations that can be acquired. Among the most important tasks that must be accomplished before claims are ready to use for outcomes analysis include creating person level files, and identifying the procedures or clinical problems of interest. In the TKR PORT, investigators from the University of Toronto, who are responsible for Canadian claims, and from the Pittsburgh

Research Institute followed all the same steps in creating analysis files as did the team members at Indiana University and the Research Triangle Institute, who primarily were responsible for use of the U.S. Medicare claims.

The strategy for creating a person level file using Medicare claims, which will allow prevalence and incidence of events to be determined, is to first identify hospitalizations associated with the condition of interest, identify the person who had the hospitalizations, and then attach outpatient claims. Hospital procedure data are the best source of information on individuals with specific conditions. This is because hospital procedures are reported better than diagnoses, and all Part A claims are regarded as more reliable than Part B claims. Because of the inaccuracy of diagnosis codes on outpatient claims, it is virtually impossible to use claims data to analyze treatment patterns for patients whose problems are treated solely on an outpatient basis. As an example, while the TKR PORT wanted to identify a cohort of individuals with severe knee arthritis, this was not possible from Part B data.

To use Part A data, researchers generally begin by searching among ICD-9-CM codes to identify those of potential interest. The process does not end there, however, because data files must then be searched to see whether, in fact, the codes have identified the procedure of interest. For example, the interest of the TKR PORT was to identify all patients who had had a TKR or osteotomy since 1985. After identifying the appropriate codes, the team looked for obvious miscoding; some codes 81.41 for TKRs upon inspection of the adjunct clinical data were determined to be 31.41s (tracheoscopies). There is the additional problem of whether an identified hospital episode really included a TKR that was performed; several of our hospitalizations were for stays less than 4 days and cost $5,000 or less (in 1985 dollars). Clinicians on the team though it impossible that a TKR could actually have been completed within these parameters, unless the patient had died. These stays were deleted. Similarly, additional inspection revealed that many stays that appeared to be genuine were not, because of the presence of a "V" code indicating that because of an in-hospital complication, the surgery was never performed. Additionally, when used in conjunction with procedure codes, diagnostic information can help to improve the validity of the data. An example from the TKR PORT is requiring the presence of a diagnosis code indicating arthritis or other joint problem in all patients undergoing a TKR or osteotomy.

After hospital stay data are "clean," it is time to create the person file. Each claim indicates the patient's unique Medicare identification number. This claim number can then be matched with another file to obtain simple demographic information including age, race, sex, whether the person is a member of a health maintenance organization, qualifies for Medicare because they have end-stage renal disease, or also qualifies for Medicaid. Once hospital claims are sorted by the Medicare identifier, additional claims of interest can be attached in order to create episode files. The construction of episode files is crucial for addressing complications and readmissions. The claims data do not indicate which hospital admission is related to the one prior. This must be decided on the basis of clinical decision rules developed by the research team and applied to delete some hospitalizations and keep others. Other unique problems may also confront researchers using claims data. Two examples from the TKR study regard the desire to differentiate primary knee replacements from revisions and identifying re-hospitalizations. Prior to October of 1989, there was no unique procedure code for revision; both primary and revision surgery were lumped together. Thus, an algorithm was developed to identify revisions based on the ICD-9-CM codes and other clinical data and was validated using the data collected after October 1989. Equally importantly, none of the claims data provide a code for differentiating surgery on the left versus right knee. Thus, the analysis of revision data must make a series of assumptions linking primary and revision TKRs. A sensitivity analysis will be performed to determine the effect of these assumptions on the results.

Analyses of claims data are nearly complete with respect to modeling of postoperative mortality, LOS, and TKR rates. The overall 30-day mortality rate for Medicare patients undergoing TKR between 1985 and 1989 was 0.62%. Logistic regression analysis was used to examine the effects of demographic characteristics, year of discharge, arthritis type, co-morbidities, and Medicaid eligibility. Only age, race, gender, and the co-morbidity index were predictive of 30-day mortality. Men and African-Americans had significantly higher mortality rates than women and whites, respectively. LOS for Medicare patients is highly skewed, with a mean of 12.24 days and a median of 11 days. Least-squares regression models on the natural logarithm of LOS were used. Candidate independent variables include demographic characteristics, health status at admission, hospital characteristics, and community resources. Results show that women, blacks, counties with a lower ratio of orthopedic surgeons to MDs, and teaching hospitals all are associated with longer LOS. A similar analysis was recently begun for total charges. Variations in procedure rates are being analyzed for both large and small areas using a log-linear Poisson regression model with an extra Poisson variance term.[6] The first analysis examined the effect of patient demographic characteristics and HCFA region on TKR rates. Rates were found to be significantly lower for men and for blacks and to have steadily increased over the 6-year period from 1985 through 1990. In addition, rates were lowest in the Middle Atlantic states and highest in the Rocky Mountain states. The largest racial differences were observed in the South and the Plains states. The second analysis models the effect of economic and health resources measures on county rates, adjusting for age, race, and sex. Preliminary results show a positive association with the number of orthopedic surgeons per capita and a negative association with unemployment rate.

Another but rarely used feature of Medicare part A claims is that there is a data field indicating the patient's hospital record number. An important potential contribution of the TKR PORT is the information that will result from its request for hospital records, which is described immediately below.

SURVEY DATA

Survey data are used by PORTs to provide information that cannot be gleaned from claims, but claims can provide the sampling frame for patient surveys. Most PORTs are using surveys of patients to obtain information on important outcomes such as functional status, pain after surgery, and quality of life. They are also gathering information on patient preferences toward health status by collecting information on patient utilities. The obvious problems that have occurred with other surveys hold true for outcomes research. Among the most important regard expense and patient recall. Here, for example, the TKR PORT faced a real dilemma. It is particularly important to obtain information on quality of life and function five or more years after the initial surgery. On the one hand, there was concern that patients could not remember their functional status prior to surgery or in the years immediately afterward. On the other hand, neither the available funding nor the 5-year time horizon of the TKR PORT permitted these data to be acquired through a prospective cohort study. In the end, both options were used by the TKR PORT. A lengthy retrospective survey was mailed to patients who had received their TKR anywhere between 2 and 7 years prior. The sampling frame was developed using Medicare claims. Each respondent was asked for permission to acquire their hospital records. More than 90% of all respondents granted this request; medical records were then obtained from the relevant hospital by identifying the hospital record number available on the Part A claims. The PORT team hopes to gain information on blood loss, intra-hospital complication, and prosthesis from this medical records request.

Also, a cohort of individuals undergoing surgery and a comparison group of patients with osteoarthritis have been identified. The cohort study is used to gain important information on how specific maneuvers that take place in the operating room (e.g., type of prosthesis, whether the cruciate ligament is spared) might be related to proximal outcomes and how outcomes in operative patients compare with those who do not get the surgery. Participating surgeons are asked to fill out an intraoperative assessment form and patients are asked to complete surveys on functional status every 6 months for 2 years. Gaining physician participation and acceptance in the cohort study has not been difficult, but finding eligible patients has. Recruitment has been lower than expected because of the decreased frequency of elective surgery during holiday periods and an overestimate, by the surgeons, of the number of procedures they perform. Obtaining an adequate response rate in physician surveys has been much more challenging.

The TKR PORT included a survey of orthopedists, rheumatologists, and primary care physicians in order to understand beliefs about the indications for surgery and to test hypotheses relating the volume of surgical operations performed to perceived outcomes. Identifying and achieving a satisfactory response rate was much more difficult for primary care physicians than those in the other specialties. First, identifying primary care physicians was difficult since state licensing records were the only sampling frame available. Specialty information is based on self-report and is missing for more than one-quarter of the physicians. Second, many of the listed addresses were out of date or incorrect. Finally, of those that were delivered, only about 20% have been returned after the second mailing. This may be due to a lack of interest concerning TKR among primary care physicians.

CONCLUSION

Each PORT is attempting to examine all possible aspects of a single clinical problem. The immense scope of this simple directive was probably not fully understood by the AHCPR or by those of us who blithely planned 5-year time lines to finish this enormous series of tasks. However, it already seems clear that the PORTs are a fitting continuation of the work in small area variations and guideline development. They will ultimately add more than the information they present in their particular area of focus. Each PORT has been forced to address issues in the areas of meta-analysis, cleaning and analysis of claims data, statistical methods for examining variation, survey sampling, utility assessment, and dissemination of information to both patients and physicians. Their experiences cannot help but prove valuable to other researchers concerned with these areas in the future.

REFERENCES

1. WENNBERG, J. E. & A. GITTELSOHN. 1973. Small area variations in health care delivery. Science **183:** 1102–1108.

2. PERRIN, E., C. HOMER, D. BERWICK, *et al.* 1989. Variation in rate of hospitalization of children in three urban communities. N. Engl. J. Med. **320:** 1183–1187.
3. WENNBERG, J. E., N. ROOS, L. SOLA, *et al.* 1987. Use of claims data systems to evaluate health care outcomes: Mortality and reoperation following prostatectomy. JAMA **257**(7): 933–936.
4. PARK, R., A. FINK, R. BROOK, *et al.* 1989. Physician ratings of appropriate indications for three procedures: Theoretical indications vs. indications used in practice. Am. J. Public Health **79**(4): 445–447.
5. PARK, R. E., A. FINK, R. H. BROOK, *et al.* 1986. Physician ratings of appropriate indications for six medical and surgical procedures. Am. J. Public Health **76**(7) 766–772.
6. BRESLOW, N. E. 1984. Extra Poisson variation in log linear models. Appl. Stat. **33:** 38–44.

DISCUSSION

ALAN MORRIS (*LDS Hospital, Salt Lake City, Utah*): I have a comment about judgment that relates to the last two presentations. I'm concerned about this evaluation of appropriateness of therapy by physicians. Remember that these are the same physicians who felt that gastric freezing was appropriate for gastrointestinal hemorrhage and who were enthusiastic about internal mammary artery ligation among other things. In constructing computerized protocols to control mechanical ventilation of profoundly ill patients we found that experienced physicians were very poor generators of the actual rules used for decision making. So when consensus is derived from their judgment and put back in the form of a protocol applied to prospectively controlled patient care, most commonly that judgment turns out to be inadequate. So I'm asking a very pertinent question about feedback. Will the PORTs be associated with a mechanism to garner the information that relates the specific reasons for which physicians have refused to follow guidelines? That way the information could be fed back to make the guidelines into something that in fact will be useable. I'm concerned that if this provision for feedback is not included, then the central element necessary for making a market-ready guideline or protocol will doom the whole process to failure.

BARRY KATZ (*Indiana University, Indianapolis, Indiana*): That's a tough question. Our goal in getting the opinions of the physicians was not to make guidelines, but to identify areas of variation, particularly among the primary care rheumatologists and the orthopedists so that we could identify the things that they don't agree on. Our PORT is, if I understood your question, not going to be issuing guidelines at this point.

BARBARA MCNEIL (*Harvard Medical School, Boston, Mass.*): I could expand on that. Our PORT is at least interested in that issue because we're very concerned about organizational factors that are associated with adherence to what is believed to be good care. So, in conjunction with investigators in Minneapolis, we're looking at organizational characteristics on the physicians' and on the providers' sides that are associated with adherence to guidelines for myocardial infarction as well as for care related to breast cancer patients and with care parameters defined by NIH consensus conferences. So our answer to Dr. Morris's question is yes, but our response is generally outside of the original PORT grant.

RICHARD PETO (*University of Oxford, Oxford, U.K.*) This conference is supposed to be on the evaluation of interventions and I can't see anything in either this paper or the preceding one that actually does anything towards evaluating the interventions. If this PORT costs five million dollars, the money would be better spent on a serious trial. The ISIS trials cost five million dollars each. This is not just a question of evaluating interventions with questionnaires. The same applies to the question of appropriateness. You use a word like *appropriateness,* which is a sort of attractive concept, and then say such and such a percentage of interventions is appropriate, and another such isn't, which just reflects the definition of the word; it's not actually saying, in the previously used meaning of the word, that the interventions were appropriate or not. It really isn't evidence. This isn't a serious way of trying to work out what works and what doesn't.

KATZ: I tend to agree with you on the trial question, but I don't think that trials are feasible for many of the PORT situations. We're not going to get surgeons who all believe that total knee replacement is a very good procedure to run a randomized clinical trial. But I feel that we are shedding some light on the usefulness of the procedure and at least getting better descriptions of what's going on. I won't comment on whether this was a good way to spend five million dollars.

Randomized Control Trials and Meta-Analyses in Gastroenterology: Major Achievements and Future Potential

THOMAS C. CHALMERS[b] AND JOSEPH LAU

Technology Assessment Group
Harvard School of Public Health, and the
Center for Health Services Research and Study Design
New England Medical Center
Boston, Massachusetts 02111

INTRODUCTION

Although the perinatal field leads the pack in the organization of randomized control trials (RCTs) and meta-analyses into clinically useful printed and electronic texts,[1] gastroenterologists probably lead in sheer numbers of RCTs that should have an important impact on the care of patients. The problem is that no one has yet organized the latter into a format that could change medical practice on a continuing basis. It is certainly hoped that the Cochrane Collaboration will successfully compile all of the important RCTs in the field of gastroenterology into clinically useful and updated meta-analyses. Two and a half years ago one of us (TCC) tried to persuade the authors of the most popular textbook of gastroenterology[2] to convert to the meta-analytic format of *Effective Care in Pregnancy and Childbirth*,[3] but failed. Apparently the effort was ahead of its time. The conference for which this manuscript was prepared[4] should go a long way towards bringing all specialties in medicine into the modern world of information synthesis and transmission to the practicing doctor for the benefit of the patients.

NOTABLE LANDMARKS

If hepatology can be considered a part of gastroenterology, an RCT of the available treatments of viral hepatitis, carried out in 1951–1952, can be considered a notable landmark.[5] Thanks to the late Dr. William B. Reynolds, it incorporated for the first time in clinical trials in humans many of the principles espoused by

[a] This work was supported in part by grants R01 HS-05936 and R01 HS-07782-01 from the Agency for Health Care Policy and Research. U.S. Public Health Service, Department of Health and Human Services

[b] Address for correspondence: Thomas Chalmers, M.D., New England Medical Center, Center for Health Services Research and Study Design, 750 Washington St., Boston, Massachusetts 02111.

the great Sir Ronald Aylmer Fisher[6]: in the first part, two popular treatments, bed rest and diet, were tested in a two-by-two factorial design. The patients, American soldiers contracting what is now called hepatitis A in Korea and Japan, were randomized in blocks of four to control for changes in severity over time; the principal endpoint, duration of illness from admission to the hospital in Kyoto, Japan, was adjusted for the initial serum bilirubin concentration, found in preliminary analyses to be an important outcome predictor; analyses of variance were carried out after conversion to logs because of the skewed distribution of the responses; the three dropouts were explained in detail and replaced as missing values in the analyses; the covariates on admission were analyzed to establish the validity of the randomization process. After bed rest and diet were found to be beneficial in the first study, a two-by-two by two-by-two factorial study was carried out: the protein in the diet proved to be the most effective, the calories somewhat, and the vitamin supplements not at all; half of all the patients sent for vigorous physical reconditioning as soon as their liver function tests were relatively normal illustrated the safety of what was at the time drastic treatment. Detailed examination of a segment of the patients as they left Japan within one year, and of the rest wherever they were throughout the United States, revealed no signs that they were harmed by early ambulation, a treatment considered radical at the time. Five years later a search of Army death records revealed no evidence of liver damage when the former patients were compared with suitable controls.

The RCTs of the symptomatic treatment of viral hepatitis are presented above in some detail to illustrate the fact that symptomatic treatments can be properly compared in humans when the need exists, no matter what the cost. The reduction in indirect costs of the illness resulting from the demonstration that strict bed rest was unnecessary can be enormous in terms of time lost from normal activities. It is a good example of how much can be accomplished by the investment of public funds in clinical trials.

Another example of gastroenterologic leadership is the exploration of surgical methods of preventing recurrent hemorrhage and death in patients who have esophageal varices complicating cirrhosis of the liver. The Boston Inter-hospital Liver Group was formed 35 years ago for the specific purpose of carrying out RCTs in patients with cirrhosis.[7] The Copenhagen Liver Group was formed around the same time for the same purpose.[8] An important reason for a dearth of patients entered into such studies was suggested by a response to an inquiry made as to why 98% of the patients in the first Boston study were from three of the six participating hospitals: "If we at the *blank* hospital cannot tell which patients would benefit from operation and which not, and therefore have to randomize, what hope is there for the rest of the world"? As it turned out, the patients with varices that had not yet bled lived as long as those undergoing surgery[9]—and longer when combined with a similar study carried out in the West Haven Veterans Administration Hospital.[10] So one-half of the randomized patients were better treated than the consecutive series treated in the non-contributing hospitals. Although there was almost universal agreement that portacaval shunts would save lives after a patient had survived the first episode of hemorrhage, the later Boston Inter-hospital Liver Group study and a cooperative one carried out in Veterans Administration hospitals showed that the operation did prevent future episodes of bleeding, but the patients lived little if any longer.[11,12] Again a characteristic of these studies was that 100% of the patients had alcoholic cirrhosis in spite of the fact that up to 40% of the patients with cirrhosis in the United States had non-alcoholic cirrhosis. Presumably the latter were paying patients, in contrast to most of the alcoholics, and their private doctors were opposed to randomization.

A meta-analysis of the RCTs of portacaval shunts in patients with cirrhosis and esophageal varices revealed data very pertinent to the comparison of randomized and historically controlled trials.[13] Survival of the patients operated upon in the historically controlled trials was the same as both the surgically and medically treated patients in the RCTs, but the historical controls had a significantly worse survival. Among the many possible explanations is the fact that historical controls do not have to give informed consent for a life-threatening operation, resulting in a built-in shortened survival, even when *post hoc* efforts to match the patients by apparent prognostic factors is attempted.

The story of survival after surgical attempts to correct portal hypertension is a pithy example of the ethical advantages of randomization over acting as if the relative outcomes are known when they are not. In the case of the early uncontrolled and historically controlled series of patients, success in the long-term outcome of patients operated upon for portal hypertension was attributed to the surgery, whereas when the impact of selection bias was minimized by random assignment to treatment, it became apparent that surgically treated patients had survived longer because healthier patients had been selected for surgery. This has profound implications whenever a selected treatment is in itself potentially hazardous.

Another example of the leadership of gastroenterology in employing RCTs is the evolving progress made in determining which type of vagotomy is the best for patients with intractable peptic ulcer. Vagotomy had been established as effective in preventing relapses of peptic ulcer, but the side effects of the operation were most distressing—diarrhea, the dumping syndrome, and gastric obstruction. Laboratory work suggested that the side effects might be due to cutting the whole nerve, whereas a careful dissection of the nerves going to the acid- and gastrin-secreting cells might decrease acid production without the side effects of cutting the rest of the nerve. Fairly early in the history of the experimental operation it was compared with classical vagotomy in a number of small RCTs, all too small to give answers in themselves. A meta-analysis has accumulated and combined data to show that the new operation has the obvious advantage of reducing untreatable side effects at the expense of more frequent relapses,[14] which are treatable by medical or surgical means.

The vagotomy story thus demonstrates how RCTs and meta-analyses are an essential part of the chain of knowledge progressing from experimental observations in animals to proper treatment of the patient in need.

The discovery of a highly effective treatment of patients with bleeding peptic ulcer for the first time has become a landmark in demonstrating the efficacy of early RCTs and meta-analyses, and at the same time the experience could have far-reaching consequences of both an ethical and a statistical-theory nature. For almost 50 years the hospital fatality rates of patients with bleeding peptic ulcers averaged 10% in spite of the fact that the rate of emergency surgical intervention, as portrayed in 61 articles reporting both death rates and surgical intervention rates, involving 21,130 patients, rose steadily from under 5% to more than 50%.[15] Surgical intervention was saving a lot of lives, but the undertakers were remaining just as busy.

There is, however, a suggestion in these uncontrolled experiences that the therapies were improving throughout the 40-year span. The average age of the patients admitted to the hospital with bleeding peptic ulcer was increasing significantly, and the death rate was higher the older the patient. So something was keeping the overall death rate from rising. It could have been the increased rate of surgical intervention, or it could have been improvements in the non-surgical interventions. RCTs could have determined which, but only three were performed over this time period,[16–18] and they were inconclusive. Too many patients randomly assigned to medical therapy were operated upon as an emergency because of continued bleeding, and too many patients assigned at random to surgery were not operated upon, presumably because they stopped bleeding. The only way for experimentation to determine the advantages and disadvantages of early surgical intervention would be to assign patients on admission to a medical or surgical floor. Even though cross consultation might occur in all difficult cases, there would surely be a difference, on the average, in the time of surgical intervention between the medical and surgical services. Such a trial has been advocated for many years, but no one has yet reported one.

In the meantime the advent of emergency endoscopy has changed the whole picture. Illustration of this fact might be considered the best possible demonstration of the utility of meta-analysis. Five RCTs of emergency diagnostic endoscopy failed to reveal benefit in terms of hospital mortality, and when they were pooled there was a distinct trend towards an increase in death rate in the intervention group.[19] But this was before anyone tried obliterating the "bleeder" through the endoscope. Now five methods have been used: two types of heater probes, two types of laser treatment, and the injection of a sclerosing agent. When compared with no endoscopic treatment, these five methods have been equally effective against bleeding vessels of all categories of severity.[20] For the first time in 50 years there has been a significant reduction in hospital mortality from bleeding peptic ulcer, demonstrable only by meta-analysis because the individual trials, with a few exceptions, did not have enough power to demonstrate the improvement. Also for the first time the rate of surgical intervention dropped appreciably.

These data also unfurl a very important lesson to be learned from the meta-analysis of RCTs of the same treatment repeatedly carried out over time. Cumulative meta-analyses, the process of performing a new meta-analysis every time a new RCT appears,[21] can demonstrate the effectiveness or lack thereof of a new treatment long before an RCT with sufficient power to do so can be undertaken. The most dramatic example of the waste of lives waiting for the big trial to be performed is in the treatment of acute myocardial infarction and the prevention of death from reinfarction.[22] These are only three of at least ten such examples to be found in the medical literature.

Even in 1993, 10 years after cumulative meta-analysis could have revealed endoscopic therapy to be effective in reducing continued or recurrent bleeding (and as a result decreasing the need for surgical intervention and eventual in-hospital mortality), RCTs were still being reported in which patients were assigned at random to a control group without treatment. FIGURE 1 presents the mortality data as an odds ratio with each study presented only with its confidence interval; FIGURE 2 presents the same data in a cumulative fashion so that the date at which the reduction in mortality became statistically signficant can be seen; and FIGURE 3 presents (on the left) the classical and (on the right) the cumulative meta-analysis of the rate of emergency surgical intervention in the patient with bleeding peptic ulcer. These data are about the same as the rate of continuing hemorrhage reported elsewhere.[15] The only ethical use of an RCT in this situation is in studies without an untreated control group that are designed to show which endoscopic therapy is most successful.

The fifty-year story of attempts to lower mortality from bleeding peptic ulcer

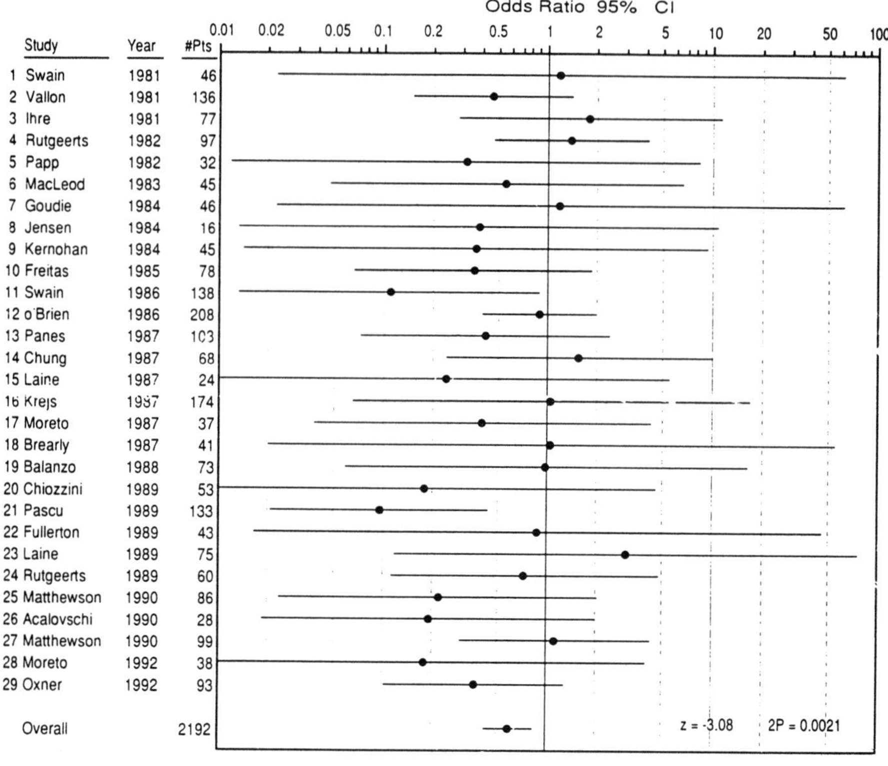

FIGURE 1. Impact of endoscopic therapy on total number of deaths in patients with bleeding peptic ulcer: random effects model (from Der Simonian and Laird).

is a potent example of mistreatment resulting from the lack of early RCTs, and more recently, the power of cumulative meta-analysis to demonstrate early efficacy without waiting for a very large trial to be organized.

Of course an early large trial would be the most efficient way to obtain an answer about innovative therapies, but it has not been feasible to get such trials under way. Even if we succeed in our long-standing battle to persuade clinicians to randomize the first patient in whom an outcome resulting from a new treatment is to be measured,[23–25] the first such examples will likely be small RCTs requiring a subsequent meta-analysis to make up for lack of power. That is one of the many reasons why the quality of RCTs must be improved to facilitate eventual meta-analyses. Eventually almost every RCT will have to be included in a meta-analysis, if not to increase power for the main effects, certainly to demonstrate the sub-group effects.

FUTURE POTENTIAL

RCTs are so necessary to evaluate the small incremental changes in the treatment of gastrointestinal and hepatic diseases evolving out of basic research that their future potential is enormous. As the suggested improvements in treatment become smaller and the use of a no-active-treatment group less ethically acceptable, individual trials will seldom be large enough. Cumulative meta-analyses will be increasingly important as one contributor to the decision needing to be made in a timely fashion as to whether a new treatment is better, worse, or the same as the standard.

Acute viral hepatitis is so variable in its course that RCTs will be crucial to the proper evaluation of the many new antiviral agents coming out of the laboratory in the next few years. Present medical and surgical therapies for portal hypertension and its complications are so unsatisfactory that many innovative techniques can be expected in the next few years. The presently popular proximal or selected vagotomy for peptic ulcer is not entirely satisfac-

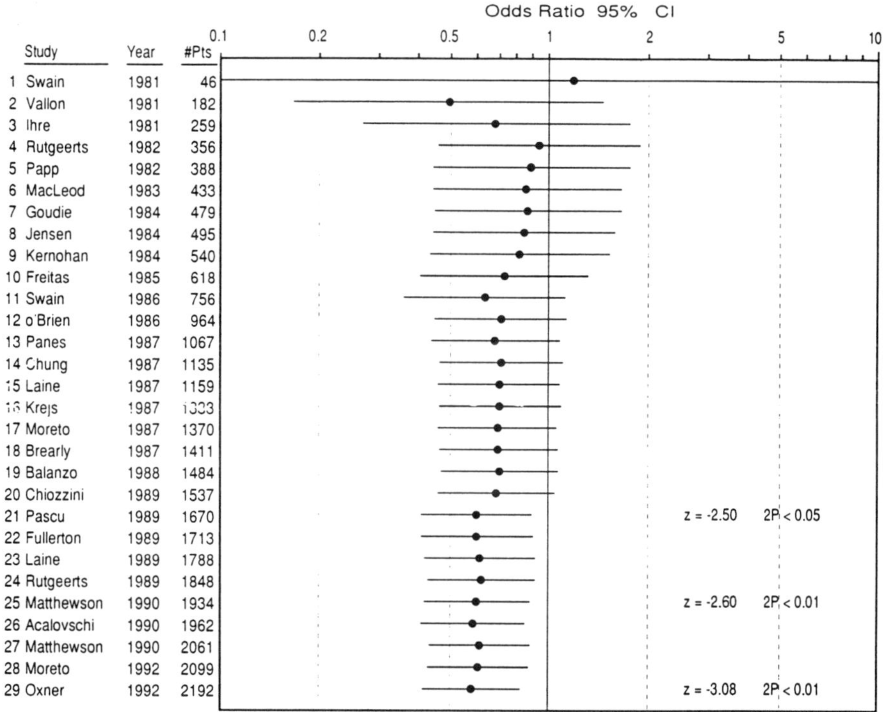

FIGURE 2. Impact of endoscopic therapy on total number of deaths in patients with bleeding peptic ulcer: cumulative meta-analysis with random effects model (from Der Simonian and Laird).

tory, and many attempts at improvement can be expected. Finally, the five methods of treating bleeding peptic ulcer through the endoscope need to be compared in well-controlled studies.

The four examples detailed above are a very small sample of the innumerable treatments of gastrointestinal and hepatic diseases that are now being evaluated in RCTs and that will need to be evaluated in the future. It is fervently hoped that in each instance randomization will begin early to avoid the paralysis caused by the three typical outcomes of uncontrolled pilot studies: the new

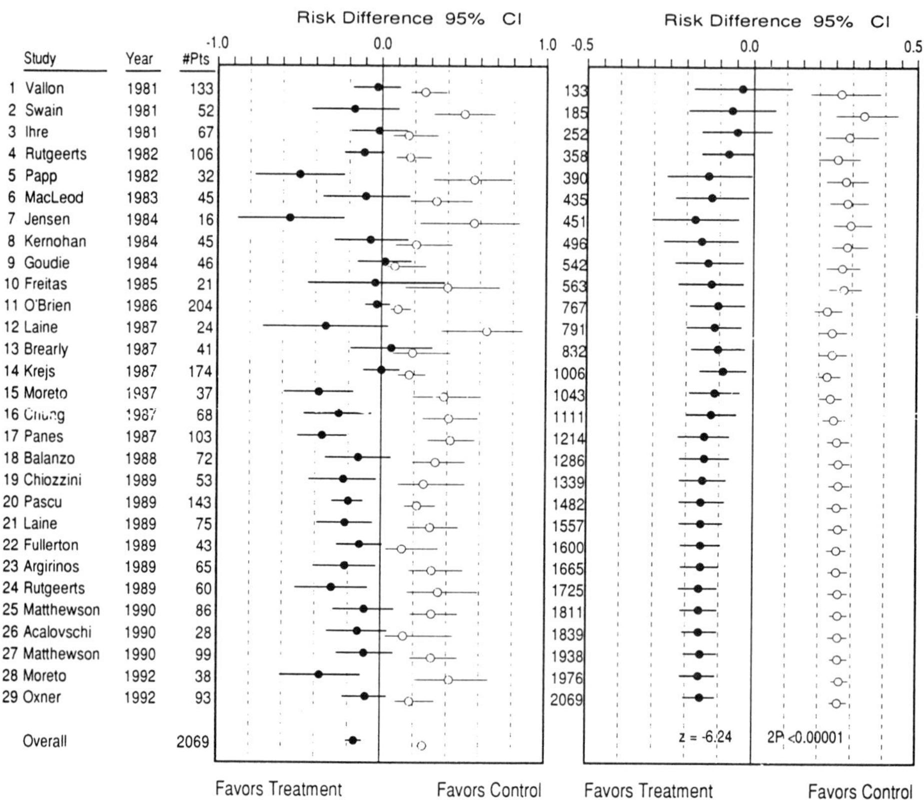

FIGURE 3. Impact of endoscopic therapy on rate of emergency surgery in patients with bleeding peptic ulcer: random effects model (from Der Simonian and Laird). *Left*: standard meta-analysis; *right*: cumulative meta-analysis.

treatment *appears* to be so effective that a randomized assignment to a no-treatment control group would be unethical; the new treatment *appears* to be so ineffective that it would be unwise to study the agent any more; the new agent *appears* to be so similar to the standard that it would be a waste of time to study it further.

If the proposed policy of randomizing the first patient in whom clinical outcome is to be measured is adopted widely, other changes in the way we treat patients and conduct clinical trial research will have to occur. To keep clinicians up to date and avoid publication bias we will need an effective system for registering clinical trials as soon as they are begun. Institutional review boards should be required to notify the registry when all trials are approved. The present double standard of requiring peer review and informed consent for randomization, but not for "trying out" new treatments as part of the practice of medicine will have to be corrected. Similarly, the equally wasteful double standard of third parties refusing to pay for studies incorporating randomization because they are considered to be research, and freely paying for uncontrolled "innovative" practice, needs to be reversed. Trials that do not seem to advance knowledge need to be published just as freely as the exciting positive studies.

For future trials to achieve their optimal potential, more attention has to be paid to their quality. Randomized assignments need to be concealed from the clinicians accepting patients for study and obtaining informed consent. Blinding of therapies, although not as important as blinded randomization, needs to be accomplished whenever possible. Patients and treatments need to be described in detail. Investigators making decisions about withdrawing or removing patients must be blinded to the treatment group. In addition, clinicians admitting patients to studies must be blinded to the trends in outcome, or their decisions or the vigor with which they obtain informed consent will be biased. Data should be presented in a format that will facilitate the almost universal meta-analyses to follow.[27] Subgroup responses such as age groupings should be presented in detail. Continuous variables should be presented as the differences in the mean changes, rather than changes in the means.

Most important of all in the planning of new RCTs in the gastroenterologic as well as all other fields, we should abandon the entrenched idea that the null hypothesis must be repeatedly tested as if there were no previous trials in the field. If a meta-analysis of past similar trials is performed before the start of all new ones, sample size estimates will be shrunk if trends favor the experimental, lengthened if they favor the control. The preliminary meta-analysis may even indicate that the contemplated trial is unnecessary. Corrections for multiple looks, based on disproving the null hypothesis as they are, should be modified or abandoned. Two prospective surveys of all clinical trials approved by separate institutional review boards have revealed more than 70% of the total of published and unpublished trials report statistical significance at the 0.05 level.[28,29] This raises important questions about the ethical propriety of asking patients to volunteer for trials that include randomization to an untreated control group when past RCTs suggest that the treatment is effective.

CONCLUSIONS

Physicians specializing in gastroenterologic and hepatic diseases have been fortunate in having available very large numbers of RCTs and meta-analyses to help them in their clinical decisions. However, they need to appreciate the nuances of quality of the individual trials and the opportunities and pitfalls made possible by the advent of meta-analyses, often performed in a cumulative fashion. They need to cogitate and enter into dialogues about how to tell when a treatment has been adequately investigated. They might well adopt the following motto: when in doubt, randomize.

REFERENCES

1. CHALMERS, I., J. HETHERINGTON, M. NEWDICK, L. MUTCH, A. GRANT, M. ENKIN, E. ENKIN & K. DICKERSIN. 1986. The Oxford Database of Perinatal Trials: developing a register of published reports of controlled trials. Controlled Clin. Trials **7**(4): 306–324.
2. SLEISENGER, M. H. & J. S. FORDTRAN. 1983. Gastrointestinal Diseases, 3rd ed. W.B. Saunders. Philadelphia, PA.
3. CHALMERS, I., M. ENKIN & M. J. N. C. KEIRSE. 1989. Effective Care in Pregnancy and Childbirth. Oxford University Press. Oxford, England.
4. Doing More Good than Harm: The Evaluation of Interventions. Conference held by the New York Academy of Sciences, March 22–25, 1993, New York, N.Y. This volume.
5. CHALMERS, T. C., R. D. ECKHARDT, W. E. REYNOLDS, R. W. REIFENSTEIN, N. DEANE, C. W. SMITH, J. G. CIGARROA & C. S. DAVIDSON. 1955. The treatment of acute infectious hepatitis. Controlled studies of the effects of diet, rest, and physical reconditioning on the acute course of disease and on the incidence of relapses and residual abnormalities. J. Clin. Invest. **34**: 1163–1234.
6. FISHER, R. A. 1948. Statistical Methods for Research Workers, 10th ed. Oliver and Boyd. Edinburgh, Scotland.
7. CHALMERS, T. C. 1969. The Boston Inter-hospital Liver Group as an experiment in cooperative research. Gastroenterology **57**(3): 339–341.
8. COPENHAGEN STUDY GROUP FOR LIVER DISEASES. 1969. Effect of prednisone on the survival of patients with cirrhosis of the liver. A report from the Copenhagen Study Group for Liver Diseases. Lancet **1**(586): 119–121.
9. GARCEAU, A. J., R. M. DONALDSON, E. T. O'HARA, A. D. CALLOW, H. MUENCH, T. C. CHALMERS, & BOSTON INTER-HOSPITAL LIVER GROUP. 1964. A controlled trial of prophylactic portacaval shunt surgery. N. Engl. J. Med. **270**: 496–500.
10. CONN, H. O. & W. W. LINDENMUTH. 1962. Prophylactic portacaval anastomosis in cirrhotic patients with esophageal varices: Preliminary report of a controlled study. N. Engl. J. Med. **266**: 743–749.
11. RESNICK, R. H., F. L. IBER, A. M. ISHIHARA, T. C. CHALMERS, H. ZIMMERMAN, & BOSTON INTER-HOSPITAL LIVER GROUP. 1974. A controlled study of the therapeutic portacaval shunt. Gastroenterology **67**(5): 843–857.
12. JACKSON, F. C., E. B. PERRIN, & A. DEGRADI. 1965. Clinical investigation of the portacaval shunt: I. Study design and preliminary survival analysis. Arch. Surg. **91**: 43–54.
13. SACKS, H. S., T. C. CHALMERS, & H. SMITH, JR. 1983. Sensitivity and specificity of clinical trials: Randomized vs. historical controls. Arch. Intern. Med. **134**(4): 753–755.
14. CHALMERS, T. C., D. T. GRAY, A. BLUM, J. BERLIN, M. J. ORZA, R. NAGALINGAM, & P. HEWITT. 1988. Data analysis in gastroenterology: Vagotomy for recurrent duodenal ulcer. Gastroent. Intern. **1**(1): 41–48.
15. CHALMERS, T. C., C. S. SEBESTYEN & S. LEE. 1970. Emergency surgical treatment of bleeding peptic ulcer. An analysis of the published data on 21,130 patients. Trans. Am. Clin. Climatol. Assoc. **82**: 188–199.
16. ENQUIST, I. F., K. E. KARLSON, A. M. TANAKA, C. DENNIS, S. FIERST, & L. A. YOUNG. 1957. Statistically controlled evaluation of three methods of management of upper gastrointestinal bleeding: A progress report. Gastroenterology **32**: 619–632.
17. SPICER, F. W., J. V. CARBONE, & C. G. LYON. 1961. Acute massive hemorrhage from gastroenteroduodenal ulceration. Am. J. Surg. **102**: 153–157.
18. READ, R. C., H. C. HUEBL, & A. P. THAL. 1965. Randomized study of massive bleeding from peptic ulceration. Ann. Surg. **162**: 561–577.
19. ERICKSON, R. A. & M. E. GLICK. 1986. Why have controlled trials failed to demonstrate a benefit of esophagogastroduodenoscopy in acute upper gastrointestinal bleeding? A probability model analysis. Dig. Dis. Sci. **31**(7): 760–768.
20. SACKS, H. S., T. C. CHALMERS, A. L. BLUM, J. BERRIER, & D. PAGANO. 1990. Endoscopic hemostasis: An effective therapy for bleeding peptic ulcer. JAMA **264**(4): 494–499.

21. Lau, J., E. M. Antman, J. Jimenez-Silva, B. Kupelnick, F. Mosteller & T. C. Chalmers. 1992. Cumulative meta-analysis of therapeutic trials for myocardial infarction. N. Engl. J. Med. **327:** 248–254.
22. Antman, E. M., J. Lau, B. Kupelnick, F. Mosteller, & T. C. Chalmers. 1992. A comparison of results of meta-analysis of randomized control trials and recommendations of clinical experts. JAMA **268**(2): 240–248.
23. Chalmers, T. C. 1975. Randomization—perils and problems. N. Engl. J. Med. **292**(19): 1036–1039.
24. Chalmers, T. C. 1975. Randomization of the first patient. Med. Clin. N. Amer. **59**(4): 1035–1038.
25. Chalmers, T. C. 1975. Randomize the first patient! N. Engl. J. Med. **296**(2): 107.
26. Chalmers, T. C. & J. Lau. 1993. Meta-analytic stimulus for changes in clinical trials. Stat. Med. Med. Res. **2**(2): 161–173.
27. Chalmers, T. C. 1993. Clinical trial quality needs to be improved to facilitate meta-analysis. Online J. Current Clin. Trials. Document #89.
28. Dickersin, K. 1990. The existence of publication bias and risk factors for its occurrence. JAMA **263**(10): 1385–1389.
29. Easterbrook, P. J., J. A. Berlin, R. Gopalan, & D. R. Matthews. 1991. Publication bias in clinical research. Lancet **337**(8746): 867–872.

DISCUSSION

Unidentified Speaker: I feel a bit uneasy asking any question of a person who has made more contributions to randomized trials in the United States than anyone, but here goes: In 1982 my colleagues and I published a paper in the *New England Journal of Medicine* demonstrating a clear benefit of streptokinase in treating acute myocardial infarction, and then later collaborated in an overview paper with the Oxford group in 1985 in the *European Heart Journal* demonstrating even more conclusive benefits and a much narrower confidence interval. In the late 1980s Rory Collins and Desmond Jullian did a survey of hospitals in the United Kingdom and found that 2% of these hospitals were using thrombolytic therapy. Gene Braunwald and Mark Pfeffer performed a survey in the United States and found that about 20% were using thrombolytic agents. After the results of GISSI-1 and ISIS-2 the U.K. data went from 2% to about 68%, with about 80% utilization of streptokinase, and the U.S. rates went curiously from about 20% to 33.3%, with 80% utilization of TPA.

So my feeling is that without GISSI-1 and ISIS-2 there would have been no impact of the meta-analysis on practice in the U.K. and a deleterious impact in the U.S. because physicians would have continued to use TPA, which we now know costs ten times as much and doubles the risk of cerebral hemorrhage. So, in practice, unless we have large trials that will influence clinicians' judgments, meta-analysis will remain a tool of the academics. I'd like your views on that.

Thomas Chalmers (*New England Medical Center, Boston, Mass.*): If I were a patient with acute myocardial infarction there might be a 1% chance that I would be willing to volunteer to enter ISIS-2 if I were shown the data and told clearly that this has been an established therapy and the reason a big trial was being done is because doctors were not paying attention to it. I think that is the crux of the matter, and I think that we should not be using big trials to convince doctors how to practice. Admittedly we may not have a better method at the moment, but we have to find one. We can't rely on a method that asks people to sacrifice themselves so that other patients can be saved by doctors who finally pay the attention that they should have paid before. This is my response to the argument that one has to do big trials because it's the only way you convince doctors. It's a terrible thing to have people lose their lives or get less effective therapy because doctors haven't responded. Again, we need to find a better method and discovering that method is where we should be putting our emphasis, but it's not a reason for a big trial. The reason for a big trial is to obtain subgroup data, and the only way to get these data is by either planning them in the small trials or doing big trials early.

ALAN MORRIS (*LDS Hospital, Salt Lake City, Utah*): I'm quite interested in the approach that you've taken, but I'm concerned about the perception of physicians that a central authority dictating therapy would be anathema, particularly in the American environment where freedom and sidearms are felt to go side by side. Do you propose that we could set up a central authority that would provide definitive direction for care? I'd rather have it come from someone like you than from a financially driven system, as in the federal government, which appears to be a likely source.

CHALMERS: My proposal requires that patients continue to be randomized until a peer review group decides that the therapy is effective enough to stop that randomization. And, by a central authority I mean a group of peers who would be advising, but not with many many months' delay. We would have to speed up the process and set up a system whereby, in addition to the center that gathers all of the data and makes them available to people, another kind of center is set up in which organized groups peer review the data and decide whether or not we should stop paying for patients in randomized trials and start paying for patients to receive the therapy routinely. And I believe that that transition requires a peer review group. I admit that it's terrible to have doctors told what to do by the government, but how else are you going to cut down on unnecessary deaths? I suppose the malpractice business will help that in a way in that once a peer review group says that this therapy is effective, then it's hard for a physician to produce in court a defensible reason for using or not using it.

UNIDENTIFIED SPEAKER: I'd like to raise a question about decision analysis. We focused on the use of quantitative techniques to summarize the evidence, but there's an important step in how we apply that quantitative estimate of effect to making a clinical decision. In some overviews that I've been involved in, there have been instances of therapies that are effective for the endpoints that have been measured by the meta-analysis, and yet the ultimate recommendation may be not yet to institute that treatment routinely. On the other hand, there are therapies that are not effective for which possibly the correct clinical decision would be to institute it, as in prevention of intracranial hemorrhage in the newborn where both phenobarbital and indomethacin may be effective even though possible effects on cerebral blood flow and blood pressure haven't been studied yet. And since there's no data on long-term outcome, clinicians have been reluctant to take the point estimate of efficacy on intracranial hemorrhage and apply that clinically.

CHALMERS: I agree, and I think that the message at this conference is that meta-analysis is just one of the tools by which one reaches a therapeutic decision, and when you're considering all the other tools you need a reliable quantitative assessment of what data you can get out of the literature; that is where meta-analysis makes a contribution. But I don't think that we should assume that once a meta-analysis is done, the problem is settled.

Randomized Trials in Perinatology: Major Achievements and Future Potential

ADRIAN GRANT

Perinatal Trials Service
National Perinatal Epidemiology Unit
Radcliffe Infirmary
Oxford OX2 6HE, United Kingdom

SYSTEMATIC IDENTIFICATION AND REVIEW OF PERINATAL TRIALS

The achievement for which perinatal medicine must stand out from other specialties is its development of a mechanism for the identification and systematic review of relevant randomized controlled trials.[1,2] This database was initiated by Iain Chalmers in the mid 1970s, when he was working in Cardiff, Wales, using an informal card-based system. After his move to Oxford to become the first director of the National Perinatal Epidemiology Unit this was formalized during the early 1980s following a hand-based search of all relevant journals back to the 1950s. The card-based filing system was cumbersome and the advent of the microcomputer naturally led to the transfer of this information onto an electronic database.[3] The database was subsequently expanded to include systematic reviews of relevant trials. This latter component consists of formal overviews (meta-analyses) with structured commentaries to aid interpretation.[4]

In 1988, as the result of collaboration involving many people, these reviews were brought together to form the basis of a 1,500-page, two-volume book entitled *Effective Care in Pregnancy and Childbirth,*[5] edited by Iain Chalmers, Murray Enkin, and Mark Keirse. In recognition of the fact that this expensive book would not be easily accessible to many of those providing care to pregnant women *Effective Care in Pregnancy and Childbirth* was subsequently summarized in an inexpensive paperback entitled *A Guide to Effective Care in Pregnancy and Childbirth.*[6] More recently, the overviews of trials of neonatal interventions have formed the basis of a second, 650-page book entitled *Effective Care of the Newborn Infant,*[7] edited in North America by Jack Sinclair and Michael Bracken. Over time, these books will become out of date and so the intention is to make updated overviews available in an electronic publication. As Iain Chalmers discusses later in this volume, the database of perinatal trials is now a component of the Cochrane Collaboration Project. The popularity of the inexpensive summary *A Guide to Effective Care in Pregnancy and Childbirth,* however, has encouraged the authors of that book to plan an update because, in the foreseeable future, this is the form in which the information is likely to be most accessible for many people providing and receiving perinatal care.

The issues of dissemination and application of evidence in practice are considered later in this volume; nevertheless, there are good reasons for believing that these systematic reviews of controlled trials in perinatal medicine are proving useful to policymakers, practitioners, and trainees.

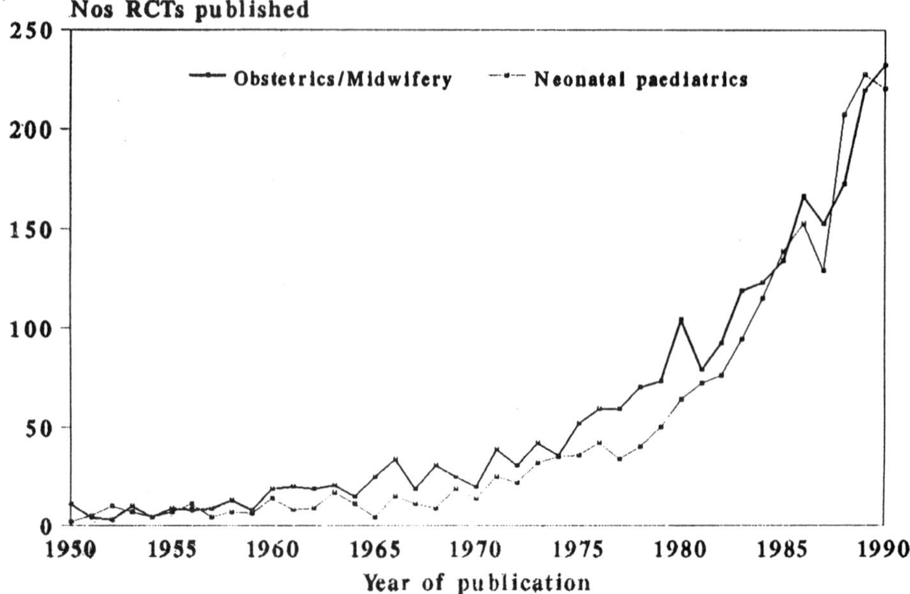

FIGURE 1. Annual numbers of published reports of perinatal trials.

THE GROWTH OF TRIALS IN PERINATAL MEDICINE

The systematic identification and review of perinatal trials can be employed
to describe the use of randomized controlled trials in perinatal medicine. The
number of perinatal trials has risen steadily since the early 1950s (FIG. 1), providing
clear evidence of the increasing popularity of this methodology for research in
the perinatal period. The numbers of trials of interventions in the neonatal period
has increased particularly rapidly in recent years, in part reflecting the growth of
the specialty of neonatology, such that there are now similar numbers of reports
of trials in the field of neonatal pediatrics as in obstetrics/midwifery. The largest
number of reports (44%) are of trials conducted in the United States, but in view
of the number of reports published per thousand annual births we see that the
methodology has been most enthusiastically embraced in Denmark. Sample size
is only a crude index of a trial's statistical power. The database indicates, however,
that median sample sizes have not increased, but the number of large trials ($>$1,000
participants) has. Randomization has thus been widely accepted as a method of
generating groups for comparison, but the need for large sample sizes[8] is still
poorly understood.

There are some classic trials amongst those conducted during the 1950s. The
comparative trial of retrolental fibroplasia and the use of oxygen[9] that demonstrated the toxic effects of neonatal managements that included high concentrations
of inspired oxygen showed the value of trials to minimize harm. The trials of

diethylstilbestrol in early pregnancy that failed to identify any benefit (and taken together suggest poorer pregnancy outcome) were largely ignored, particularly in North America. The later identification of genital tract abnormalities including vaginal carcinoma is perhaps the most notorious example of an iatrogenic disaster. The lessons of diethylstilbestrol will always be relevant to perinatal care. For example, recent large-scale trials showed that first-trimester chorion villus sampling did have disadvantages that had not been recognized by some of its proponents (although it does have the psychosocial advantage of affording earlier diagnosis in most cases), and now there is growing evidence of a link between this invasive procedure during very early pregnancy with serious oromandibular-limb hypogenesis malformations.[10]

EFFECTIVE BUT UNDERUSED TREATMENTS

In contrast, some of the most effective interventions identified in the systematic review of perinatal trials are currently underused. More than 40 trials provide convincing evidence of the effectiveness of giving antibiotics prior to cesarean section to reduce the risk of puerperal infection.[11,12] Despite this evidence, antibiotics are not routinely prescribed prior to cesarean section, presumably reflecting a variety of concerns, including the possible emergence of antibiotic resistance. Equally surprising is the fact that trials of prophylactic antibiotics are still being conducted and reported, despite the clear evidence of benefit that currently exists.

Similar confusion about the status of current evidence seems to prevail in respect of the administration of corticosteroids to women prior to the birth of a very immature baby. A review of 14 controlled trials provides very clear evidence that this intervention reduces the risks of neonatal mortality and morbidity. Publication of the results of this overview in a peer-reviewed journal in 1990[13] has led to a greater awareness of the effectiveness of this treatment. Nevertheless, it is still not used consistently, with wide variation both within and between countries.[14,15] This reflects amongst other things confusion caused by small trials that do not give clear-cut answers, inappropriate subgroup analyses (for example, suggesting that the intervention is only effective in black female babies or at certain gestational ages[15]), and theoretical concerns about possible long-term harmful effects (which were not substantiated in long-term follow-up of cohorts of children from the trials[13]). The data from corticosteroid trials provide an object lesson in the dangers of trials of insufficient size, of inappropriate subgroup analysis, and of the necessity of looking at the totality of evidence when considering the effectiveness of an intervention.

INEFFECTIVE OR HARMFUL INTERVENTIONS

Systematic overviews of perinatal trials have also identified interventions that are either ineffective or even harmful. There is no evidence to support routine weighing during pregnancy[16] or a policy of elective cesarean section after one previous cesarean.[17] In some places as many as 50% of all women require surgical repair of trauma sustained during vaginal delivery. Use of one particular suturing material—glycerol-impregnated catgut—in the repair of perineal trauma sustained during childbirth appears to double the risk of dyspareunia three years after the delivery.[18]

LARGE TRIALS BASED ON OVERVIEWS OF SEVERAL SMALL TRIALS

Richard Peto and his colleagues have led the way in using overviews of relatively small trials as a basis for deciding what interventions should be tested in large-scale trials.[19] There are examples of this approach in the perinatal field. In what was probably the first overview of perinatal trials ever conducted, Chalmers noted that there were fewer cases of neonatal seizures amongst the babies of women randomly allocated to more intensive continuous electronic monitoring of the fetal heart rate during labor.[20] The numbers were small (0 versus 6), but this observation, together with other considerations, was the basis of the design of the substantially larger trial that was subsequently conducted in Dublin.[21] This trial remains the largest perinatal trial ever conducted using randomization of individual women. The hypothesis that more intensive electronic monitoring reduced the risk of neonatal seizures was tested and sustained.

A major criterion for deciding whether our group conducts a large multicenter trial is the evidence available from previously conducted smaller trials. This is the basis for our current plans, for example, to mount a large multicenter European trial of thyrotropin-releasing hormone (TRH) given to women prior to the birth of a very immature baby. Evidence from five small trials suggest that TRH administration may substantially reduce the risks of neonatal respiratory morbidity.[22] But this is not certain, and TRH could have unrecognized adverse effects.

Evolving evidence from an overview can also lead to a modification of a trial protocol in the light of the new evidence. This occurred recently in the Canadian TERM PROM trial, where new evidence of differential effects of alternative methods of induction of labor[23] led to a change of emphasis in the protocol.

In other circumstances, a much larger trial has been conducted because an overview of several small trials failed to give any clear indication of the likely treatment differences. The issue of whether or not to induce labor when a pregnancy goes post-term has long been a matter for fierce debate. Although a number of trials had tried to address this issue, they were all small and did not provide a clear answer, even when considered together. This situation changed in 1991 with the publication of the Canadian Post-Term Pregnancy Trial,[24] a substantially larger trial, which indicated that induction from about a week after term does have benefits for the mother. Furthermore, when the data from this trial were added to the overview, benefits for the baby also emerged.

The potential dangers of basing practice on data from a few small controlled trials have recently been highlighted by trials of low-dose aspirin therapy in pregnancy. Published data from a series of 11 small trials suggested that daily low-dose aspirin may be very effective in reducing the complications of pre-eclampsia and intrauterine growth retardation.[25] However, data from two larger, but still moderate-sized, trials have recently become available.[26,27] These failed to demonstrate any beneficial effect of low-dose aspirin. The place of low-dose aspirin in perinatology is now uncertain. Fortunately, some larger trials are nearing completion (see below) and these should help to clarify the place of low-dose aspirin, if any, in pregnancy.

OVERVIEWS ARE OF NO VALUE UNLESS THE NECESSARY PRIMARY RESEARCH HAS BEEN CONDUCTED

Systematic overviews of perinatal trials have therefore been invaluable in clarifying the value of some interventions in pregnancy. Nevertheless, perhaps the most striking feature in the Oxford Database of Perinatal Trials is that many interventions have never been tested in the context of a formal randomized controlled trial, and for many others the evidence is so limited as to provide no sound basis for clinical practice. Overviews depend on the results of primary research and for most interventions in the perinatal field the data available for meta-analysis are insufficient, either because the trials conducted have been too small, or because they have never been conducted at all.

RANDOMIZATION IS NOT SUFFICIENT AND LARGE SAMPLE SIZES ARE REQUIRED

There are indications from research on new interventions in the perinatal period that the requirement for substantially larger sample sizes in trials is being realized. Interventions are being thoroughly evaluated as they move from the laboratory to clinical practice. Low-dose aspirin administration in pregnancy is likely to be the most thoroughly evaluated intervention in obstetric practice. The Collaborative Low-Dose Aspirin Study in Pregnancy (CLASP)[28] is the largest trial of drug treatment ever conducted in pregnancy. It has involved more than 9,000 women recruited in 226 centers in 17 countries (including four centers in Russia[29]). Results will be available early in 1994.

The program of research to evaluate exogenous surfactant administration to prevent or treat respiratory distress in the neonate will also stand as an exemplar for future research. After painstaking laboratory investigation, a series of more than 30 well-conducted randomized controlled trials has provided unequivocal evidence of the effectiveness of exogenous surfactant administration in reducing the risk of mortality and certain types of morbidity.[30,31] Subsequent follow-up assessment of the surviving children from some of these trials has provided reassuring evidence that these benefits in the neonatal period are not reflected in an increased number of survivors with severe disabilities. More recently, the introduction of exogenous surfactant into practice has been used as an opportunity to evaluate this treatment more fully. Trials have assessed the optimal time to start treatment, the optimal frequency of administration, and the optimal preparation. The OSIRIS trial[32] coordinated from Oxford demonstrated that for high-risk babies early administration, before respiratory problems develop, is a more effective policy than delayed, selective administration to those babies who subsequently develop breathing problems. This trial involved nearly 7,000 very immature babies recruited from more than 200 hospitals in 21 countries. The death rate was more than 20% and a further 30% of the infants had long-term dependence on oxygen. This trial proved that it is possible to recruit sufficiently large numbers of high-risk babies to be able to identify moderate, but clinically important, differences in mortality and serious morbidity, and this may be its most enduring quality.

Exogenous surfactant is expensive: the average cost per baby is about $1,500. Extra use of surfactant therefore has significant resource implications, an indication of the growing importance of health economics in perinatal trials.[33] An ongoing study in the U.K. is estimating the cost of different levels of neonatal care. These estimates will be applied to the results of the OSIRIS and other neonatal trials to estimate cost-effectiveness. Cost-effectiveness studies have been valuable in emphasizing the relative effectiveness of antenatal corticosteroids in comparison with neonatal administration of exogenous surfactants,[34] but have also shown that neonatal surfactant administration compares favorably in its cost effectiveness with many other medical interventions that have been subjected to cost-effectiveness analysis.

THE SPECIAL CIRCUMSTANCES OF PERINATAL CARE AND THE NEED FOR A MULTIDISCIPLINARY APPROACH TO EVALUATION

It is important to recognize that there are some special circumstances that apply in perinatology. Most pregnancies are a normal physiological event leading to a healthy mother and baby. Pregnant women have been persuaded to attend regularly for antenatal care in what is essentially a largely unevaluated screening program. Issues of safety and satisfaction with care therefore predominate. So-called "softer" measures of outcome, such as women's views of care, carry particular weight in the field of perinatal medicine. Social scientists therefore have an important part to play in perinatal trials, and their involvement is likely to increase, this aspect of evaluation having been incorporated in some trials[35,36] in the perinatal period. This angle of insight has helped to identify important aspects of care that would not have been recognized otherwise, and has also indicated the weights that women attached to different types of outcome.

The importance of women's views of the care they receive has also been reflected in the involvement of representatives of the users of the maternity services in perinatal research. A striking example of the importance of this was the Medical Research Council's European Chorion Villus Sampling Trial.[37] Representatives of voluntary organizations were involved in the planning of this study and actively promoted its successful conduct. In the U.K., at least, groups representing users of the services have been particularly helpful in ensuring that the information given to women and parents in multicenter perinatal trials is appropriate. We have found this partnership extremely helpful and profitable. For example, representatives of consumer groups wrote the first draft of the patient information booklet for the Collaborative Low-Dose Aspirin Study in Pregnancy.[28] And more recently, they have been actively involved in ensuring that parents of children recruited to a multicenter trial of Extra-Corporeal Membrane Oxygenation are sympathetically and properly informed about the study. An exciting new development in this regard has been an initiative taken by one of these groups, the National Childbirth Trust, to conduct the first multicenter trial organized by a voluntary organization concerned with maternity service.[38] This latter study was a component of a larger midwifery-led initiative to evaluate treatments given to women whom it was anticipated would have breastfeeding problems, the so called MAIN trial[38] (Multicentre Trial of Alternative Treatments for Inverted and Flat Nipples in Pregnancy). Midwives both within the U.K. and worldwide are showing an increasing confidence in research and in randomized controlled trials in particular. Midwifery interventions are a major component of the Cochrane Collaboration Pregnancy and Childbirth database. Attitudes amongst midwives to research and research-based practice have changed dramatically over the last few years in the U.K. The Department of Health funded a midwifery research initiative based at the National Perinatal Epidemiology Unit in Oxford, and this has acted as a catalyst for change.

The MAIN trial is in fact the first international collaborative trial run by midwives; already further trials are planned or ongoing.

PERINATAL TRIALS IN LESS-DEVELOPED COUNTRIES

Perhaps the biggest challenge facing those working in perinatology is to identify safe and effective interventions that can be used in less-developed countries. As many as half a million women die each year from causes associated with pregnancy and childbirth, of whom 99% live in developing countries.[39] Only a small minority of perinatal trials have been conducted in such countries. In part this reflects the particular problems of research in such countries, but it also reflects attitudes that the issue is one of implementation of forms of care that are known to be effective rather than one of further evaluation.[40] Our experiences are that there is enthusiasm and goodwill for trials in developing countries if suitable support is available. Hypertensive disease in pregnancy, and eclampsia in particular, is one of the major causes of maternal death.[41] The Eclampsia Trial, co-ordinated by my colleague Lelia Duley, is trying to identify the most effective way to control eclamptic seizures in women in developing countries; it involves 19 centers in seven countries across three continents. This trial should provide the most reliable evidence on which to base the management of this uncommon but life-threatening complication of pregnancy.

NEED FOR MULTICENTER COLLABORATION AND THE EMERGENCE OF COLLABORATIVE NETWORKS

Enthusiasm is increasing for randomized controlled trials in perinatal medicine. There is a willingness to randomize treatments, as evidenced by the increasing number of trials that are being conducted and the large numbers of clinicians who are willing to participate in multicenter randomized controlled trials. The challenge remains to mount sufficiently large trials in sufficient numbers to identify relatively moderate, but clinically useful effects of practicable treatments for the most common problems in perinatal care. These usually require surprisingly large numbers. The inevitable implication of this is that multicenter collaboration is required either because the condition for which the treatment is being tested is statistically uncommon, or because the outcome of interest is statistically rare. There are encouraging developments to facilitate such multicenter collaboration. The Canadian Perinatal Trials Network[42] involves the majority of larger perinatal centers in that country. That network and the philosophy that it encourages have already fostered some landmark trials in Canada. Within the United States, the National Institute of Child Health and Human Development is providing substantial support for two perinatal trials networks, one obstetric and the other neonatal. Each of these networks contains only about 12 university centers, however, and so will never be able to mount the really large trials that are required to provide clear evidence in respect of the most important outcomes on which to base perinatal practice. Our experience has been that community hospitals have often been the most important contributors to multicenter trials. Developments within the United States to involve such hospitals, such as through the network that has been established by neonatologists based in Vermont,[43] should be encouraged. There are signs that a loose network is also evolving amongst obstetricians in Australia. A trial of antenatal TRH administration[44] is nearing completion and plans for a new multicenter Australian trial are being actively considered. Within the U.K., the British Association of Perinatal Medicine has established a Perinatal Clinical Trials Group.[45] This is proving an efficient mechanism for identifying potential collaborators in perinatal trials and for canvassing their views during protocol development. A biannual newsletter keeps members informed about developments in perinatal trials. Within Europe more broadly, the European Community promises to provide an infrastructure for European collaborative trials.[46]

THE PERINATAL TRIALS SERVICE BASED AT THE NATIONAL PERINATAL EPIDEMIOLOGY UNIT

When the National Perinatal Epidemiology Unit was established in 1978, randomized controlled trials were identified by Iain Chalmers as one of four principal components of the Unit's future program of work. I was appointed to the Unit in 1980 with the specific remit to establish a program of perinatal trials. Over the subseqent 13 years the emphasis has shifted from single-center studies to multicenter international trials.[47,48] We are indebted to Richard Peto, Rory Collins, and their colleagues in the Clinical Trial Service Unit for their generous support. More importantly, they have had an immense influence on perinatal medicine where large, simple-in-design, randomized trials are increasingly accepted as the way to identify moderate, but clinically important, effects of promising new treatments. More recently, the success of this program of randomized controlled trials in perinatal medicine co-ordinated from Oxford has been recognized by the Department of Health in London with the granting of support for the Perinatal Trials Service,[48] based at the National Perinatal Epidemiology Unit. Salary support for a team of five people with complementary skills (clinical, epidemiological, statistical, social science, computing, administrative, secretarial, and clerical) provides the core support for a program of trials. About two new trials start recruitment each year. Each study attracts project grant support providing funds for necessary additional staff and to cover non-salary expenses. Many of these trials involve follow-up in childhood, cost-effectiveness analysis, and an assessment of the views of parents and caregivers. Evaluation of midwifery practices is of increasing importance. We are fortunate that the Perinatal Trials Service is based within a larger multidisciplinary research group (the National Perinatal Epidemiology Unit[47]) with expertise in all these domains.

Arguably, the risk-minimizing approach of randomized controlled trials is particularly appropriate for perinatal medicine, where actions taken may alter prospects for the next 70 years. Nevertheless, there are constraints to progress that are particular to this field. The first is that this is not perceived as a large potential market for pharmaceutical companies; more importantly, however, the current litigious climate is leading some companies to decide as a matter of policy to withdraw from research and development in this field. The second constraint is that when our patients die they do not leave large sums of money to charities to support research to find a way to prevent others dying from the illness that killed them. We are therefore particularly dependent on public money. These considerations should be taken into account when decisions are taken about priorities for future research.

CONCLUSION

In summary, I see the major achievement in respect of randomized trials in perinatology as the formal identification and systematic review of perinatal trials. This has allowed the reliable identification of some treatments that are effective, some that are ineffective, and some that are even harmful. Most interventions have been the subject to little formal evaluation by controlled trial. Clarification of the value of these, particularly those that show promise on the basis of a few small trials, requires further primary research, using a broad multidisciplinary approach. There is enthusiasm for multicenter collaboration, but an infrastructure is required if this is to be harnessed efficiently, and this will be largely dependent on public money.

REFERENCES

1. CHALMERS, I. 1986. A register of controlled trials in perinatal medicine. WHO Chron. **40:** 61–65.
2. CHALMERS, I., J. HETHERINGTON, M. NEWDICK, L. MUTCH, A. GRANT, M. ENKIN, E. ENKIN & K. DICKERSIN. 1986. The Oxford Database of Perinatal Trials: Developing a register of published reports of controlled trials. Controlled Clin Trials **7:** 306–324.
3. MUGFORD, M., A. GRANT & I. CHALMERS. 1982. Developing a register of randomized controlled trials in perinatal medicine. *In* Lecture Notes in Medical Informatics. Proceedings of Medical Informatics Europe 1982. D. A. B. Lindberg & P. L. Reichertz, Eds. **16:** 162–167. Springer-Verlag. Dublin.
4. CHALMERS, I., ED. 1986. The Oxford Database of Perinatal Trials. Oxford University Press. Oxford, U.K.
5. CHALMERS, I., M. ENKIN & M. J. N. C. KEIRSE, EDS. 1989. Effective Care in Pregnancy and Childbirth. Oxford University Press. Oxford, U.K.
6. ENKIN, M., M. J. N. C. KEIRSE & I. CHALMERS, EDS. 1989. A Guide to Effective Care in Pregnancy and Childbirth. Oxford University Press. Oxford, U.K.
7. SINCLAIR, J. C. & M. B. BRACKEN, EDS. 1992. Effective Care of the Newborn Infant. Oxford University Press. Oxford, U.K.
8. YUSUF, S., R. COLLINS & R. PETO. 1984. Why do we need some large, simple randomized trials? Stat. Med. **3:** 409–420.
9. KINSEY, V. E. 1956. Retrolental fibroplasia. Comparative study of retrolental fibroplasia and the use of oxygen. Arch. Ophthalmol. **56:** 481–543.
10. FIRTH, H. V., P. A. BOYD, P. CHAMBERLAIN, I. Z. MACKENZIE, R. H. LINDENBAUM & S. M. HUSON. 1991. Severe limb abnormalities after chorion villus sampling at 56–66 days' gestation. Lancet **337:** 762–763.
11. SMAILL, F. 1992. Prophylactic antibiotics in caesarean section (all trials). *In* Oxford Database of Perinatal Trials. I. Chalmers, Ed. Version 1.2, Disk Issue 8, Autumn 1992. Record 3690.
12. MUGFORD, M., J. KINGSTON & I. CHALMERS. 1989. Reducing the incidence of infection after caesarean section: Implications of prophylaxis with antibiotics for hospital resources. Br. Med. J. **299:** 1003–1006.
13. CROWLEY, P., I. CHALMERS & M. J. N. C. KEIRSE. 1990. The effects of corticosteroid administration before preterm delivery: An overview of the evidence from controlled trials. Br. J. Obstet. Gynaecol. **97:** 11–25.
14. KHANNA, R. & S. RICHMOND. 1993. OSIRIS Trial. Lancet **341:** 174.
15. GRANT, A., D. ELBOURNE, A. WILKINSON, M. WEINDLING & R. COOKE. 1993. OSIRIS Trial. Lancet **341:** 173–174.
16. CHALMERS, I., M. ENKIN & M. J. N. C. KEIRSE. 1989. Effective care in pregnancy and childbirth: A synopsis for guiding practice and research. *In* Effective Care in Pregnancy and Childbirth. I. Chalmers, M. Enkin & M. J. N. C. Keirse, Eds.: 1465–1477. Oxford University Press. Oxford, U.K.

17. ENKIN, M. 1989. Labour and delivery following previous caesarean section. *In* Effective Care in Pregnancy and Childbirth. I. Chalmers, M. Enkin & M. J. N. C. Keirse, Eds.: 1196–1215. Oxford University Press. Oxford, U.K.

18. GRANT, A., J. SLEEP, H. ASHURST & J. A. D. SPENCER. 1989. Dyspareunia associated with the use of glycerol-impregnated catgut to repair perineal trauma: Report of a three-year follow-up study. Br. J. Obstet. Gynaecol. **96:** 741–743.

19. ISIS-2 (Second International Study of Infarct Survival) Collaborative Group. 1988. Randomized trial of intravenous streptokinase, oral aspirin, both, or neither among 17,187 cases of suspected acute myocardial infarction: ISIS-2. Lancet **ii:** 349–360.

20. CHALMERS, I. 1979. Randomized controlled trials of fetal monitoring 1973–1977. *In* Perinatal Medicine. O. Thalhammer, K. Baumgarten & A. Pollak, Eds.: 260–265. Georg Thieme. Stuttgart.

21. MacDONALD, D., A. GRANT, M. SHERIDAN-PEREIRA, P. BOYLAN & I. CHALMERS. 1985. The Dublin randomized controlled trial of intrapartum fetal heart rate monitoring. Am. J. Obstet. Gynecol. **152:** 524–539.

22. CROWTHER, C. A. & A. M. GRANT. 1992. Antenatal thyrotropin releasing hormone prior to preterm delivery. *In* Oxford Database of Perinatal Trials. I. Chalmers, Ed. Version 1.2, Disk Issue 8, Autumn 1992. Record 4749.

23. HANNAH, M. E. 1992. Prostaglandins vs. oxytocin for prelabour rupture of membranes at 37+ weeks. *In* Oxford Database of Perinatal Trials. I. Chalmers, Ed. Version 1.2, Disk Issue 8, Autumn 1992. Record 3273.

24. HANNAH, M. E., W. J. HANNAH, J. HELLMANN, S. HEWSON, R. MILNER, A. WILLAN & CANADIAN MULTICENTER POST-TERM PREGNANCY TRIAL GROUP. 1992. Induction of labor as compared with serial antenatal monitoring in post-term pregnancy. A randomized controlled trial. N. Engl. J. Med. **326:** 1587–1592.

25. COLLINS, R. 1992. Antiplatelet agents for IUGR and pre-eclampsia. *In* Oxford Database of Perinatal Trials. I. Chalmers, Ed. Version 1.2, Disk Issue 8, Autumn 1992. Record 4000.

26. Italian Study of Aspirin in Pregnancy. 1993. Low-dose aspirin in prevention and treatment of intrauterine growth retardation and pregnancy-induced hypertension. Lancet **341:** 396–400.

27. SIBAI, B. M., S. N. CARITIS, E. THOM, M. KLEBANOFF, D. McNELLIS, L. ROCCO, R. H. PAUL, R. ROMERO, F. WITTER, M. ROSEN, R. DEPP & THE NATIONAL INSTITUTE OF CHILD HEALTH AND HUMAN DEVELOPMENT NETWORK OF MATERNAL FETAL MEDICINE UNITS. 1993. Prevention of pre-eclampsia with low-dose aspirin in healthy nulliparous pregnant women. N. Engl. J. Med. **329:** 1213–1218.

28. DE SWIET, M. 1990. Aspirin-towards 2000. Ed. *In* Royal Society of Medicine International Congress and Symposium. G. R. Fryers, Ed. Series Number **168:** 9–14.

29. VIKHLYAEVA, E. & I. CHALMERS. 1992. Russian collaboration in the collaborative low-dose aspirin study in pregnancy (CLASP). Maternal and Child Health **1:** 57–62.

30. SOLL, R. F. & M. C. McQUEEN. 1992. Respiratory distress syndrome. *In* Effective Care of the Newborn Infant: J. C. Sinclair & M. B. Bracken, Eds.: 325–358. Oxford University Press. Oxford, U.K.

31. HALLIDAY, H. L. 1992. Other acute lung disorders. *In* Effective Care of the Newborn Infant. J. C. Sinclair & M. B. Bracken, Eds. 359–384. Oxford University Press. Oxford, U.K.

32. OSIRIS Collaborative Group. 1992. Early versus delayed neonatal administration of a synthetic surfactant—the judgment of OSIRIS. Lancet **340:** 1363–1369.

33. MUGFORD, M. & S. HOWARD. 1993. Cost-effectiveness of surfactant replacement in preterm babies. PharmacoEconomics **3:** 362–373.

34. MUGFORD, M., J. PIERCY & I. CHALMERS. 1991. Cost implications of different approaches to the prevention of respiratory distress syndrome. Arch. Dis. Child. **66:** 757–764.

35. GARCIA, J., M. CORRY, D. MacDONALD, D. ELBOURNE & A. GRANT. 1985. Mothers' views of continuous electronic fetal heart monitoring and intermittent auscultation in a randomized controlled trial. Birth **12:** 79–85.

36. ELBOURNE, D., M. RICHARDSON, I. CHALMERS, I. WATERHOUSE & E. HOLT. 1987. The Newbury maternity care study: A randomized controlled trial to assess a policy of women holding their own obstetric records. Br. J. Obstet. Gynaecol. **94:** 612–619.

37. MRC Working Party on the Evaluation of Chorion Villus Sampling. 1991. Medical Research Council European trial of chorion villus sampling. Lancet **337:** 1491–1499.
38. RENFREW, M. J. & R. McCANDLISH. 1992. With women: New steps in research in midwifery. *In* Women's Health Matters. H. Roberts, Ed.: 81–98. Routledge. London.
39. MAHLER, H. 1987. The safe motherhood initiative: A call to action. Lancet. **i:** 668–670.
40. DULEY, L., A. GRANT & I. CHALMERS. Promoting safe motherhood. Lancet **339:** 812.
41. DULEY, L. 1992. Maternal mortality associated with hypertensive disorders of pregnancy in Africa, Asia, Latin America and the Caribbean. Br. J. Obstet. Gynaecol. **99:** 547–553.
42. HEWSON, S. 1992, ED. Canadian Clinical Trials Network. Newsletter 6. McMaster University. Hamilton, Canada.
43. LUCEY, J., J. D. HORBAR & R. F. SOLL, EDS. 1992. Vermont-Oxford Trials Network. Newsletter, September 1992. Neonatal Research & Technology Assessment Inc. Burlington, Vermont.
44. CROWTHER, C. A. 1992. ACTOBAT: Australian collaborative trial of betamethasone and TRH. *In* Oxford Database of Perinatal Trials. I. Chalmers, Ed. Version 1.2, Disk Issue 8, Autumn 1992. Record 5212.
45. GRANT, A., ED. 1992. British Association of Perinatal Medicine Perinatal Clinical Trials Group. Newsletter 1. National Perinatal Epidemiology Unit. Oxford, U.K.
46. DELLAGRAMMATICAS, H., D. ELBOURNE, J. FOOKS, A. GRANT & M. LELOUP. 1992. First report of the EC collaborative randomized controlled trial of prophylactic ethamsylate in very preterm infants: Mortality and morbidity by three months of age. J. Perinat. Med. **20:** 28.
47. CHALMERS, I. 1991. The work of the National Perinatal Epidemiology Unit. One example of technology assessment in perinatal care. Int. J. Tech. Assess. Health Care. **7:** 430–443.
48. GRANT, A. 1992. Rationale for and work of the Perinatal Trials Service. Early Hum. Dev. **29:** 305–308.

DISCUSSION

RORY COLLINS (*Radcliffe Infirmary, Oxford, U.K.*): Dr. Grant, you have shown very encouraging results from the overview published in 1990 of corticosteroids, results that are perhaps the most encouraging of all of the overviews done in ECPC. Yet as I recall in the OSIRIS study, which was run after that period, a minority of the mothers were given corticosteroids despite the fact that they had pre-term premature babies. What should be done in a situation where there are very encouraging data that corticosteroids would be beneficial and yet you know that even your collaborators are not taking those results to heart in their practice?

ADRIAN GRANT (*Radcliffe Infirmary, Oxford, U.K.*): Anecdotally I have the impression that corticosteroids are being used more widely, certainly in the U.K. But you are right, Dr. Collins: in the OSIRIS trial conducted in 1990/91 the use of corticosteroids given to the mothers before the birth of the babies in this trial was surprisingly low and varied widely from country to country. For example, in New Zealand, where the first and largest trial was conducted, the use was greater than 50%, whereas it was as low as 10% elsewhere. And you have to remember that some of these babies are born so quickly there isn't an opportunity to give corticosteroids. I'm not sure why these results are not being incorporated in some people's practice, but then I might ask you the same question about streptokinase treatment in suspected myocardial infarction. However, I do believe that confused interpretation of the data is one reason, and another is that there are worries about long-term adverse effects that have not been substantiated by follow-up studies of some cohorts of children.

ALAN MORRIS (*LDS Hospital, Salt Lake City, Utah*): This would seem to provide a wonderful opportunity for exploring the applicability of a PC-based algorithm that could be distributed to large numbers of centers, particularly community hospitals. Have you considered trying to formulate a set of rules for decision-making in order to reduce "noise" introduced in the management of these large clinical trials? I think it would satisfy Dr. Peto's need for a simple trial in the sense that an algorithm that was validated would be rather simple to use at the bedside and provide consistent instructions to all operators.

GRANT: Do you mean in the context of the trial?

MORRIS: Yes—in the context of the rules used to move from one therapy to another such as how long to treat and when to stop. These trials are run by physiologic variables that are measured. There are a lot of quantifiable indicators in the management of these babies that would be useful as determinants of action.

JOHN FERGUSON (*NIH, Bethesda, Md.*): The low use of steroids in the appropriate patient population in the United States of 18% of those at risk has led the National Institute of Child Health and Human Development to have a consensus development on this issue even though it seems to have been solved in the literature by the work that you've presented. We hope that the message will get out.

GRANT: A letter from Iain Chalmers was published in the *Lancet* two weeks ago in which he wondered how long it would be before women sued obstetricians after a tragedy when they hadn't been given corticosteroids.

General Discussion: I

JOHN CLARKE (*Medical College of Pennsylvania, Philadelphia, Pa.*): Many of you who have done meta-analysis are aware of the fact that surgeons have never gotten past case reports and case series into randomized control trials. One of the problems with doing such randomized trials is because of the fact that the patient is selected before the surgeon even sees him. And before he even becomes a candidate for surgery, there's an investment cost in a person's undergoing a randomized control trial one arm of which involves being in the hospital for 3 weeks and undergoing a lot of pain and risk of death; in addition, there is a lot of variation in these very complex procedures. Then there is the whole business of compliance—some people may sign up for the study, may be randomized to a particular group and very likely may choose another one. The study is obviously not blinded and surgeons vary in ability to perform different procedures; it's not like giving someone a pill. So it seems easier to do a randomized control trial with drugs, but very difficult to do it with surgical procedures, even though it is important to do so. How can we get around some of those difficulties?

DAVID SACKETT (*McMaster University, Hamilton, Ontario, Canada*): I hope that Richard Peto can speak about the European carotid surgery trial. Surgical trials *are* different from medical trials. Surgeons learn; drugs don't. There are issues of what happens intraoperatively among other challenges to determining efficacy regardless of whether the methods are subexperimental or experimental. But the problems are all solvable. There has been a rapid rise in the introduction of random allocation in sorting through issues of surgical therapy, and as a group the surgeons are much more heroic than the internists involved in trials—and I say that speaking as an internist, since with ECIC we put some of our collaborators out of work by showing that the procedure that they were famous for was not efficacious. Surgeons also lose half the patients that they otherwise might be operating upon and profiting from so we have to credit them for their courage in subjecting themselves to this sort of review.

RICHARD PETO (*University of Oxford, Oxford, U.K.*): I think that the key concept for getting surgery trials done is what we have christened the "uncertainty principle." Basically, it means that a patient is eligible for randomization into a trial of some particular type of surgery *if, and only if, the doctor and patient are both substantially uncertain whether to go for such surgery.* If either of them are, after appropriate consideration of the options, reasonably certain that such surgery is advisable, then they discuss it and decide what to do, but they are not eligible for randomization. If either the doctor or the patient is reasonably certain that such surgery is not advisable, then again the patient is not eligible. Only if both are substantially uncertain is randomization to be allowed. So eligibility is defined not by the patient's real need for surgery, but by the doctor's and patient's *opinion* about that need. Uncertainty in the mind of the doctor is needed for eligibility. Now if you're a surgeon who's having patients referred to you, and you don't have any choice as to whether you operate, then the randomization takes place among the doctors who are choosing whether or not to make the referral. It's at the point where the choice as to whether or not surgery is going to be performed that the randomization can take place. We used this concept of certainty and uncertainty in randomizing 2,500 patients for carotid artery surgery, which will be described subsequently by Peter Sandercock. We got such large numbers just by saying that eligibility for the trial is defined by uncertainty, a criterion that seems to work in both medical and surgical circumstances. We're now randomizing 200 patients a month between different types of breast cancer surgery in China using that same principle.

KENNETH WARREN (*Picower Institute for Medical Research, Manhasset, N.Y.*): There are a spate of different ways of evaluating interventions, and a lot of money is being spent on such evaluations, but I've been wondering how these different methods compare. Are they all good and useful in different ways? Or are some better than others and some relatively useless? Also, the relative costs of each of these methods is an exceedingly important issue in today's economic and political climate.

DIXIE SNIDER (*Centers for Disease Control and Prevention, Atlanta, Ga.*): My question concerns another kind of intervention that we are very concerned with, especially as it relates to HIV and chronic disease, and that is *behavioral* interventions. I would ask the experts to comment on trials which involve behavioral interventions as opposed to drug or surgical therapies.

SACKETT: I can make two quick comments on that issue based on research that Brian Haynes led in our group a decade and a half ago, where the behavior that we were attempting to change was that of getting hypertensive patients to take their medications. First, there was a need for *attention* since one element of altering patient behavior may simply be the fact that someone is paying attention to the patient and is expressing a caring attitude toward him or her. Second, there is a need to recognize that different patients respond to different sorts of behavioral interventions, something our colleagues in the social sciences would call marketing segmentation. You can get patients on antihypertensive drugs to take their medications much better if you first teach them how to measure their own blood pressure, have them record it with their pill-taking, see them every two weeks, and provide them with positive feedback when they behave in ways that you wish. Each of those four different elements is going to affect a different patient, and yet those elements can't be easily teased apart.

PETER SANDERCOCK (*Western General Hospital, Edinburgh, Scotland*): I'd like to come back to the question of cost. There are two philosophies of clinical trials and, while I don't want to use the Atlantic Ocean as the dividing line, it does seem that the philosophy is different on either side of the Atlantic. Because the clinicians participating in the European carotid surgery trial did so for love, so to speak, not money, the trial could be done relatively cheaply—it cost about 4 or 5 million U.S. dollars over the long term. The corresponding trial done in North America, on the other hand, cost about 16 million dollars for NASET, which is about three-quarters more expensive. An issue that has to be addressed is whether collaborators should be paid for putting patients into a trial.

The same situation is true in the context of the acute stroke studies on which we are currently working. We're seeking North American collaboration in this international stroke trial and on our side of the Atlantic doctors are doing it for love, but on the U.S. side they are demanding money to put patients into this trial, which is not a pharmaceutical-sponsored trial. This leads to the question of whether trials should be designed so that they must be expensive. Trials can be made simple and cost-effective, but often one of the components of the cost is paying the doctors to put the patients into the trial and making the trial architecture extremely expensive. I maintain that simple, low-cost trials can randomize large numbers of patients without the cost of paying doctors to enter patients.

FREDERICK MOSTELLER (*Harvard University, Boston, Mass.*): Is the doctor actually paid much money compared to the cost of the treatment?

Sandercock: The ISIS trials offered some modest support to the centers to pay for photocopying, but that was all. Yet for other trials, such as one on therapies for acute stroke, the doctors received some $5,000 per patient randomized. There is a view that randomized trials are necessarily very expensive, and I'm questioning that view.

Iain Chalmers (*U.K. Cochrane Centre, Oxford, U.K.*): One of the most important things that has been achieved by the people involved in the so-called outcomes movement is that they have drawn attention to results that the patients regard as important but which haven't necessarily been studied by researchers. But I am puzzled about their position on the control of bias in the assessment of the relative effects of alternative treatments. Let me give a specific example: The New Hampshire Group has made a very impressive interactive videodisc designed to help people who have symptoms of benign prostatic hypertrophy to choose between alternative forms of care. One effect of using this format was that a smaller proportion of the patients ended up choosing surgery than was the case prior to the introduction of the disc. But, as far as I remember from watching the disc, I was not told that if I did choose surgery and I accepted an invitation to have a *transurethral* operation I would incur a 20% higher risk of ending up dead prematurely than if the operation was done by open surgery. Such a lapse puzzles me because of the enormous effort that has been made by that and other groups to assess the relative risks of premature death after these two different types of surgery.

I imagine that millions of dollars have been spent on those analyses, yet the fact that the group is not presenting that information in a patient information packet suggests to me that they're uncertain about the validity of the comparisons. They're uncertain about whether or not they've excluded bias in rather the same way Barbara McNeil was earlier when she depended on the results of randomized controlled trials to identify where effective forms of care lay and therefore which forms of practice to audit. So I am left unclear about the extent to which the people who are engaged in and who propose database analyses rely on them when it comes to the crunch. Otherwise why not present the results of those analyses to patients so that they can see that, as far as I can make out, there is a 20% higher mortality with the most common form of surgery for benign prostatic hypertrophy.

Peto: I'd like to speak to the same question. Hundreds of millions of dollars has been mandated for the nonrandomized assessment of whether treatments work or not. There are lots of other questions that can be asked about treatments, but one of the most important is the question of whether or not they work. If you compare two treatments you have to ask whether one is better than the other in terms of major outcome or treatment versus nothing. Does treatment do something? Does it do nothing? And the arguments that often you're going to be looking for moderate differences and that therefore anything other than randomization is useless—especially if there is a large number of endpoints—simply haven't been answered.

Every decade there's something new in the way of alternatives—it was historical controls in the mid 1970s and it had some other name in the 1980s and now it's called outcomes research in the 1990s. People keep trying to avoid proper randomization and they never come up with any serious reason for letting us believe that they have anything worthwhile to offer. Instead, they are diverting attention from the need for serious randomization of large numbers. I don't agree with a comment made earlier about being sort of courteous to the people who hold different views if by such courtesy serious discussion is bypassed. I think the different views on this are nonsense—recurrent nonsense—and I would like a serious answer. Why is money being spent on outcomes research on the pretense that it is going to assess whether things work or not, because it will not do so.

GEORGE SILVERMAN (*Government Accounting Office, Washington, D.C.*): This is the third or fourth meeting at which this issue has been raised and the discussion is often frustrating because people are speaking at cross purposes. First, the core of the proposition that what we really need are large-scale randomized simple trials and the part that draws the most attention is the part that deserves the least argument, and that is the issue of randomization. There is no one in this room that I have encountered, nor at any other meeting, who does not want randomization when it can be achieved. It then becomes a question of what you do if randomization means that you have to give up size.

Now what we have done in this country typically is to continue with the randomization and to ignore the size. Dr. Chalmers' earlier question about whether there are any situations in which database analyses have been used for definitive therapy can be turned to inquire how many questions have been answered definitively for marginal therapies with small-scale randomized trials. So the issue is not whether or not we should randomize, but rather what we should do when randomization means inordinate costs or the inability to achieve large-scale size. We have to ask whether we can do some other form of research, not for definitive answers but for hypothesis generation—for getting some sense of where to put our trial money—and that is largely what database analyses are for. They will never give definitive answers, but that doesn't mean that they're useless in getting an understanding of the etiology of disease or of the subgroups in which the putative therapy should be tested most efficiently.

Richard Peto argues that simple large-scale inexpensive trials are possible in the United States and we actually have a bet on whether this is true. And while his idea is a wonderful one we must admit that randomized trials in this country leave a lot of questions open. For example we have had many trials in adjuvant therapy for breast cancer as well as a multiplicity of consensus conferences, each of which gets less and less certain about the appropriate therapy for subgroups of patients. Trials, as they have been structured, have not been able to answer our questions.

BARRY KATZ (*Indiana University, Indianapolis, Indiana*): I'd like to echo some of what was said. What is coming out of the PORTs—and I'm speaking as a "fundee" not a funder—is not an evaluation of the intervention in the way discussants are thinking of it. We are able to see what's going on and shed some light on the effect of the intervention on mortality rates and utilization rates, but we're not able to say the treatment is better than doing no intervention or doing another intervention. We would all agree that only a randomized trial can do that. Does every situation call for a randomized trial? I'm not sure. Can we even get the doctors treating the patients to cooperate in a randomized trial in every case? The answer to that is a resounding *no*—there isn't enough uncertainty in the minds of many physicians to warrant that. But there are issues that we can shed light on so I don't think that the money spent is being thrown down the drain.

THOMAS CHALMERS (*Harvard School of Public Health, Boston, Mass.*): I'd be glad to answer Iain Chalmers' question: I don't think anybody in his right mind thinks for one minute that you can learn how patients should be treated by observing how doctors are treating them and the PORTs have accomplished a great deal in showing that. Barbara McNeil did not claim that the Boston Myocardial Infarction PORT was learning from outcome data how patients should be treated. I hate to hear, however, of the either/or of outcomes research versus only very large trials because such dichotomizing only defeats our purposes. Very large trials are hard to get, and what we need is many small trials. We need early randomization, and we need to find some way in which patients can be attracted into trials very early in the development of new technology. I have a solution to that problem which goes over like a lead balloon, but I keep pushing it. Third parties should not reimburse for new technology that has not yet been proven to be effective or ineffective unless the patient is part of a randomized control trial designed to determine efficacy. We have trouble adopting that philosophy for political reasons, and yet it seems to be the only solution to the problem. The thing that determines whether patients get into a trial or not is whether they think there is an advantage, or a possible advantage, in getting the new treatment. And if they can only get the new treatment by being part of a randomized control trial, they'll all flock into the trials and their doctors will collaborate.

KAY DICKERSIN (*University of Maryland, Baltimore, Md.*): In response to George Silverman's comment about how we haven't learned much that's important from clinical trials so far as to be able to affect treatment, I'd like to note that it's not possible because few agencies have been willing to fund systems such as the one devised by Iain Chalmers for finding out what randomized trials have been done in all of medicine and then also some sort of system for keeping account of what's being done currently. If we don't have either of those, then how can we evaluate the treatments that are being investigated?

FREDERICK MOSTELLER (*Harvard University School of Public Health, Boston, Mass.*): The issue of dissemination of information has not been thoroughly explored here. Dissemination is a big job in itself and different from what most of us who work on the science side are used to.

BARBARA MCNEIL (*Harvard Medical School, Boston, Mass.*): It was never our intent for the PORT to replace a randomized clinical trial. We thought instead that there were a number of very clear-cut situations where we could get data that were unavailable by conventional means in populations currently excluded from randomized trials. We can get better information on complication rates, for example, than would be available from traditional clinical trials. For example, we've recently finished looking at the incidence of hemorrhagic stroke in patients who were treated since the introduction of thrombolysis. Now there may be all kinds of problems with the data, but it does look as if the incidence of hemorrhagic strokes that we have is several-fold greater than the 1.4% figure that was mentioned earlier that arose from clinical trials. Some generalizations or extrapolations can be made from claims data, but we're not saying that those data can be used to determine whether one therapy is better than another. I also think that perhaps we can get a better handle on such things as quality of life and complications. We can get more information on the cost of care and how those costs vary by site and provider. We can work in the area of information dissemination and in essence do trials of the kinds of dissemination efforts that are believed to be useful. And finally we can look at the extent to which adherence to certain practices or guidelines for care actually improves outcomes. All of these areas are worthwhile in refining the way medicine is practiced. I would put them in a side bar to the issue of randomized trials. There are niches for everything and I believe the PORTs have a place in the discussion.

JEROLD LUCEY (*University of Vermont, Burlington, Vt.*): I'd like to respond to the issue of paying investigators for participating in trials. We were inspired by Iain Chalmers' and Adrian Grant's work in Oxford to create a trials network here of neonatal intensive care units which we've called the Vermont Oxford Trials Network. We now have about 80 participating neonatal intensive care units, the vast majority of which represent private-practice neonatologists who are not in university practices. About 30 of those centers are currently participating in our first trial and none of the investigators is paid; in fact, the members have actually supported the network with a small annual membership fee.

ARGYE HILLIS (*Scott & White Hospital, Temple, Texas*): My whole career as a statistician has been in trials in eye surgery. One problem is that there is no public pressure for surgical trials like there is for drug trials. But there are also some advantages because you have to choose the first patients one by one to do surgery on and it's easy to apply randomization in that context. Otherwise you would have a built-in bias in choosing which patients to try in your surgical series. That leads into the possibility for getting large randomized inexpensive trials if you can get an agreement on introducing new devices and new surgery through selecting the first patients to try them because you have to try these on a limited number of patients anyway in a random formal way instead of choosing which ones you happen to feel like that day.

PETO: I don't think that any of these replies have actually come anywhere near suggesting that methods other than randomization can be used to evaluate treatments. I don't see any reason to believe that the acute myocardial infarction PORT is going to give reliable answers to questions as to whether adherence to a protocol improves outcomes and the stroke rate of 1.4% and the fact that you get much higher rates than that in patients over 65 was already found in the trials. The trials have shown a strong age-dependence on the risk of stroke reduced by thrombolytic therapy so if you look at the appropriate age group that's not a new finding. And with regard to George Silverman's comment that since there are various subgroups if you divide and subdivide and resubdivide the breast cancer patients until you eventually get to a point where the trial evidence is inconclusive for that particular subgroup, that does not mean that the analysis of nonrandomized data is going to give anything very useful in that subgroup. Sure, there are questions that haven't been answered, but I think the solution is to try and do the trials better rather than to look for alternatives to randomization. I don't think there's been any answer to suggest anything otherwise.

The Science of Reviewing Research[a]

ANDREW D. OXMAN[b,c,d] AND GORDON H. GUYATT[d,e]

Departments of [c]Family Medicine
[d]Clinical Epidemiology and Biostatistics, and [e]Medicine
Faculty of Health Sciences
McMaster University
Hamilton, Ontario, Canada L8N 3Z5

AUTHORITY, SUPERSTITION, AND SCIENCE

Medical practitioners enjoy positions of authority. Considerable economic resources are directed to the practice and improvement of medicine. Courts of law recognize qualified medical practitioners as being expert witnesses on many matters. Witchdoctors and other alternative health care providers do not receive comparable resources or recognition. Why is this? Modern medicine is based on science, whereas witchcraft and other alternatives are based on "superstition."[1] But what is it that distinguishes science from superstition, and to what extent can medical practitioners claim to be scientific?

Most medical practitioners are not likely to have given much thought to questions such as these. According to Thomas Kuhn, the same can be said of practitioners of other scientific disciplines.[2] Kuhn has described scientific paradigms as encompassing all that which the practitioners of a particular scientific discipline take for granted. The paradigm constitutes the framework within which the scientists reason when they try to solve their scientific problems. It represents the premises of scientific thinking and therefore is not usually considered a scientific problem in itself. As Kuhn points out, as a general rule, scientists do not learn concepts, laws, and theories in the abstract. Instead, they gradually learn to use these intellectual tools by reading and by listening. As a consequence, scientists may "learn easily and well about the particular individual hypotheses that underlie a concrete piece of current research," but in spite of that "they are little better than laymen at characterizing the established basis of their field."[2]

When defects in an existing paradigm accumulate to the extent that the paradigm is no longer tenable, the paradigm is challenged and replaced by a new way of looking at the world. Kuhn, a physicist, is particularly interested in physics, chemistry, and astronomy, and uses examples from the history of these sciences to illustrate his ideas. It is not clear that science always develops in leaps and bounds as described by Kuhn. It is particularly uncertain to what extent Kuhn's theory correctly describes the development of medicine, which encompasses both clinical research and the practice of medicine. Moreover, medicine comprises a variety of subdisciplines. The paradigm underlying medical thinking is likely to vary, for example, from pathologist to psychiatrist.[3]

[a] This work was supported by Grant No. 01969 from the Ontario Ministry of Health. Drs. Guyatt and Oxman are Career Scientists of the Ontario Ministry of Health.

[b] Address for correspondence: Dr. Andy Oxman, Department of Family Medicine, McMaster University Medical Centre 1200 Main Street West, Room 2V10, Hamilton, Ontario, Canada L8N 3Z5.

Nonetheless, it is tempting to describe changes that have occurred over the past 30 years as a paradigm shift.[3,4] In the 1960s, an increasing number of clinicians began to demand empirical proof of the effectiveness of medical interventions. Led by pioneers such as Archie Cochrane, Austin Bradford Hill, Richard Doll, and more recently by people like Richard Peto and Iain Chalmers, the randomized controlled trial has emerged as the ideal—or paradigm—of clinical research.

Kuhn's view is that scientists working within a scientific paradigm need not necessarily engage in philosophical debate regarding the paradigm so long as their activity within the paradigm is productive. Others, such as Popper, argue that this is dangerous. According to Popper, a scientist who is not critical of the paradigm within which s/he works "has been taught in a dogmatic spirit" and is "a victim of indoctrination."[3]

In this paper we will briefly describe the shift from "authoritative reviews" of medical problems to systematic reviews that place particular emphasis on the role of "experts" in the process of synthesizing the results of research. This shift can be viewed as an extension of the shift from a paradigm that relied heavily on unsystematic clinical experience and pathophysiologic rationales to one that stresses rigorous clinical evaluations of medical interventions. Finally, we would like to reiterate that we need to be critical of the "new paradigm," even though it is highly productive.

AUTHORITATIVE REVIEWS VERSUS SYSTEMATIC REVIEWS

Traditionally, review articles which survey an area of scientific inquiry or clinical practice have been written by experts in the field. When seeking critiques of review articles (peer review), editors have looked to other experts in the field for help. These policies are illustrated by the two following responses to a small survey of editors of medical journals undertaken in 1986:[5]

> From the point of view of an editor of a journal, the acceptability of research reviews depends greatly on the advice given by experts in the field. Reviews should give an adequate coverage of the literature and it is only those who know the field who would be able to advise on whether this had been done. The assessment of original articles of course is another matter and criteria for this activity have been published in a number of places.

> The people chosen to serve on the Editorial Committee are those who we believe have a good grasp on their particular subfields within medicine. At a yearly meeting, each Committee member proposes certain topics with specific authors to be invited. An invitation to prepare a review on a particular topic is then sent to the chosen author. From this procedure I think you can see that we rely heavily on the expertise of our individual Committee members as guided by the whole group to choose qualified reviewers. We thus monitor the quality of the manuscripts before they are even written!

These policies may appear intuitively reasonable and appropriate. However, there are reasons for serious skepticism. It is possible that experts might lack the objectivity desirable in preparing or critiquing a review article. For example, personal experience in primary research is highly salient and considerably more vivid than the research of others, and therefore likely to be overweighted in judgments.[6] This is also true for personal clinical experience.

When the consistency of expert ratings of journal articles has been examined, it has been found to be poor. Ten articles from which quantitative estimates of

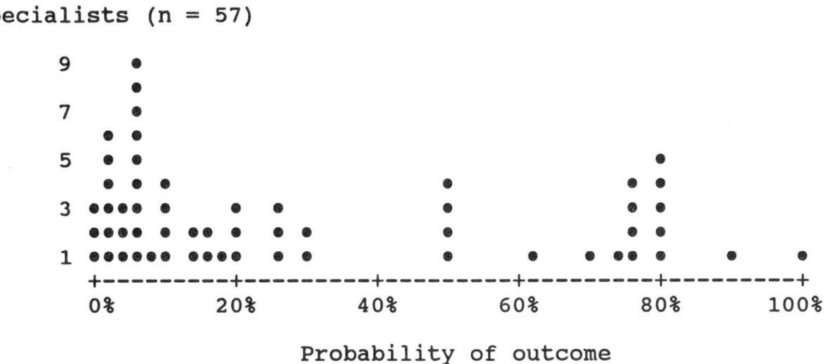

FIGURE 1. Specialists' beliefs about the probability of a particulaly important outcome for a common and important intervention. (The specialty society that convened the meeting at which the estimates were obtained requested to remain anonymous.) (Adapted from Eddy.[17])

consistency (inter-judge agreement) are available found correlation coefficients of from 0.19 to 0.54, with most results clustering around the lower values.[7-16] While the need for agreement among peer reviewers has been challenged, and its desirability has been questioned,[19,20] agreement is important, though not sufficient, to ensure the quality of the peer review process. If peer reviewers cannot agree, the quality of their judgments must be considered unreliable.

Similarly, experts often disagree about the results of a review. Eddy has provided the following example of this problem: A group of medical specialists met to develop a guideline for a common and important intervention. When they were asked to write down their beliefs about the probability of a particularly important outcome in patients receiving this intervention their answers ranged from 0% to 100% (FIG. 1).[17] Whatever mental processes the experts used to arrive at their beliefs, they had very different perceptions.

The problem with not knowing the reasoning that was used is that it is impossible to critique the methods that were used. There is no way to tell which answer is most correct. Moreover, when information is synthesized and probabilities are estimated informally, there are a number of factors that can lead to systematic errors in the judgments that are made.[18] One such bias is a tendency to overlook small but clinically important effects when research is synthesized subjectively. Cooper and Rosenthal demonstrated this experimentally by randomly assigning reviewers to either use or not use meta-analysis to combine the results of several studies. The studies, which included some that did not show significant results, demonstrated an overall significant effect ($p = 0.016$). The reviewers not using meta-analysis were significantly more likely to find little or no support for the hypothesis being tested.

THE RELATIONSHIP BETWEEN EXPERTISE AND METHODOLOGIC RIGOR

In the process of developing criteria for formal evaluation of the methodologic rigor of review articles,[19-21] we addressed two issues related to the role of expertise

TABLE 1. Criteria for Assessing the Methodologic Rigor of Research Reviews

1. Were the search methods reported?
2. Was the search comprehensive?
3. Were the inclusion criteria reported?
4. Was selection bias avoided?
5. Were the validity criteria reported?
6. Was validity assessed appropriately?
7. Were the methods used to combine studies reported?
8. Were the findings combined appropriately?
9. Were the conclusions supported by the reported data?
10. What was the overall scientific quality of the review?

in the process of preparing and critiquing review articles. We compared the consistency of assessments of the methodologic rigor of review articles using our criteria by experts in the field (given instructions, but no training) with that of non-experts (trained to apply our criteria in a standardized way). In addition, we examined the relationship between the expertise of the author and the methodologic rigor of the review article.

Methods

The results of our assessment of the reliability and validity of the criteria have been reported elsewhere.[20,21] Twelve judges evaluated the methodologic rigor of 36 published review articles using the criteria shown in TABLE 1. The review articles were drawn from three sampling frames: articles highly rated by criteria external to the study; meta-analyses; and articles selected from a broad spectrum of medical journals. Four categories of judges assessed the articles: research methodologists, clinicians with research training, research assistants, and content-area experts, with three judges in each category. The non-experts all received training in the application of our criteria.

Authors of the review articles were surveyed. Respondents were asked to categorize their level of expertise using the following seven-point scale:

1	2	3	4	5	6	7
Limited Background		Knowledgeable		Very Knowledgeable		Expert

Expert = Prior to writing the review, you had already read extensively in this area, *and* done research or written articles on the same topic.

Very Knowledgeable = You had already read extensively on this topic, but *not* done research in this area.

Knowledgeable = You kept up with the literature in this general area routinely, *and* were familiar with *most* of the primary research in this area.

Limited Background = You had *not* read most of the primary literature directly relevant to the topic of this review.

Respondents were also asked to estimate the amount of time they spent preparing their reviews, and to rate the strength of their prior opinions on the topic of the reviews as follows:

Please indicate the *strength of your opinion prior* to preparing this review, with respect to the primary question that the review addresses.

Respondents were asked to categorize the strength of their opinions using the following seven-point scale:

1	2	3	4	5	6	7
Decided		Strong Opinion		Week Opinion		Undecided

An intraclass correlation coefficient (ICC), which is the ratio of the variance between review articles to the total variance, was used to measure agreement among judges.[22] The ICC's and their 95% confidence intervals (CIs) were calculated according to Shrout and Fleiss' guidelines.[23] The analyses were done using BMDP.[24]

Spearman rank order correlations between the degree of expertise of the author and the author's strength of prior opinion, the amount of time spent preparing the review article, and the quality of the review were calculated. For the correlation of degree of expertise with the quality of the review, the quality of the review was determined by taking the mean global rating of the reviewers (groups 1, 2, and 3) who reviewed all 36 articles (there is a summary question which asks for a global rating of the methodologic quality of the review).

Results

The intraclass correlation coefficients for each of the four groups of raters are summarized in FIGURE 2. Consistency of ratings was higher for groups 1 to 3 than for the experts on each of ten questions. The gradient between groups 1 to 3 and the experts was considerably greater for questions which required substantial judgment (questions 2, 4, 6, 8, 9, 10) than for questions which did not require as much judgment (questions 1, 3, 5, 7). For the overall rating of methodologic rigor, the intraclass correlations were 0.79 (95% CI, 0.65–0.87) for group 1, 0.77 (95% CI, 0.51–0.79) for group 2, 0.69 (95% CI, 0.38–0.78) for group 3, and 0.23 (95% CI, 0.03–0.45) for the experts.

Thirty of thirty-six authors (83%) responded to our survey concerning their methods. The correlation between expertise and strength of prior opinion was 0.55 ($p = 0.03$); the more expertise, the stronger the prior opinion. The correlation between expertise and the amount of time spent preparing a review was -0.40 ($p = 0.045$); the more expertise, the less time. The correlation between expertise and the quality of a review was -0.52 ($p = 0.004$); the more expertise, the lower quality.

DISCUSSION

At least two possible explanations for the poorer agreement among the experts are possible: either lack of training, or expertise itself. In either case, these results cast doubt on the wisdom of relying exclusively on experts without specific training to assess the methodologic rigor of review articles.

These results also cast doubt on the wisdom of relying on experts to be solely responsible for preparation of review articles. Our data suggest that experts, on average, write reviews of inferior quality; that the greater the expertise the more likely the quality is to be poor; and that the poor quality may be related to the

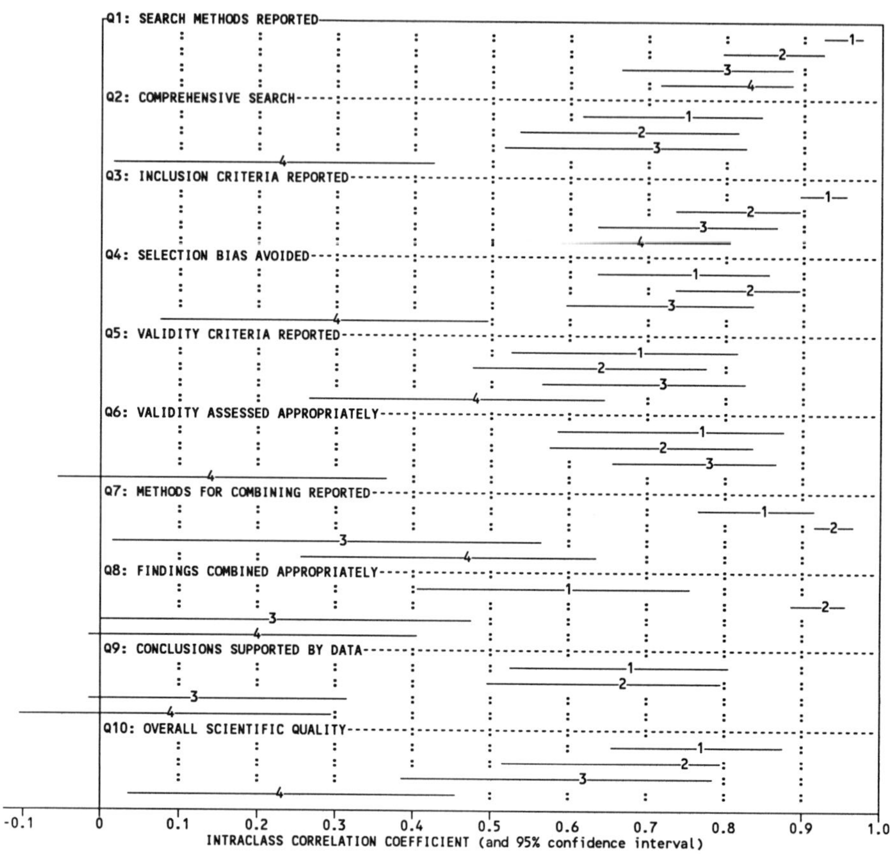

FIGURE 2. Agreement within groups of judges. 1 = experts in research methodology (group 1); 2 = MDs with research training (group 2); 3 = research assistants (group 3); and 4 = content-area experts (group 4).

strength of their prior opinions and the amount of time they spend preparing a review article.

What is it about expertise that might predispose to such difficulties in making judgments of methodologic rigor, and such problems in preparing high-quality reviews? It is natural that investigators will be biased so that they give more weight to their own work versus that of others. In addition, many investigators will have strong opinions about their area which will lead them to judge evidence differently according to whether it supports their beliefs. A third issue is the personal competitiveness and antagonism that unfortunately often plays a role in scientific endeavor and scientific debate.

An extreme interpretation of the results of this investigation might be that experts should occupy themselves with the task of producing new data, or retire from the topics of their expertise,[25] and so in either case leave judgments and summaries of their efforts to those who have specific training in the science of research reviews. A more reasonable interpretation might be to acknowledge the value of expertise in recognizing subtle, but important clues that someone without expertise might overlook while, at the same time, appreciating the risks of blind faith in the subjective thought processes of experts or anyone else.

As Louis Pasteur once wrote: "Chance favors the prepared mind."[26] Expertise might be of great value in this regard, provided experts are able to follow the injunction cited by Iain Chalmers in an article published a decade ago on scientific inquiry and authoritarianism: "Teach thy tongue to say 'I do not know' and thou shalt progress."[27]

CONCLUSION

Systematic and explicit approaches to reviewing research are essential, but not sufficient to ensure the validity of the results. "Science, no less than painting, cannot be done by numbers."[28] And, in the words of J. M. Ziman:[29]

> Our present system of rewards and incentives in science does not encourage individuals to devote themselves for years on end to these critical synthesizing activities. "Recognition," by way of professional advancement and prestige, is given solely for primary research; has any academy ever mentioned that the hero was the author of a valuable treatise or of the authoritative review that has since determined the course of research in his field?

> The trouble is, quite simply, a matter of philosophy. We are so obsessed with the notions of discovery and individual originality that we fail to realize that scientific research is essentially a corporate activity, in which the community achieves far more than the sum of the efforts of its members.

We are delighted that the New York Academy of Sciences has chosen to present the L. W. Frohlich award to Richard Peto and Iain Chalmers for their pioneering work as proponents and practitioners of systematic reviews of randomized controlled trials rather than for their "authoritative reviews." The successes that they have had, and the vision they have shown, in organizing international efforts to critically synthesize and keep up-to-date the scientific basis of medical practice are inspiring.

We would, nevertheless, like to come back to the need to remain critical of the very paradigm that they have helped to pioneer. There is still an enormous amount of productive work to be done within this paradigm. However, to capitalize on the solutions that can be derived within this paradigm, knowledge that is derived from other "paradigms" is also needed. In particular, on the level of clinical practice "hermeneutics" (interpretative reflection) is necessary to appreciate the subjective reality of individual patients; and on the level of policy, we clearly have a long way to go to ensure that the results of good clinical research actually lead us to do more good than harm.

ACKNOWLEDGMENTS

We would like to express our appreciation to the judges for their contribution to this study, particularly Drs. Charlie H. Goldsmith, Brian G. Hutchison, Ruth

A. Milner and David L. Streiner. We would also like to thank Dr. Joel Singer for his assistance with the analyses, and the authors of the review articles who responded to our survey.

REFERENCES

1. BRISKMAN, L. 1988. Doctors and witchdoctors: Which doctors are which? *In* Logic in Medicine. C. I. Phillips, Ed.: 1–16. British Medical Journal. London.
2. KUHN, T. S. 1970. The Structure of Scientific Revolutions, 2nd ed.: 46. The University of Chicago Press. Chicago.
3. WULFF, H. R., S. A. PEDERSEN & R. ROSENBERG. 1990. The paradigm of medicine. *In* Philosophy of Medicine, 2nd ed.: 1–12. Blackwell Scientific Publications. Oxford, U.K.
4. EVIDENCE-BASED MEDICINE WORKING GROUP. 1992. Evidence-based medicine: A new approach to teaching the practice of medicine. JAMA **268:** 2420–2425.
5. OXMAN, A. D. 1987. A Methodological Framework for Research Overviews. M.Sc. thesis.: 212–218. McMaster University. Hamilton, Ontario.
6. COOPER, H. M. 1986. On the social psychology of using research reviews: The case of desegregation and the black achiever. *In* Social Psychology of Education. R. S. Feldman, Ed.: 341–363. Cambridge University Press. Cambridge, U.K.
7. SMIGEL, E. O. & H. L. ROSS. 1970. Factors in the editorial decision. Am. Sociologist. **25:** 19–21.
8. INGELFINGER, F. J. 1974. Peer review in biomedical publication. Am. J. Med. **56:** 686–692.
9. SCOTT, W. A. 1974. Interreferee agreement on some characteristics of manuscripts. Am. Psychologist. **29:** 698–702.
10. CICCETTI, D. V. & H. CONN. 1976. A statistical analysis of reviewer agreement and bias in evaluating medical abstracts. Yale J. Biol. Med. **49:** 373–383.
11. HENDRICK, C. 1976. Editorial comment. Person. Soc. Psychol. Bull. **2:** 207–208.
12. LINDER, D. E. 1977. Evaluation of the Personality and Social Psychology Bulletin by its readers and authors. Person. Soc. Psychol. Bull. **3:** 583–591.
13. GOTTFREDSON, S. D. 1978. Evaluating psychological research reports: Dimensions, reliability, and correlates of quality judgements. Am. Psychologist. **33:** 920–934.
14. SCARR, S. & B. L. R. WEBER. 1978. The reliability of reviews for the American Psychologist. Am. Psychologist. **33:** 935.
15. CICCETTI, D. V. & L. D. ERON. 1979. The reliability of manuscript reviewing for the Journal of Abnormal Psychology. J. Abnorm. Psychol. **22:** 596–600.
16. MARSH, H. W. & S. BALL. 1981. Interjudgemental reliability of reviews for the Journal of Educational Psychology. J. Ed. Psychol. **73:** 872–880.
17. EDDY, D. M., V. HASSELBLAD & R. SHACHTER. 1992. Meta-analysis by the Confidence Profile Method: The Statistical Synthesis of Evidence: 3. Academic Press. San Diego, CA.
18. DAWSON, N. V. & H. R. ARKES. 1987. Systematic errors in medical decision making: Judgment limitations. J. Gen. Intern. Med. **2:** 183–187.
19. OXMAN, A. D. & G. H. GUYATT. 1988. Guidelines for reading literature reviews. Can. Med. Assoc. J. **138:** 697–703.
20. OXMAN, A. D., G. H. GUYATT, J. SINGER, *et al.* 1991. Agreement among reviewers of review articles. J. Clin. Epidemiol. **44:** 91–98.
21. OXMAN, A. D. & G. H. GUYATT. 1991. Validation of an index of the quality of review articles. J. Clin. Epidemiol. **44:** 1271–1278.
22. STREINER, D. L. & G. R. NORMAN. 1989. Health Measurement Scales: A Practical Guide to their Development and Use. Oxford University Press. Oxford, U.K.
23. SHROUT, P. E. & J. L. FLEISS. 1979. Intraclass correlations: Uses in assessing rater reliability. Psychol. Bull. **86:** 420–428.
24. DIXON, W. J., ED. 1983. BMDP Statistical Software. University of California Press. Berkeley, CA.

25. SACKETT, D. L. 1983. Proposals for the health sciences—I. Compulsory retirement for experts. J. Chron. Dis. **36:** 545–547.
26. CONANT, J. B. 1951. Science and Common Sense.: 109. Yale University Press. New Haven, CN.
27. CHALMERS, I. 1983. Scientific inquiry and authoritarianism in perinatal care and education. Birth **10:** 151–162
28. GJERTSEN, D. 1989. Science and Philosophy: Past and Present.: 113. Penguin Books. London.
29. ZIMAN, J. M. 1969. Information, communication, knowledge. Nature **224:** 318–324.

DISCUSSION

RICHARD PETO (*University of Oxford, Oxford, U.K.*): Dr. Oxman, even on reviewing evidence, you've got to start by saying what sort of relative risk you are talking about. These problems arise where you're likely to have moderate relative risks. You know you may get things wrong in terms of two-fold errors, but you're less likely to make 10-fold errors. For example, if you were reviewing the evidence as to whether smoking is massacreing vast numbers of people, then you wouldn't need the kind of methodologic quality that you've described, and it wouldn't necessarily be a fair criticism of review of evidence on smoking to say that the review didn't go into the kind of detail that you described. But if you were trying to study something, such as beta blockers in acute myocardial infarction, then you would need a great deal of attention to detail. In reviews, as in trials, the critical question is: What is the relative risk? That is, what sort of differences are we trying to discriminate between? You've shown very nicely that quite substantial biases will result if the reviewing process isn't done properly. But there are circumstances where reviews that are not done according to any of the criteria that you've described might nevertheless be scientifically sufficient. It is the relative risk that always matters in determining what is plausible.

ANDREW OXMAN (*McMaster University, Hamilton, Ontario, Canada*): For any research endeavor it's how important the problem is that determines how many resources we put into the effort. And I agree entirely with your comments earlier that a marker of importance is how common the problem is and how severe its outcomes are. From the point of view of a reviewer of research it is also important to take into consideration the quality of the available information. One needs to consider how thoroughly to look for research, what to include and what to exclude, and how to validate the information. All of this is going to be determined by the effect sizes one is looking at as well as the availability of the research, the amount of one's own resources, and the importance of the problem. I think that it's a mistake to say that these criteria don't apply to any type of problem—I think they do. What differs from problem to problem is the decisions that are made relative to each of these criteria about how many resources you use to identify research, how you assess the information, what effort you put into validating the data, and what analytic techniques you use to put them together at the end of the day.

PETO: For the evaluation of interventions, which is what this meeting is about, I think your material is totally relevant. It's just that there are other areas of review that aren't so much concerned with the evaluation of interventions, such as the effects of smoking, where you don't need to randomize to work out that it causes lung cancer.

THOMAS CHALMERS (*New England Medical Center, Boston, Mass.*): I gathered from your presentation, Dr. Oxman, that you distinguished between a systematic review and a meta-analysis by pointing out that you didn't want to put the emphasis on statistics. If one assumes that a good meta-analysis includes all of the things that you've pointed out are necessary for doing a review—such as control of bias and duplicate determination, adequate searching of the literature, and a quantitative analysis of the data as presented in the literature—is there any place for a systematic review without the quantitative analysis? Is there any place for a review of data in the literature where the data have not been statistically analyzed? Should not all qualitative reviews that do not analyze the data as data be replaced by adequately done meta-analyses?

OXMAN: This relates to the point that Richard Peto just made—that there are situations in which the applications of statistical techniques aren't warranted either because the data are so obvious that you don't need them or because the data aren't sufficient for statistical analysis. A good example of this is seen by the knee replacement PORT that was discussed earlier. If the data you have are not good enough to be combined in order to draw conclusions it is worthwhile to know that so that investigators can go out then and collect good evidence. It's not worth the sort of efforts that Richard Peto's group puts into reviews, but it's worth having gone through the steps up to the point of saying that this is the best evidence we have, this is the quality of the evidence, this is what we know at this point in time, and now let's go out and try and learn some more.

DIXIE SNIDER (*Centers for Disease Control and Prevention, Atlanta, Ga.*): The systematic reviews and meta-analyses are properly emphasized as being very important. On the other hand, as someone who's recently retired as a content expert and moved into the area of methodology, I have also seen bias on the part of persons who do systematic reviews, particularly a tendency toward iconoclastic destruction of the status quo. Perhaps that's good, but I would also like to point out that many times the content experts are knowledgeable about information that's not necessarily available in the literature; having been on some data safety and monitoring boards I've experienced that on several occasions. So instead of having two different groups—the authorities and the methodologic experts—I would suggest that teams of people with an expertise in both areas "duke it out," so to speak. Such an approach could produce a better review than one coming at it from either extreme.

OXMAN: I agree entirely; in fact, that's the approach that we've been taking with the reviews with which I've been involved. Meta-analysis or systematic reviews in general are tools for putting together what we know and like any tool can be misused. It's important that these methods be used properly, and the insights that experts can bring to a review are important and should be kept in perspective.

Publication Bias: The Problem That Won't Go Away

KAY DICKERSIN

Department of Epidemiology and Preventive Medicine
University of Maryland School of Medicine
Howard Hall
660 West Redwood Street
Baltimore, Maryland 21201

YUAN-I MIN

Department of Epidemiology
The Johns Hopkins University
School of Hygiene and Public Health
615 North Wolfe Street
Baltimore, Maryland 21205

BACKGROUND

Publication bias is any tendency on the parts of investigators or editors to fail to publish study results on the basis of the direction or strength of the study findings. The earliest complaint about publication bias of which we are aware was made in 1661 by the chemist Robert Boyle who said:

Many excellent notions or experiments are, by sober and modest men, suppressed.[1]

Later, in 1909, an editorial on the topic was written in the *Boston Medical Journal* and included the following statement:

We too commonly see references of "so many successful cases," with a certain inevitable emphasis on the word "successful". . . . There is unquestionably a false emphasis in all such publications, tending to increase the reputation of the writer, but not render the public more secure.[2]

In this century, there have been frequent references to the problem of publication bias, or "the file drawer problem," although until recently there have been few data to support expressions of concern about the problem.

The earliest study providing evidence of publication bias of which we are aware was performed in 1959.[3] Sterling reviewed four prominent psychology journals (TABLE 1) and found that, of the articles reporting results involving hypothesis testing, more than 95% reported statistically significant ("positive") findings. Dr. Sterling updated his study in 1988 and reviewed the same four psychology journals and four medical journals, for 1986 and 1987 (personal communication to K.D., March 19, 1993). There was little indication that the situation had changed in the psychology journals over the 40-year period covered, with about 95% of the articles that performed hypothesis testing reporting statistically significant results. The situation in the medical journals was found to be very similar, with about 85% of the articles reporting statistically significant results. Although it is possible that 85% to 95% of all studies undertaken have results that reject a prior null hypothesis

TABLE 1. Statistically Significant Articles in Psychology and Medical Journals[a]

	Articles Reviewed in 1986–87	% Rejecting H_0 in 1986–87	% Rejecting H_0 in 1955–56
Psychology Journals			
Experimental Psychology	165	93.5	99.1
Comparative and Physiological and Psychology	119	97.1	96.8
Consulting and Clinical Psychology	83	97.5	95.2
Personality and Social Psychology	230	95.6	96.9
Medical Journals			
American Journal of Epidemiology	141	80.9	N/A
American Journal of Public Health	97	88.1	N/A
New England Journal of Medicine	218	87.9	N/A

[a] See Ref. 3 and personal communication with K. Dickersin.

(H_0), this possibility seems remote. Since Sterling's original report, evidence has accumulated to show that studies reaching publication are a select sample of all studies conducted.[4,5]

The first evidence of publication bias with respect to clinical trials was reported in a study by John Simes.[6] He compared the results of two separate meta-analyses of chemotherapy clinical trials: one meta-analysis used only data from studies that had been published, and the other used data from studies listed in a cancer trials registry, some of which had never been reported. Simes found that when just published trials were considered, use of a combined chemotherapeutic regimen for ovarian cancer was statistically significantly superior to use of a single alkylating agent. When the results of all *registered* trials were considered, however, including those that remained unpublished, no statistically significant advantage of the combination chemotherapy was observed.

In another study,[7] authors of published reports of randomized trials were surveyed to learn which other trials they had performed, the results of these trials, and their publication status. Fifty-five percent of the published trials, compared with only 15% of the unpublished trials, had statistically significant results favoring a new therapy. Most of the unpublished trials had not detected any differences between treatments (44%) or had only shown a trend that had not achieved "statistical significance" (35%).

In this article, we will review the evidence showing that clinical trials are more likely to be reported in print if investigators find statistically significant differences between treatments. Recently, several very similar investigations of publication bias were conducted on four separate populations.[8–10] The investigations were designed to be similar; all of the primary investigators were located at Johns Hopkins University (JHU) in Baltimore. One group (our own) examined publication bias in three of the populations studied, and the other (led by Philippa Easterbrook) investigated the fourth population. All four studies used similar data-collection instruments and collected data on a common set of variables. All of the investigations were designed to address the same prior hypotheses, involving, first, the association between study results and publication, and second, the association between other study and investigator characteristics and publication.

The investigators who designed these four studies were particularly interested in clinical trials, although the populations studied were individually too small to expect reliable estimates to emerge. Publication bias was shown to exist in all four populations, although estimates of the size of the bias varied among the groups studied. Variables other than study findings (e.g., funding source, multicenter design) were also examined, but none was consistently and confidently shown to be associated with publication status. One reason for this may have been the small size of the subgroup populations examined, and this is particularly likely to be true for the analyses focussing on randomized clinical trials. This situation offered an excellent opportunity for meta-analysis.

MATERIALS AND METHODS

We have combined data from four similar investigations of publication bias in order to investigate factors that may influence publication behavior and publication bias.[8-10] Examples of factors hypothesized to be related to publication are *study characteristics,* such as funding source and funding type, multicenter design, and items thought to be related to study quality, such as use of randomization and sample size, and *author characteristics,* such as sex.

The methods used to collect the original data for each investigation are described in the primary reports of these studies. Briefly, the populations studied were as follows:

1. Studies approved in 1980 by the institutional review board for the Johns Hopkins University School of Medicine (JHU-Med)

2. Studies approved in 1980 by the institutional review board for the Johns Hopkins University School of Hygiene and Public Health (JHU-PH)

3. Clinical trials funded by the National Institutes of Health (NIH) in 1979,[11] but not including those funded by the National Cancer Institue

4. Studies approved in 1984 to 1987 by the Central Oxford Research Ethics Committee (Oxford).

The original study cohorts were followed in 1988 for JHU-Med, JHU-PH, and NIH, and in 1990 for Oxford, using telephone interviews of the principal investigators, or their surrogates, to learn of the study results, publication status and other factors associated with the studies. Only studies classified by the investigators as having completed data collection and analysis were included in our analyses.

For the meta-analysis, the original data sets created for the JHU-Med, JHU-PH, and NIH populations were used. The Oxford data were abstracted by us from the published report.[8] For the analyses restricted to clinical trials, data from only the JHU-Med, JHU-PH, and NIH populations were used since these were readily available, having been collected by the same group of investigators. Data on trials from JHU-Med and JHU-PH were combined to form the JHU population because so few trials had been performed by investigators based at the School of Hygiene and Public Health (JHU-PH).

Analyses focused initially on studies classified by the investigators as clinical trials having comparison or control groups, and subsequently on controlled trials classified as "randomized." The variables studied as possibly related to publication included: nature of results ("significant" vs. "not significant"); institutional source of original data (NIH vs. JHU); whether the study received external funding (yes vs. no); number of sites (multicenter vs. single center); sample size (≥ 100 vs.

<100); type of control group (parallel vs. other); use of randomization (yes vs. no); use of masking (yes vs. no); use of intention-to-treat analysis (yes vs. no); and sex of principal investigator (PI) (male vs. female). Findings were classified as "significant" when the investigators reported them to be "statistically significant" (in either direction) or when statistical tests were not performed, but the investigators deemed the results to be of "great importance."[9,10] "Not significant" results included those that showed a trend in either direction, but which were not statistically significant, results suggesting "no difference," and results deemed by the investigator to be of "moderate" or "little" importance when no statistical tests had been performed. NIH trials funded by the extramural route were considered to have had external funding, and those funded by the intramural route were classified as not to have had external funding.

Most analyses were performed using PC-SAS.[12] Initial analyses involved comparing the frequency distributions for each of the above variables separately for the JHU and NIH populations. Cross tabulations were made showing the relation between the study variables and publication status. Subsequent analyses were performed merging data from the two groups after a Breslow-Day test for homogeneity[13] failed to detect differences between the results obtained for the separate populations. Stratified analyses were performed to assess the effect of individual categories of variables on publication bias (the association between publication and "significant" results).

Unadjusted odds ratios and 95% confidence intervals were calculated using the Mantel-Haenszel method. When there were empty cells in the cross tabulations, 0.5 was added to each cell. The associations between publication bias and the variables of interest were assessed by Chi-square statistics and associated p values.

Adjusted odds ratios were calculated by multiple logistic regression using BMDP LR (BMDP statistical software, Los Angeles, 1990). Regression analyses used merged original data from JHU and NIH for the individual variables. The original regression model included all variables found to be significantly related to publication in the univariate analyses of the merged dataset and in the individual investigations. Missing values were imputed to the most frequent category. A backward, stepwise procedure was used to select variables that were statistically significantly associated with publication status. This process involved elimination of variables from the regression model, starting with the variable/publication association having the largest p value. The elimination process was stopped once all the remaining associations between variables and publication yielded p values of 0.05 or less.

RESULTS

A simple meta-analysis of the association between study findings ("significant" results) and publication, using data from JHU-Med, JHU-PH, NIH, and Oxford, provided a combined odds ratio of 2.88 (95% confidence interval = 2.13 to 3.90) (FIG. 1). The point estimates of the individual odds ratios associated with these four cohorts were 1.78 (95% CI 0.94 to 3.39), 3.38 (95% CI 1.93 to 5.93), 7.04 (95% CI 1.90 to 26.16), and 2.91 (95% CI 1.80 to 4.73), respectively.

Subsequent analyses, using only the Johns Hopkins and NIH populations, focused on clinical trials. Merged data are presented (TABLE 2) because, in all but one respect—sample size—JHU and NIH trials were comparable in terms of

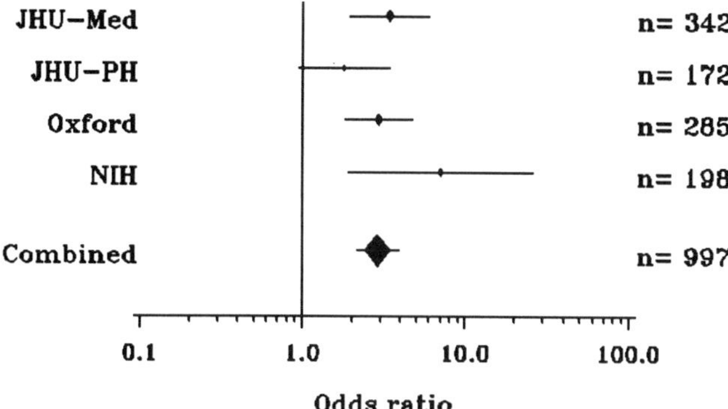

FIGURE 1. Association between significant results and publication. Unadjusted odds ratios and 95% confidence limits. (From Dickersin and Min.[10] Reprinted by permission from the *Online Journal of Current Clinical Trials.*)

study characteristics. Sample sizes greater than 100 were less common for JHU than NIH (32% versus 58%), but this is likely to reflect the way the sample size question was asked of investigators: JHU investigators affiliated with clinical sites for multicenter trials were asked to provide the sample size for the JHU site alone, while NIH investigators were asked to provide the sample size for the entire trial.

Overall, 90% of all studies classified as controlled trials were published, and almost as high a proportion were funded (87.5%) (TABLE 2). Almost half of the trials (44.3%) were multicenter. As far as study design was concerned, 83.2% were classified as "parallel," 74.6% as randomized, and 56.1% as masked. Analysis was stated to have been by "intention-to-treat" for 86.6% of the trials. Most principal investigators (91.8%) were men.

Because there were no differences observed between odds ratios calculated for the JHU and NIH populations separately, all data were merged for subsequent analyses. Despite the fact that the overwhelming majority of trials were published, there was still strong evidence of publication bias: the odds ratio (OR) for the association between "significant" results and publication was 5.96 (95% CI 2.33 to 15.22) (TABLE 3). In the univariate analyses, funding and multicenter status were the only other variables statistically significantly associated with publication status. The following variables remained in the logistic model as having a statistically significant relation to publication: significant results (OR = 6.15; 95% CI 2.24 to 16.92); funding (OR = 3.42; 95% CI 1.25 to 7.36); and use of randomization (OR = 2.84; 95% CI 1.09 to 7.36). Stratified analyses did not reveal a significant effect of any individual variable on publication bias.

Most of the time investigators stated that they did not publish their findings because the results were "not interesting" (61%) or because they "did not have the time" (7%). Other reasons were: problems with co-investigators (14%), and the desire to do additional analyses (14%). No trials remained unpublished because a submitted report had been rejected for publication.

Analyses restricted to the 200 randomized trials produced similar results (TABLE 4). Univariate analyses revealed that publication was associated only with "significant" results (OR = 8.92; 95% CI 1.96 to 40.65) and funding (OR = 3.59;

TABLE 2. Characteristics of Controlled Trials Combined in Meta-Analysis

Study Characteristics	N	Percent
Total controlled trials	280	100.0
Publication		
Yes	252	90.0
No	28	10.0
Institution		
JHU	109	38.9
NIH	171	61.1
External funding		
Yes	245	87.5
No	35	12.5
Multicenter		
Yes	124	44.3
No	156	55.7
Sample size[a]		
≥ 100	130	47.8
<100	142	52.2
Type of control		
Parallel	233	83.2
Other	47	16.8
Randomization[a]		
Yes	200	74.6
No	68	25.4
Masking[a]		
Yes	151	56.1
No	118	43.9
Intention-to-treat analysis[a]		
Yes	238	86.6
No	37	13.4
Sex of principal investigator		
Male	257	91.8
Female	23	8.2

[a] Category has missing values so does not add to 280.

95% CI 1.03 to 12.52). Stratified analyses were limited by the small numbers of studies in subgroups, but no statistically significant associations between other variables and publication bias were detected.

Because it is possible that some JHU controlled clinical trials were funded by the NIH and thus may have appeared in both datasets, we reanalyzed our data after omitting all JHU trials funded by NIH (JHU $n = 54$, NIH $n = 171$). The results were no different from those obtained using the complete dataset, except that two additional factors were positively associated with publication in the univariate analysis: institution (NIH was positively associated with publication compared to JHU), and sample size ≥ 100. After adjustment using backward stepwise logistic regression, "significant" results, use of randomization, and institution (NIH) remained positively associated with publication.

DISCUSSION

Meta-analyses using data from four prospective studies (JHU-Med, JHU-PH, NIH, and Oxford) provide strong evidence of a positive association between statistically significant results and publication (unadjusted OR = 2.88; 95% CI 2.13 to 3.90). Analyses using just controlled trials (JHU and NIH) show that this relationship is even stronger in this subset of studies (OR = 6.15; 95% CI 2.24 to 16.92), and randomized trials appear to be no different from controlled trials in general (OR = 8.72; 95% CI 1.91 to 39.81). Investigators, not referees or editors, appear to be the group responsible for failure to publish. Although the overall rate of RCT publication is slightly higher than that for other types of studies, trialists appear to be no better than others in terms of their tendency not to publish "negative" results.

There is now considerable evidence for a reporting bias throughout the various means available for reporting research results: acceptance of abstracts for presentation at meetings; subsequent full publication of studies initially presented as abstracts; full publication of initiated studies, whether first presented as abstracts or not; and reporting of published results by the lay press.

Koren *et al.*[14] examined the association between study findings and acceptance of abstracts submitted for presentation to a large scientific meeting. The authors

TABLE 3. Association of Various Study Characteristics with Publication for Controlled Trials

Study Characteristics	N	Percent Published	OR (95% C.I.)[a]
Total controlled trials	280		
Primary results			
Significant	162	96.3	5.96 (2.33–15.22)
Not significant	118	81.4	
Institution			
JHU	109	86.2	0.52 (0.24–1.13)
NIH	171	92.4	
External funding			
Yes	245	91.8	3.33 (1.34–8.30)
No	35	77.1	
Multicenter			
Yes	124	94.4	2.60 (1.07–6.34)
No	156	86.5	
Sample size[b]			
≥100	130	93.9	2.36 (0.99–5.59)
<100	142	86.6	
Type of control			
Parallel	233	91.0	1.77 (0.70–4.43)
Other	47	85.1	
Randomization[b]			
Yes	200	92.5	2.13 (0.91–4.99)
No	68	85.3	
Masking[b]			
Yes	151	89.4	0.78 (0.34–1.79)
No	118	91.5	
Intention-to-treat[b]			
Yes	238	90.8	1.90 (0.72–5.05)
No	37	83.8	
Sex of principal investigator			
Male	257	90.3	1.39 (0.39–5.02)
Female	23	87.0	

[a] 95% confidence limits by Woolf's method.
[b] Category has missing values so does not add to 280.

followed 58 abstracts describing studies that examined fetal outcome after gestational exposure to cocaine. Twenty-eight of 49 (57%) abstracts showing a positive effect were accepted, while only one of the nine (11%) abstracts showing no effect was accepted. This increased acceptance rate for abstracts describing "positive" results did not appear to be based on factors related to study quality, as the studies with "negative" results tended more often to verify cocaine use, be concerned predominantly with cocaine use, have a larger sample size, and include a control group.

TABLE 4. Association of Various Study Characteristics with Publication for Randomized Controlled Trials

Study Characteristics	N	Percent Published	OR (95% C.I.)[a]
Total randomized controlled trials	200		
Primary results			
Significant	109	98.2	8.92 (1.96–40.65)
Not significant	91	85.7	
Institution			
JHU	74	89.2	0.49 (0.17–1.40)
NIH	126	94.4	
External funding			
Yes	179	93.9	3.59 (1.03–12.52)
No	21	81.0	
Multicenter			
Yes	98	94.9	2.02 (0.67–6.14)
No	102	90.2	
Sample size[b]			
$\geq$100	106	94.3	1.85 (0.63–5.42)
$<$100	90	90.0	
Type of control			
Parallel	179	92.7	1.34 (0.28–6.41)
Other	21	90.5	
Masking[b]			
Yes	122	91.8	0.78 (0.26–2.37)
No	77	93.5	
Intention to treat analysis[b]			
Yes	176	92.1	0.55 (0.07–4.41)
No	22	95.5	
Sex of principal investigator			
Male	184	92.4	0.81 (0.10–6.59)
Female	16	93.8	

[a] 95% confidence limits by Woolf's method.
[b] Category has missing values so does not add to 200.

A number of studies have documented that even though an abstract may be accepted for presentation, the results may never be published in a full-length report.[15,16] Abstracts reporting the results of clinical trials have less than a 50% likelihood of being published in full.[15,16] Although neither the statistical significance of study findings nor study quality appear to be associated with abstracts reaching full publication, only a few studies have examined this issue.

There are now ample data, including the results presented in the current study, showing that if one follows a cohort of new and ongoing studies, those with negative findings are less likely to be published.[5] Funding by an external mechanism (such as the NIH) also appears to be positively associated with publication.

Finally, the reporting of results by the lay press is also biased: Koren and Klein[17] compared the rates of newspaper reporting for two studies published in the same 1991 issue of *JAMA:* their topics were similar, yet one had negative and one had positive results. Newspaper reports focused 10 of 19 times on both studies and 9 of 19 times on the study with positive findings. No report focused solely on the study with negative results.

Despite offering support for the existence of publication bias with respect to research studies in general and clinical trials in particular, our findings may not be generalizable to the population of all clinical trials. For example, our group of trials may have an unusually high publication rate. The trials in the JHU and NIH cohorts include a high proportion of externally funded studies (89% and 87%, respectively), and external funding has been shown to be positively associated with publication, providing support for this possibility. Evidence from follow-up studies of published abstracts, described above, also suggests that our rate may be unusually high. Lack of generalizability may also stem from the fact that the NIH cohort of trials did not include National Cancer Institute–funded trials. The JHU cohort did, however, and we have no reason to believe that cancer trials are different from other trials in terms of publication. In fact, Simes' data[6] showed a publication bias for ovarian cancer trials.

All in all, the high rate of publication we have observed, despite the existence of publication bias, is reassuring. If our publication rate were generalizable, the potential problem of publication bias might be very small.

Our analyses for the association between sample size and publication are compromised by the fact that investigators were asked the question on sample size in different ways. JHU multicenter trials for which there was a clinical center at JHU were asked to report the sample size at that center alone, rather than for the trial as a whole, because it was felt that the JHU investigators would often not know the sample size for the entire study. A Chi-square test for homogeneity, in fact, identified this variable as one that was different between the JHU and NIH cohorts.

Where do we go with the information gained from this study and others? Because the results of research in this field have been so consistent, it is probably safe to conclude that publication bias is real and widespread. Publication of trials appears to be related to being externally funded and multicenter, but not to other study variables examined. The lack of a statistically significant relationship with certain other variables (e.g., sample size ≥ 100, use of randomization) may be due to a lack of statistical power to detect a relationship that truly exists.

The results of clinical trials, and randomized clinical trials, in particular, should not be suppressed in this way. A few of us could continue, in speeches and editorials, to implore investigators to publish their results, to urge funding agencies and institutional review boards to require publication of study findings, and to encourage editors to let investigators know that publication decisions will be based on study quality, not on study findings. But these approaches seem unlikely to achieve the changes that are needed.

Another possibility is to require registration of all clinical trials prior to initiation. While this is widely agreed to be a good approach,[6,15,18–21] widespread registration has not yet been effected. There are encouraging signs of moves in this direction, however:

• An International Collaborative Group for Clinical Trials Registries has met annually for several years.[22] The group has agreed on a recommended "core content" of information to be kept on trials registries, and has helped to establish a "register of registers" of clinical trials. Members of the group have provided support to new registries getting started and are currently developing an "operating manual" for registry keepers.

- The National Institutes of Health, Office of Medical Applications of Research, is planning to sponsor a December 1993 conference that focuses on the issue of trial registration (John Ferguson, personal communication to K.D., 1993).

- *The Online Journal of Current Clinical Trials* is an entirely electronic publication, sponsored by the American Association for the Advancement of Science and edited by Dr. Edward Huth.[23] Because it is computer- and not paper-based, it has no page limitations. Its commitment is to publish the results of studies of good quality, regardless of the direction or nature of the results. This may encourage investigators to write up their "negative" or "null" results and submit them for publication.

The identification of planned and ongoing trials will be a continuing challenge until registration is required of investigators. The National Institutes of Health can effect registration of the trials it funds, which will account for a significant proportion of large trials conducted in the United States. Currently, there is no way to assure registration of trials funded by pharmaceutical firms in the U.S., although all must pass through institutional review boards (IRBs) prior to enrolling patients. IRBs would thus prove the best means in the U.S. of identifying clinical trials at inception. Spain already has such a system in place, requiring that drug trials be registered with the Ministry of Drug Evaluation.[24]

Who will take the lead? Individuals should not try to take on the task of trial registration, especially without promise of funding or future support. For one thing, it is unlikely that other investigators or industry would respond positively to approaches that do not carry the imprimatur of a government or regulatory agency. The lead is being taken by government groups in the United Kingdom and Europe. The Project Register being established as part of the Information Systems Strategy created to support the National Health Service Research and Development Programme in the U.K. is an example of the kind of initiative that will be required (J. Ennis, personal communication, 1993). We are encouraged by signs that the National Institutes of Health may also be moving to take some action.

It has been suggested elsewhere[21] that underreporting research is scientific misconduct. If those conducting reviews of evidence about the effects of health care do not have available for consideration all relevant evidence related to a given treatment, the possibility exists that the conclusions they reach regarding safety and efficacy will be wrong. The Cochrane Collaboration, which includes an international effort to identify all published trials, is currently ongoing and should assist with identification of trials conducted and published in the past.[19] Registers of ongoing and completed unpublished trials are less well developed, however, and their absence threatens the process of a systematic review. Thus, the current efforts on the part of the biomedical community to conduct more scientific research and reviews, and thereby to do more good than harm, may be frustrated by publication bias and other selective publishing practices.

SUMMARY

Conclusions about the efficacy and safety of medical interventions are based on data presented in the scientific literature. The validity of these conclusions is threatened if publication bias results from investigators or editors making decisions about publishing study results on the basis of the direction or strength of the study findings. This paper reports meta-analyses performed using data from four prospective investigations in which a total of 997 initiated studies were followed to learn of study results, publication status, and reasons for nonpublication. The analysis indicates that there is a positive association between "significant" study results and publication (OR = 2.88; 95% confidence interval [CI] 2.13 to 3.90). When the analysis was restricted to controlled trials (n = 280), an even stronger relationship between "significant" results and publication was observed (OR = 6.15; 95% CI 2.24 to 16.92), with randomized trials (n = 200) apparently no less susceptible to publication bias than controlled trials in general (OR = 8.72; 95% CI 1.91 to 39.81). In every case, failure to publish was investigator-based, and not due to editorial decisions. The results of clinical trials should not be suppressed in this way. Development of registration systems for randomized trials is essential if this problem is to be minimized in future.

ACKNOWLEDGMENT

We thank Iain Chalmers for his helpful criticism of the manuscript.

REFERENCES

1. HALL, M. B. 1965. Robert Boyle on Natural Philosophy.: 121. Indiana University Press. Bloomington, IN.
2. ANON. 1909. The reporting of unsuccessful cases [editorial]. Boston Med. Surg. J: 263–264.
3. STERLING, T. D. 1959. Publication decisions and their possible effects on inferences drawn from tests of significance—or vice versa. J. Am. Stat. Assoc. **54:** 30–34.
4. BEGG, C. B. & J. A. BERLIN. 1988. Publication bias: A problem in interpreting medical data. J. Roy. Stat. Soc. A **151:** 419–463.
5. DICKERSIN, K. 1990. The existence of publication bias and risk factors for its occurrence. JAMA **263:** 1401–1405.
6. SIMES, R. J. 1986. Publication bias: The case for an international registry of clinical trials. J. Clin. Oncol. **4:** 1529–1541.
7. DICKERSIN, K., S. CHAN, T. C. CHALMERS, H. S. SACKS & H. SMITH, JR. 1987. Publication bias and clinical trials. Controlled Clin. Trials **8:** 343–353.
8. EASTERBROOK, P., J. A. BERLIN, R. GOPALAN & D. R. MATTHEWS. 1991. Publication bias in clinical research. Lancet **337:** 867–872.
9. DICKERSIN, K., Y. I. MIN & C. L. MEINERT. 1992. Factors influencing publication of research results: follow-up of applications submitted to two institutional review boards. JAMA **267:** 374–378.
10. DICKERSIN, K. & Y. I. MIN. 1993. NIH clinical trials and publication bias [article]. Online J. Curr. Clin. Trials [serial online] 1993 Apr 28; (Doc No 50): [4967 words; 53 paragraphs]. 1 figure; 3 tables.
11. NATIONAL INSTITUTES OF HEALTH. 1979. National Institutes of Health Inventory of Clinical Trials for FY79. Form NIH-2241 (Rev 10-79). Bethesda, MD, OMB No. 68-R1492.
12. PC-SAS [computer program] Release 6.04. 1986. SAS Institute, Inc. Cary, NC.
13. BRESLOW, N. E. & N. E. DAY. 1980. Statistical methods in cancer research I: The analysis of case-control studies. International Agency for Research in Cancer Scientific Publication **32:** 192–246. Lyon, France.
14. KOREN, G., H. SHEAR, K. GRAHAM & T. EINARSON. 1989. Bias against the null hypothesis: The reproductive hazards of cocaine. Lancet **ii:** 1440–1442.
15. CHALMERS, I., W. TARNOW-MORDI, J. HETHERINGTON, C. L. MEINERT, S. TONASCIA,

K. DICKERSIN, T. C. CHALMERS & M. ADAMS. 1990. A cohort study of summary reports of controlled trials. JAMA **263:** 1401–1405.

16. SCHERER, R. & K. DICKERSIN. 1993. Full publication of results initially reported in abstracts. Presented at the Second International Congress on Peer Review, September 10, 1993, Chicago, Illinois. Unpublished manuscript.

17. KOREN, G. 1991. Bias against negative studies in newspaper reports of medical research. JAMA **266:** 1824–1826.

18. MEINERT, C. L. 1988. Toward prospective registration of clinical trials. Controlled Clin. Trials **9:** 1–5.

19. PIANTADOSI, S. & D. BYAR. 1988. A proposal for registering clinical trials. Controlled Clin. Trials **9:** 82–84.

20. DICKERSIN, K. 1988. Report from the Panel on the Case for Register of Clinical Trials at the Eighth Annual Meeting of the Society for Clinical Trials. Controlled Clin. Trials **9:** 76–81.

21. CHALMERS, I. 1990. Under-reporting research is scientific misconduct. JAMA **263:** 1405–1408.

22. CHALMERS, I., K. DICKERSIN & T. C. CHALMERS. 1992. Getting to grips with Archie Cochrane's agenda. Br. Med. J. **305:** 786–788.

23. ANON. 1991. Making clinical trialists register. Lancet **338:** 244–245.

24. PALCA, J. 1991. New journal will publish without paper (News). Science **253:** 1480.

25. DICKERSIN, K. & F. GARCIA-LOPEZ. 1992. Regulatory process effects clinical trial registration in Spain. Controlled Clin. Trials **13:** 507–512.

DISCUSSION

MICHELE ORZA (*U.S. General Accounting Office, Washington, D.C.*): Your funding variable is interesting, and the implication about funding from something like a pharmaceutical house is fairly obvious. But what about other fields where the funding source actually has an overriding interest in seeing the negative studies come out? For example, in areas like tobacco smoking or in electromagnetic fields, where the primary funding comes from industry, the funders are obviously interested in making sure that the negative studies are published. I wonder if that's another aspect of publication bias—but one in favor of negative results rather than positive results.

KAY DICKERSIN: (*University of Maryland School of Medicine, Baltimore, Md.*): That's a good point. We found in our studies that the size of the association between significant results and publication was the same for industry-supported and other studies, implying no difference in publication bias. However, studies funded by industry tended to be published much less often than other studies. In terms of the negative bias, I've heard suggestions along those lines before, but have never seen any data.

JEROLD LUCEY (*National Research and Technology Assessment, Burlington, Vt.*): As the editor of *Pediatrics* I want to thank you for exonerating some editors, saying we're not the cause of bias, but you couldn't resist a little dig later on when you said we should not reject papers with negative results. In my 20 years of editing a journal I can't ever remember rejecting a paper just because it showed negative results. The commonest cause of rejection is serious methodologic flaws and the reviewer's comment usually is this paper should never be published or something like that. There must be some studies that are simply seriously flawed and should not be published, but you seem dedicated to resurrecting these studies and ignoring the fact that they have been judged by some of their peers to have been terrible.

DICKERSIN: We tried to look at some variables in our studies that might be thought to be associated with study quality and these factors did not seem to be associated in our studies with publication. What I was trying to say was that *quality* and not results should be what's looked at by journal editors. We have all seen papers published on new treatments that have just involved a few patients but showed striking results. I was thinking more in terms of that with respect to the responsibility of the editors.

LUCEY: The other area I'd like you to comment on is studies done by drug companies. These companies abort many of the trials that they launch and I wonder whether they are judged to be headed in the wrong direction and are aborted for commercial reasons. Do you have any feeling on that?

DICKERSIN: No, I don't, although that's part of the problem with the NCI trials. We didn't include them because they change very quickly; for example, what they call a single protocol may be a shift from a certain chemotherapy cocktail to another because one isn't producing the desired results or something new comes along.

KENT JOHNSON (*Federal Drug Administration, Rockville, Md.*): Given those two major factors and the inability to really be able to quantitate those, do you think the p value used to indicate significance in a meta-analysis should be ratcheted down from 0.05 and made tougher? Since we have a convention for a single trial and eventually we're going to probably come to an implicit consensus anyway about a test for significance for meta-analyses, what do you think that test should be given the fact that you have these major biases?

DICKERSIN: I don't know.

JOHN CLARKE (*Medical College of Pennsylvania, Philadelphia, Pa.*): I wonder whether the publication bias might not just be an anomaly of the difficulty of proving a negative result or no difference versus a positive result. If I have a hundred patients and I can show a difference, then I can be fairly confident at publishing at 100, but if I don't show any difference in order to really be secure that there is in fact no difference, I've got to extend that study to maybe 1,000 patients, and if funding or time gets in the way, then I may abandon the project because it must become a bigger project if I'm trying to show no significance.

DICKERSIN: The analyses that we did tried to take that idea into account. First, the reasons that some investigators gave for not publishing were that they didn't think it was a very good study at the end, perhaps because the group of patients was too small. We also did stratified analyses where we looked at publication bias, that is, the association between significant results and publication by sample size and we didn't see any difference. So it doesn't look like that's what is happening there.

RICHARD DOLL (*Imperial Cancer Research Fund, Oxford, U.K.*): May I make a proposal that we abolish the term "statistically significant" and never use it again—that we just give p values and enable people to attach what importance they think is appropriate to that value.

DICKERSIN: That sounds good to me. This is always a terrible group of studies to report because I'm using "statistically significant" as a study variable and then also talking about the results of the study itself. I'd be happy to dump it.

ARGYE HILLIS (*Scott & White Hospital, Temple, Texas*): In all diffidence and humility I would suggest we commend that suggestion and just use confidence intervals instead of p values.

RICHARD PETO (*University of Oxford, Oxford, U.K.*): What are they going to be—95%, 99.9%? You're going back to exactly the same thing. I was actually quite encouraged, Dr. Dickersin, by the lack of publication bias. If you actually take the randomized trials, you've got 7.5% of them unpublished and those were the smaller ones. That means you've got more than 95% of the studies of randomized patients published, which actually says that as far as the randomized trials were concerned, if the group of trials that you've looked at were representative, which you say it isn't, then actually you've shown that if there is a problem it is fairly trivial as far as adding up the trials and seeing what the grand total looks like.

Someone else asked about industry-funded trials. I think there are quite a lot of trials that have been done, but are not turning up. The FDA is now demanding that those studies are also made available, and industry is actually trying to comply with that when they try to add their cases into registration. So I think, Dr. Dickersin, that you should be emphasizing that as far as randomized evidence is concerned in this particular group of studies there really isn't any big problem. More then 95% of the randomized patients finish up as part of published studies. You're putting it the wrong way around for this group of studies.

DICKERSIN: I think that you're right, at least in terms of this group of studies. Most of them were published, which is pretty encouraging. But if we're talking about a possible selection bias in the data collection methods used for meta-analysis, then I would say that this is one element where we might have some concern. It doesn't mean that it is the biggest problem there is with meta-analysis.

Collaborative Worldwide Overviews of Randomized Trials

PETER SANDERCOCK

Department of Clinical Neurosciences
Western General Hospital
Edinburgh, Scotland EH4 2XU

INTRODUCTION

Formal overviews, or meta-analyses, are often used to derive an estimate of treatment effect from a collection of randomized trials which have addressed a broadly similar therapeutic question. Because the statistical methods involved in such overviews are relatively simple, clinicians may be tempted to assemble the publications from a few well known trials, extract the key data from the published reports, and perform a statistical analysis. If only a few trials (or perhaps only a few tens of trials) are available for review, such overviews are within the capabilities of a single person or a few individuals working in a single department. However, a formal review of all the published and unpublished literature may often be a daunting task indeed. There have been several thousand publications relating to clinical studies of antiplatelet agents in man over the past forty years, and well over 400 randomized trials have been identified by the Antiplatelet Trialists' Collaboration.[1,2] Other forms of therapy to treat or prevent vascular disease are also associated with very large amounts of randomized trial data (for example, fibrinolytic therapy for acute myocardial infarction, cholesterol reduction, and antihypertensive therapy). There are large numbers of trials relating to the treatment of early breast cancer, colorectal cancer, advanced ovarian cancer, and leukemia. As a means of reviewing these large bodies of data, several international collaborative review groups have been established. In this article I will mainly deal with the Antiplatelet Trialists' Collaboration[1,2] and the Early Breast Cancer Trialists' Collaborative Group.[3]

WHY SYSTEMATIC OVERVIEWS?

It is hard to quantify a clinician's sense of "information overload" when faced with 50 randomized controlled trials all addressing the same subject. So, at the simplest level, clinicians find overviews helpful since they provide a succinct summary of a huge mass of trial data (within which individual trials may have results that, at first glance, seem to conflict with each other). The main statistical reason for undertaking systematic overviews is to derive an estimate of treatment effect that is as free as possible from bias (by avoiding undue data-dependent emphasis on particular trials), and has least random error by including a larger number of events.

DISADVANTAGES OF SIMPLE OVERVIEWS

Overviews can operate at several levels. At the lowest level, a few publications which relate to randomized trials of a particular treatment in a particular category of patient are assembled. After some efforts, a number of published studies are assembled, and summary data (for example, the number of deaths in each treatment group) are then extracted from each publication for statistical analysis. The analyses that can be performed on such data are limited. Any one of a number of different statistical techniques can be used to derive an estimate of treatment effect (for instance, the reduction in mortality). When the analyses are complete, a report may then be published in the name of one or two authors, but not generally in the name of the trialists who undertook the original studies being reviewed. Such relatively simple overviews have many attractions: they are quick, cheap, and do not require much in the way of rigorous data checking, complex statistical analysis, or expensive data handling.

However, there are some drawbacks: publications of randomized controlled trials regrettably do not appear in an exactly standardized format, so not all data items are available for all trials; some trials may not report detailed information on all of the patients excluded after randomization and may not give detailed tabulations of the numbers of events in each treatment group by allocated treatment (thus making an "intention-to-treat analysis" impossible). An additional problem is incomplete follow-up. In several trials in vascular disease, follow-up ceased in patients who had a non-fatal event, which thereby prevented a complete (and unbiased) analysis of the effects of treatment on mortality.

Simple overviews generally do not include unpublished trials (often because of worries that the study report has not been submitted to peer review by an independent journal referee) even though the trial may have been conducted to high methodologic standards. Failure to include unpublished results may bias the estimates of treatment effect.

A major disadvantage of simple analyses of summary data is the difficulty of undertaking survival analyses over several years. For example, an analysis at a fixed point in time, say two years after randomization, might obscure the fact that some treatment benefits become increasingly obvious with longer-term follow-up. A good example is found in the trials of ovarian ablation in women with breast cancer. The benefits from ovarian ablation became greatest between years 5 and 10,[3] but these benefits only emerged from an international collaborative overview which utilized individual patient data from each trial. In the case of the trials of antiplatelet therapy in patients at high risk of vascular events, where mean duration of follow-up was one or two years, it is important to know whether any early benefits are maintained over the long term.

In many trials (both in cancer and in vascular disease), it is important to look at the effect of treatment in particular categories of patient (males and females, old and young, pre- and postmenopausal, diabetic and nondiabetic, etc.), yet trialists may not report their data in a form that allow such subgroup analyses.

GENERAL FEATURES COMMON TO A LARGE INTERNATIONAL COLLABORATIVE OVERVIEW GROUP

Forming a Collaborative Group

Most overview groups have been founded because trialists recognized that there was a huge mass of data from randomized trials which all addressed approximately the same therapeutic question. The main international overview groups are concerned with common diseases (cancer and vascular disease) and simple widely practicable treatments (antiplatelet therapy, adjuvant therapy for breast cancer, cholesterol reduction by drugs). When the principal investigators of similar trials recognize that the trials address the same question, there is usually little difficulty in obtaining agreement that a formal overview of all of the data should be undertaken.

Holding a Meeting of the Trialists

In 1986, the principal investigators of the major trials of antiplatelet therapy met in Oxford to review the data from 25 trials (which had recruited some 29,000 patients) of antiplatelet therapy in patients with recent myocardial infarction, recent transient ischemic attack (TIA), stroke, or unstable angina. During the preparations for the meeting, it rapidly became evident that there existed perhaps one or two hundred additional trials of antiplatelet therapy in patients with other forms of symptomatic vascular disease (stable angina, intermittent claudication, and patients undergoing a variety of vascular surgical procedures).

Furthermore, it appeared that there were at least fifty randomized trials of antiplatelet therapy in the prevention of deep vein thrombosis. At the meeting, the group decided to constitute itself formally as the Antiplatelet Trialists' Collaboration, and undertook to publish a formal overview of the 25 trials of antiplatelet therapy in patients with recent myocardial infarction, unstable angina, TIA, or ischemic stroke. One important feature of the meeting was that a major study of antiplatelet therapy in survivors of myocardial infarction was identified that had been undertaken in East Berlin, a study which had not previously been widely reported (it had appeared in published form only once, in a book of conference proceedings). The meeting also provided a very useful forum for comment and discussion on the principal findings of the initial overview, and these comments were incorporated into the group's first report. The draft report was then circulated to all members for further comment and the final version was published two years later in 1988.[1] At the first meeting, the group also decided that the collaboration should be broadened to include the trials in other categories of patients and should also include a review of the randomized trials of antiplatelet therapy in the prevention of deep venous thrombosis. The Clinical Trials Service Unit and the Neurosciences Trials Unit in Edinburgh agreed to coordinate this overview. It was agreed that any publications would be in the name of the group as a whole and not in the names of any one individual or in the names of those in the secretariats. By March 1990, more than 400 studies had been identified. On closer review, some trials were either still being planned or were in progress, some were not truly randomized, and others measured only laboratory parameters (and did not study clinical events).

Obtaining Individual Patient Data

Where possible, trialists were asked to provide a few items of data on every patient randomized. The data which were sought included: identifier, data of birth, gender, allocated treatment, date of randomization, essential baseline data, and occurrence of major events during follow-up (with dates). These data were provided in whichever form was most convenient for the trialists and were collated and checked by the statistical and clinical secretariats (in Oxford and Edinburgh, respectively). Data were checked for internal consistency and were also checked against any published reports. The process often involved extensive correspondence with the trialists. Data errors and inconsistencies—which had not previously been identified by the trialists—were discovered and clarified by this meticulous process. Appropriate analyses of prespecified subgroups and analyses of survival were undertaken. These analyses revealed further errors and inconsistencies, which were then corrected. The analyses were presented at a second meeting in 1990 of the group (now much enlarged), which included more than 100 trialists from around the world. Extensive discussions were held and comments noted. Further trials were identified at the meeting and further analyses suggested, and the secretariat incorporated these comments when preparing the manuscripts. With such a very large volume of data, data checking has been extensive and the final publications will appear in print shortly.[2] A further meeting of the group is provisionally planned for 1995. The analyses presented at their meeting will be updated to include all trials completed between 1990 and 1994, and will include analyses of trials of antiplatelet therapy in acute ischemic stroke (two large trials, each planning to randomize a few tens of thousands of patients, should be completed by then).

WHAT ARE THE BENEFITS OF INTERNATIONAL COLLABORATIVE OVERVIEWS (AS OPPOSED TO SIMPLE SINGLE-CENTER OVERVIEWS) AND ARE THEY WORTH THE EFFORT?

The benefits of international collaboration may be listed as follows:

1. Clear evidence of benefit emerges that would not have been apparent from less-detailed reviews. The analyses made possible by the different overview groups have demonstrated that, for some treatments, a much wider variety of patients can be offered effective therapy than was previously recognized. Similarly, for other forms of therapy, evidence emerged that fewer patients should be exposed to the treatments which had proved more hazardous or less beneficial than was previously thought. It is worth emphasizing that such clear evidence of these benefits would not have emerged from "lower-level" overviews, and could have only emerged from the detailed analysis of individual patient data.

2. All the relevant trials are more completely ascertained. International collaborative overview groups are much more likely to identify most, if not all, the relevant trials. Experience with the Antiplatelet Trialists' Collaboration and with the Breast Cancer Trialists shows that some very large trials can remain unknown to a wider community of trialists. It is absolutely crucial that such trials are identified and included in the overview.

3. Collaborative reviews promote data donation. Trialists are much more likely to contribute their data to a collaborative overview which will be published in all of their names jointly than to an overview where particular individuals will receive credit and the contributing trialists do not receive due recognition.

4. Collaborators' meetings help develop consensus (where appropriate) and define research priorities. The meetings of the trialists' groups are an important component of the overview process since they provide a forum at which one can achieve consensus on the issues where the trial data provides proof beyond all reasonable doubt about particular therapeutic questions. Equally, such meetings provide a unique forum at which new areas of uncertainty can be more clearly defined, and thereby allow priorities for future research to be determined.

5. Results are disseminated more quickly and widely. Overview groups comprise the principal investigators of all the major trials, persons who are important figures within the research community in their own country. Consequently, the participants in such meetings provide a well-informed nucleus from which the results can be particularly widely and rapidly disseminated.

6. Data quality are better and there is more flexibility of analysis. Simple overviews using summary tabulations of data extracted from publications which have been submitted only to peer review by a journal reviewer are based on data that may still contain some important errors. A statistical referee, when assessing an article reporting a randomized trial, has only limited information by which to judge the quality of the data. Summary tabulations and a selection of statistical tests may be presented, but these do not allow the original data to be reviewed in detail. International collaborative overviews, where individual patient data are available for review can (and do) check (1) the internal consistency of the data, (2) whether there are any errors not noted by the trialist, and (3) for any evidence of systematic differences between treatment groups (e.g., for improprieties of randomization).

Such checks are simply not possible on tabular data in a manuscript. Access to individual patient data allows substantially greater flexibility in analysis, for example, in analyses of subgroups; short- and long-term survival; survival, censoring different events; and of different clusters of events. These (and other analyses) are all feasible when the original individual patient data are available.

7. Data archiving is provided. Finally, an international overview group also provides an absolutely essential archive of the original trial data. Trialists may not have the space to store their data and may therefore be under pressure to destroy it or get rid of it (this has certainly happened to some of the old Antiplatelet Trials). Trialists themselves get old, get tired of trials, and eventually die. If their data are not archived at some central resource, they may be lost for future overview analyses.

CONCLUSIONS

International collaborative overviews are needed when a simple, widely practicable treatment for a disease of major public health impact has been tested by a large number of similar randomized controlled trials.

At first sight, international collaborative overviews may seem expensive and time-consuming, but the marginal costs involved are small in comparison to the money, time and effort involved in undertaking the original trials, and trivial in comparison to the overall expenditure on health care for the diseases in question. Policymakers will always seek to maximize the public health impact of different forms of therapy and to achieve greatest impact at the lowest cost. In this context, clinical trials and collaborative overviews of trials are an extremely cost-effective investment, giving clear guidance not only for current health policies, but also for future research priorities.

SUMMARY

Formal overviews (or meta-analyses) are now widely accepted as the most reliable way to evaluate the evidence from several randomized controlled trials that have all assessed a particular form of therapy. If a limited amount of trial data has accumulated, overviews can be undertaken at a relatively simple level, assembling just summary data extracted from published reports. Such overviews are likely to be incomplete and biased and may (because of the restricted number of analyses that are possible) not answer all the clinically important questions that might be addressed. Where a particularly large body of data from randomized trials has accumulated, more thorough and detailed overview analyses are needed. Such detailed reviews are greatly facilitated if a collaborative group of all the trialists is formed. Such groups have sought to collate individual patient data (a very few key items for every patient randomized). A central statistical secretariat then coordinates the process of data collection, checking, and analysis. Analyses are presented to the whole group for discussion and final reports are published in the name of the whole group. Experience from two very large groups that have followed this model, the Antiplatelet Trialists' Collaboration and the Early Breast Cancer Trialists' Collaborative Group, has shown that detailed collaborative overviews have many benefits: the results are particularly clear and therefore have substantial public health impact; the areas of statistical and medical agreement on the evidence can be defined; the areas of uncertainty (and hence future research priorities) are clarified; and the group can disseminate the results particularly widely and rapidly.

REFERENCES

1. ANTIPLATELET TRIALISTS' COLLABORATION. 1988. Br. Med. J. **296:** 320–331.
2. ANTIPLATELET TRIALISTS' COLLABORATION. Collaborative overview of randomized trials of antiplatelet treatment. Part I. Prevention of death, myocardial infarction and stroke by prolonged antiplatelet therapy in various categories of patient; Part II. Maintenance of vascular graft or arterial patency by antiplatelet therapy; Part III. Reduction in pulmonary embolism and venous thrombosis by antiplatelet prophylaxis among surgical and medical patients. Br. Med. J. In press.
3. EARLY BREAST CANCER TRIALISTS' COLLABORATIVE GROUP. 1992. Lancet **339:** 1–15, 71–85.

DISCUSSION

THOMAS CHALMERS (*New England Medical Center, Boston, Mass.*): Except for the plans for the international stroke study, Dr. Sandercock, you have not mentioned the possible increased efficacy of combining antiplatelet and anticoagulant drugs and the potential for increased toxicity. Your registry of such collaborative trials might have some data along that very important line since both anticoagulant and antiplatelet drugs seem to work in a number of situations. We'd all like to know whether these drugs work better in combination. Also, it's unfair to attribute the increased cost of $10 million of the American study to the fact that it was done in America, when in fact you're comparing an anticoagulant study with an antiplatelet study. Presumably in the anticoagulant study there is the cost of measuring the effect of the drug by the prothrombin time or clotting time, whereas in the antiplatelet drugs the measurement of effects is so complex that they're never included in trials.

Peter Sandercock (*Western General Hospital, Edinburgh, Scotland*): Yes, the comparison is not entirely fair. I only mentioned it to show that $10 million is being spent on a trial that won't produce a clear mortality result—it's just not the way to go. In fact, the International Stroke Trial is testing both antiplatelets and anticoagulants simultaneously in a factorial design, which will yield the only serious data so far on anticoagulants in acute stroke. Thus far, a review of the evidence on anticoagulants in acute stroke amounts to 10 trials with 1,000 patients and 173 deaths—these are not serious data.

Brian Haynes (*McMaster University, Hamilton, Ontario, Canada*): The work that you're doing in collaborative overviews, Dr. Sandercock, is very important. Along the lines of what Tom Chalmers said, I'd like to put in a plea for big expensive trials, whether they're done in North America or anywhere else, because the work you're doing on subgroups is hampered by the limited amount of data that you're collecting in these streamlined trials. For example, in the area of stroke, in terms of planning health services, it's important to know the extent of functional impairment of patients and the amount of disability, and you can't get that information if you don't have the data.

Also, you need to look a bit further into cost comparisons because in the streamlined trials the actual expenses of the trial are basically distributed to the investigators in the field. I'm not arguing against that approach, but it's a different way of accounting for who's paying for the work to be done. Many trials in North America are unnecessarily burdened by superfluous data collection and they are far too expensive for the things that they do. They then lack focus and we've been responsible for contributing that superfluity in some of our trials. Partly this is because of the ethos of the peer review committees that insist that the trial be encumbered with their questions. I don't think that the analysis that you're presenting is a fair one for the benefits and costs of the trials that are done.

Sandercock: We must reduce the amount of work that must be done in a particular trial. The reason that the International Stroke Trial (IST) is cheap is because there is almost no work involved. Follow-up is central and there's just one form to complete at 2 weeks. As far as subgroups and disability is concerned we've addressed both of those issues in the stroke trial, first by measuring disability and functional outcome and the completeness of recovery at 6 months so we will have functional outcome data. It is not just a mortality trial. And the second thing is that in terms of subgroups—that is, who benefits—we've identified different categories of patients who will be easily clinically identifiable so that the IST will provide clear evidence, not just on whether antithrombotic treatment saves lives, but also whether it improves functional outcome in survivors and for what categories of stroke patients. So simple trials can be done, provided you reduce the work for the collaborators, and they can be done to provide evidence on who benefits.

The Cochrane Collaboration: Preparing, Maintaining, and Disseminating Systematic Reviews of the Effects of Health Care

IAIN CHALMERS

The UK Cochrane Centre
NHS R&D Programme
Summertown Pavilion
Middle Way
Oxford OX2 7LG, England

WHO WAS ARCHIE COCHRANE?

Archie Cochrane is best known for his influential book, *Effectiveness and Efficiency: Random Reflections on Health Services,*[1] published in 1972. The principles he set out in it so clearly were straightforward: he suggested that, because resources would always be limited, they should be used to provide *equitably* those forms of health care which had been shown in properly designed evaluations to be *effective*. In particular, he stressed the importance of using evidence from randomized controlled trials (RCTs) because these were likely to provide much more reliable information than other sources of evidence. Cochrane's simple propositions were soon widely recognized as seminally important—by lay people as well as by health professionals.

Although Cochrane's ideas have received increasingly explicit support from a wide range of commentators, progress in applying his principles in practice has been very slow. In part, this reflects the fact that strong evidence about the effects of health care often threatens a variety of vested interests. A more basic problem, however, is that valid evidence about the effects of health care, even though it may have been published, is not readily accessible to those who wish to use it in making decisions.

THE NEED FOR MORE RELIABLE REVIEWS OF RESEARCH EVIDENCE

It is unreasonable to expect people such as clinicians, policymakers, or patients who want reliable information about the effects of health care to unearth all the relevant evidence from reports of original research. These are far too numerous and too dispersed to be of practical use. Most people must rely on reviews of the primary research as a way of coping with the information overload confronting them. Reviews thus occupy a key position in the chain that should link the results of research at one end to improved outcomes of health care at the other.

Unfortunately, the quality of reviews in the past has left much to be desired. This is because most reviewers have not approached their task systematically, with a respect for scientific principles.[2] For example, most textbook and journal reviews of evidence about the care of patients with myocardial infarction have not reflected the strong evidence that has emerged in systematic reviews of the relevant RCTs.[3] As a result, advice on some life-saving therapies has been delayed for more than a decade, while other treatments have continued to be recommended long after controlled research has shown them to be either ineffective or actually harmful.

Cochrane recognized that people who wanted to take more informed decisions in health care did not have ready access to reliable evidence. In 1979, he wrote: "It is surely a great criticism of our profession that we have not organised a critical summary, by specialty or subspecialty, adapted periodically, of all relevant randomized controlled trials."[4]

SYSTEMATIC, UP-TO-DATE REVIEWS OF RCTs OF HEALTH CARE

During the 1980s, health professionals began to respond to Cochrane's criticisms. International collaborative efforts to review the results of RCTs of treatments for breast cancer[5,6] and ovarian cancer,[7] for example, and systematic reviews of trials assessing the effects of antiplatelet drugs on coronary artery disease and stroke,[8,9] have provided very important information for guiding treatment and future research. Further, these particular systematic reviews remain yardsticks against which the quality of other reviews continues to be judged. In addition, international collaboration has led to the preparation of systematic reviews of all of the RCTs relevant to the care of women during pregnancy and childbirth,[10] and of newborn infants.[11]

Cochrane lived long enough to appreciate these developments. In 1987, the year before he died, he referred to the systematic review of RCTs of care during pregnancy and childbirth as "a real milestone in the history of randomized trials and in the evaluation of care," and suggested that other specialties should copy the methods used.[12]

As Cochrane emphasized, systematic reviews of RCTs must be kept up to date to take account of new evidence. If this is not done, important effects of health care (good and bad) will not be identified promptly, and people using the health services will be ill-served as a result. In addition, without systematic, up-to-date reviews of previous research, plans for new research will not be well-informed. As a result, researchers and funding bodies will miss promising leads, and embark on studies asking questions that have already been answered.

Arrangements already exist for updating collaborative reviews of RCTs in several areas of cancer and cardiovascular disease. Similarly, reviews of RCTs in pregnancy and childbirth have also been maintained and extended as new evidence has become available. Updated analyses have usually been published using traditional media (journals, books, drug bulletins, etc.), and they will continue to be published in these ways in future. Electronic media, however, offer a particularly appropriate means of modifying and disseminating systematic reviews of RCTs as new evidence accrues, as has been demonstrated with electronically published reviews of RCTs of care in pregnancy and childbirth.[13]

THE COCHRANE COLLABORATION

The Cochrane Collaboration has developed in response to Cochrane's call for systematic, up-to-date reviews of all relevant RCTs of health care. His hope that the methods used to prepare and maintain systematic reviews of RCTs in pregnancy and childbirth would be adopted and developed by other specialties was reflected in the decision to establish a center named after him, as part of the new Research and Development Programme established to support the National Health Service in the United Kingdom. In the months after the opening of the center at the end of 1992, people all over the world expressed strong support for its aims. The concept and the reality of the Cochrane Collaboration has thus emerged naturally as a result of this support for Cochrane's ideas.

The task of the Cochrane Collaboration is to prepare, maintain, and disseminate systematic, up-to-date reviews of RCTs of health care, and, when RCTs are not available, reviews of the most reliable evidence from other sources. Although a massive effort is required to build, maintain, and disseminate the database of systematic reviews of health care which Cochrane envisaged, it has become clear that the collaborative spirit required to make efficient progress already exists. A willingness to collaborate with others is a fundamental prerequisite for coming to grips with Cochrane's agenda, and individuals and institutions contributing to the Collaboration are clear about this. Thus, although the names of those contributing to the Collaboration are made clear in its electronically published output, the Cochrane Collaboration itself belongs to all of the contributors, collectively.

As with any new field of activity, experience of preparing and updating systematic reviews on the scale needed remains limited. Further, the time required to prepare valid reviews is often grossly underestimated. Lack of experience and time often forces good scientists to produce scientifically inadequate reviews. The key to the success of the Collaboration is thus to find means of harnessing the specific interests and enthusiasm of individuals who support the overall objectives of the Collaboration, and to find ways of providing the support of various kinds which they need to prepare and maintain systematic reviews.

Although the Cochrane Collaboration is still at an early stage of its development, its basic structure and methods of working have been established. Each **reviewer** is a member of a **collaborative review group,** which consists of individuals sharing an interest in a particular topic (stroke, for example). Collaborative review groups have often grown out of an *ad hoc* meeting of people who have recognized that they share an interest in preparing and maintaining systematic reviews of RCTs within a particular field; but review groups have also emerged in other ways. Members of the review group seek funding and other support for their activities from whichever specific sources they consider appropriate. Each of the collaborative review groups is coordinated by an **editorial team.** The editorial team is responsible for preparing an **edited module** of the reviews prepared by members of the review group for dissemination through the **Cochrane Database of Systematic Reviews** (see below).

The pregnancy and childbirth collaborative review group, for example, comprises about 30 reviewers who, collectively, are currently responsible for maintaining between 500 and 600 systematic reviews of RCTs, and for dealing with between 200 and 300 new reports of trials every year. The group includes reviewers in Australia, Canada, Ireland, the Netherlands, South Africa, the United Kingdom, and Zimbabwe. The individual reviewers are responsible for obtaining the resources (of which their time is often the most important) which are needed to prepare and maintain the reviews that fall within their respective areas of expertise. The editorial team coordinating the group consists of four editors, an administrator and an administrative secretary, and the work of the team is supported by a grant from the Department of Health for England. Together with members of the collaborative review group, the editorial team is responsible for preparing an edited

Pregnancy and Childbirth Module for incorporation in the **Cochrane Database of Systematic Reviews.**

THE COCHRANE DATABASE OF SYSTEMATIC REVIEWS

To ensure that the results of their work can be widely and freely disseminated, reviewers contribute their reviews to the Cochrane Database of Systematic Reviews on the understanding that these will not be subject to any exclusive copyright arrangements. Each review incorporated in the Database consists of:

- a "cover sheet," giving the title and citation details of the review; the names, addresses, and other contact details, both of the reviewer(s) and of the editorial team responsible for the collaborative review group to which the reviewer(s) belong(s); and the sources of support for preparing and updating the review;
- a structured report of the review, consisting of an Introduction/statement of objectives, information about the Materials and Methods used, the Results of the systematic review, and a Discussion section;
- full citations of reports of the studies incorporated in the review, and of reports of those studies that were potentially eligible, but which the reviewer(s) decided to exclude (with reasons for the exclusions);
- tabulation of the characteristics of the trials included in the reviews, including information relevant to an assessment of the methodologic quality of each of the studies included; and
- tabulation of the results of the review, with presentation of statistical syntheses (meta-analyses), when these were both possible and appropriate.

Because the Cochrane Database is updated and amended as new evidence becomes available and errors are identified, electronic media offer obvious advantages for disseminating and interrogating its contents. The complete Database will be distributed online and on CD-ROM. Smaller, specialized databases derived from the main database will also be compiled and published on floppy disk. Sometimes these specialized databases will simply contain all of the reviews prepared by a particular collaborative review group (the "edited module" which has been contributed by the group to the main Database). In addition, however, specialized databases will be compiled from reviews drawn from more than one of the edited modules contributed to the main Database. For example, a specialized database of reviews relevant to people providing primary health care will be compiled from reviews prepared under the aegis of several different collaborative review groups.

It is important to make efficient arrangements for criticizing the reviews prepared by investigators contributing to the Cochrane Collaboration, and for amending reviews in the light of valid criticisms. Developing these arrangements will be facilitated if the potential of electronic publication is exploited imaginatively. At present, opportunities for criticism before publication of reviews in print are restricted by the numbers and competence both of the referees selected by journal editors and of journal editors themselves. After a review has been printed, opportunities for published criticism are usually limited to the few letters that editors can accept for publication. There is also no straightforward way in which the authors of printed reviews can amend their reviews to take account of valid criticisms. Over the coming years, the Cochrane Collaboration aims to create an iterative system through which successive versions of each review will reflect not only the emergence of new data, but also valid criticisms, solicited or unsolicited, from whatever source. Successive versions of a particular review, together with any intervening criticisms, will be archived electronically.

COCHRANE CENTRES

So far four Cochrane centres—in the U.K., Canada, Scandinavia, and the United States—have been established to facilitate the work of the review groups contributing to the Cochrane Collaboration. The centres are responsible for:

- maintaining a register of existing systematic reviews, and of reviews currently being prepared or planned, so that, within the Cochrane Collaboration, unnecessary duplication of effort can be minimized and collaboration promoted;
- helping to establish a register of all RCTs, completed and ongoing, to assist reviewers to identify relevant studies;
- organizing workshops and seminars to develop mutually acceptable working practices and to help reviewers to adopt these;
- preparing protocols and software, to make the task of preparing and updating systematic reviews less onerous, and to facilitate electronic transfer of data and reviews within the Collaboration;
- developing policies and setting standards to maximize the reliability of information disseminated through the Cochrane Database of Systematic Reviews; and
- promoting research to improve the quality of reviews.

GOOD DECISIONS ABOUT HEALTH CARE RELY ON MORE THAN GOOD REVIEWS OF THE RESULTS OF RESEARCH

As the Cochrane Collaboration develops, it will make the results of research assessing the effects of health care more easily available to those who want to take better decisions. As Cochrane made clear in *Effectiveness and Efficiency,* however, reliable evidence about the effects of health care, although essential for improving decisions about health care and research, is only one of the elements needed for better decision-making.

If people are to receive care that is appropriate, then policymakers and decision-takers, ranging from ministers of health to individual clinicians and patients, must consider their needs, the availability of resources, and priorities. Furthermore, if better decisions are to lead to improved health, then effective mechanisms are needed for implementing them efficiently. Forms of care that have been shown to do more good than harm should be encouraged, while those that do more harm than good need to be discarded. And the many forms of care that have unknown effects should, as far as possible, be provided only as part of research studies to find out whether they help or do harm.

But careful assessment of the needs of people using the health services will remain of paramount importance. An episode during Cochrane's years as a prisoner of war, when he was trying to care for a young Soviet prisoner who was dying, illustrates dramatically the challenges which will continue to face those trying to provide effective care:

> The ward was full, so I put him in my room as he was moribund and screaming and I did not want to wake the ward. I examined him. He had obvious gross bilateral cavitation and a severe pleural rub. I thought the latter was the cause of the pain and screaming. I had no morphia, just aspirin, which had no effect. I felt desperate. I knew very little Russian then and there was no-one in the ward who did. I finally instinctively sat down on the bed and took him in my arms, and the screaming stopped almost at once. He died peacefully in my arms a few hours later. It was not the pleurisy that caused the screaming, but loneliness. It was a wonderful education about the care of the dying. I was ashamed of my misdiagnosis and kept the story secret.[14]

With this anecdote Archie Cochrane reminds us that decisions about how best to care for patients are often complex, and that undue reliance on evidence from formal investigations will sometimes be inappropriate. Nevertheless, during his last illness, he was pleased to discover a randomized trial comparing the effects on the quality of life of different ways of trying to provide supportive care for the dying and their families. In this, as in most other components of health services, systematic reviews of well-designed evaluations provide information that is essential for improving policies and decisions in health care and research.

SUMMARY

In an influential book published more than twenty years ago,[1] Archie Cochrane drew attention to our great collective ignorance about the effects of health care, and explained how evidence from randomized controlled trials (RCTs) could help us to use resources more rationally. He recognized that people who want to take more informed decisions about health care do not have ready access to reliable reviews of the available evidence. In 1979, he wrote: "It is surely a great criticism of our profession that we have not organised a critical summary, by specialty or subspecialty, adapted periodically, of all relevant randomised controlled trials."[4]

The Cochrane Collaboration has evolved in response to this challenge and will eventually cover all areas of health care. Contributors in many countries and specialties are preparing and maintaining systematic reviews of RCTs, and reviews of other evidence when appropriate. These reviews will be disseminated using electronic media through the Cochrane Database of Systematic Reviews.

ACKNOWLEDGMENTS

It is a pleasure to acknowledge the willingness to collaborate shown by the many people who have helped to get the Cochrane Collaboration off to a good start and to Professor Michael Peckham, Director of the NHS Research & Development Programme, for supporting the creation of the first Cochrane centre. I am grateful to Andrew Herxheimer, Brian Haynes, Andrew Oxman, and Chris Silagy for helpful comments on earlier drafts of this manuscript.

REFERENCES

1. COCHRANE, A. L. 1972. Effectiveness and Efficiency. Random Reflections on Health Services. Nuffield Provincial Hospitals Trust. London. (Reprinted in 1989.)
2. MULROW, C. D. 1987. The medical review article: State of the science. Ann. Intern. Med. **106:** 485–488.
3. ANTMAN, E. M., J. LAU, B. KUPELNICK, F. MOSTELLER & T. C. CHALMERS. 1992.

A comparison of results of meta-analyses of randomized control trials and recommendations of clinical experts. Treatment for myocardial infarction. JAMA **268:** 240–248.

4. COCHRANE, A. L. 1979. 1931–1971: A critical review, with particular reference to the medical profession. *In* Medicines for the Year 2000. G. Teeling-Smith, Ed.: 1–11. Office of Health Economics. London.

5. EARLY BREAST CANCER TRIALISTS' COLLABORATIVE GROUP. 1990. Treatment of Early Breast Cancer. Volume 1: Worldwide Evidence 1985–1990. Oxford University Press. Oxford.

6. EARLY BREAST CANCER TRIALISTS' COLLABORATIVE GROUP. 1992. Systemic treatment of early breast cancer by hormonal, cytotoxic, or immune therapy. Lancet **339:** 1–15.

7. ADVANCED OVARIAN CANCER TRIALISTS' GROUP. 1991. Chemotherapy in advanced ovarian cancer: An overview of randomised clinical trials. Br. Med. J. **303:** 884–893.

8. ANTIPLATELET TRIALISTS' COLLABORATION. 1988. Secondary prevention of vascular disease by prolonged antiplatelet treatment. Br. Med. J. **296:** 320–331.

9. ANTIPLATELET TRIALISTS' COLLABORATION. 1993. Collaborative overview of randomised trials of antiplatelet treatment. Br. Med. J. In press.

10. CHALMERS, I., M. ENKIN & M. J. N. C. KEIRSE, Eds. 1989. Effective Care in Pregnancy and Childbirth. Oxford University Press. Oxford.

11. SINCLAIR, J. C. & M. BRACKEN, Eds. 1992. Effective Care of the Newborn Infant. Oxford University Press. Oxford.

12. COCHRANE, A. L. 1989. Foreword. *In* Effective Care in Pregnancy and Childbirth. I. Chalmers, M. Enkin & M. J. N. C. Keirse, Eds. Oxford University Press. Oxford.

13. CHALMERS, I. 1991. Improving the quality and dissemination of reviews of clinical research. *In* The Future of Medical Journals. S. Locke, Ed.: 127–146. British Medical Journal. London.

14. COCHRANE, A. L. (with M. Blythe). 1989. One Man's Medicine.: 82. British Medical Journal (Memoir Club). London.

APPENDIX

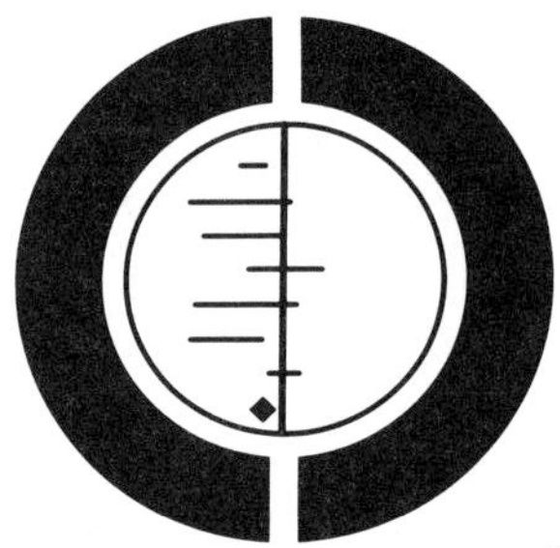

The Cochrane Collaboration logo (above) is a diagrammatic representation of a systematic review of data from seven RCTs. Each horizontal line represents the results of one trial (the shorter the line, the more certain the result); and the diamond represents their combined results. The vertical line indicates the position around which the horizontal lines would cluster if the two treatments compared in the trials did not differ in their effects; and if the horizontal line touches the vertical line, it means that that particular trial found no clear difference between the treatments. The position of the diamond to the left of the vertical line indicates that the treatment studied in the trials is beneficial.

This particular analysis shows the results of a systematic review of RCTs of a short course of an inexpensive drug (a corticosteroid) given to women expected to give birth prematurely. The first of these RCTs was reported by Liggins and Howie in 1972. The picture in the logo summarizes the evidence that would have been revealed had the available RCTs been reviewed systematically a decade later: it indicates strongly that corticosteroids reduce the risk of babies dying from the complications of immaturity. By 1991, a further seven trials had been reported, and the picture in the logo had been strengthened still further. Corticosteroids given to women expected to give birth prematurely reduce the odds of their babies dying from the complications of immaturity by between 30 and 50 per cent.

Because no systematic review of these trials had been published until 1989, most obstetricians had not realized that this treatment was so effective. As a result, tens of thousands of premature babies have probably suffered and died unnecessarily (as well as costing the health services more than was necessary). This is just one of many examples of the human costs resulting from failure to perform systematic, up-to-date reviews of RCTs of health care.

DISCUSSION

UNIDENTIFIED SPEAKER: Obviously the major ingredient in achieving your goal is obtaining the funds to do it with. I know that your budget is generous within a local context, but is hardly enough to get the work under way and keep it going around the world. How can efforts to gather and summarize evidence be done efficiently and effectively?

IAIN CHALMERS (*The UK Cochrane Centre, Oxford*): It depends on the stage at which the collaborative review group finds itself. Peter Sandercock will correct me if I'm misinterpreting the situation, but let's take stroke as an example. Stroke was designated a priority for the National Health Service Research and Development Programme so I had to take notice of it from within the UK Cochrane Centre. I knew that there was a very strong group based in Edinburgh who had many international contacts who might be willing to take on the responsibility for producing up-to-date reviews. So I contacted Charles Warlow and Peter Sandercock as the leaders of that group and asked them whether they were interested in this idea. Their reaction was actually quite interesting: They said that as self-respecting researchers in this field they had a duty to keep on top of the evidence anyway. They regarded doing proper reviews as part of their normal work so that they could design better primary research. Just as some investigators regard proper reviews as a duty, funding agencies should also regard it as their duty to insist that researchers applying for funds to do new research should do systematic reviews to make sure that their research is justified and well-designed.

Charles Warlow and Peter Sandercock then called an *ad hoc* meeting of persons from various countries—the Netherlands, Sweden, Canada, France—and from other parts of the U.K., to discuss whether the workload could be shared. The people who came to that meeting agreed that it could, then went and found the funds that they needed to support their part of the review, while the coordinating group sought funds to support a coordinating function. In other words the resources required for doing different bits of this work are being obtained by the people responsible for those bits. That way there's no enormous load on any one funding agency.

By contrast with stroke, there's very little in the way of systematic reviews available in the field of mental health. In the *British Journal of Psychiatry* alone there are 600 reports of randomized controlled trials. Getting on top of what must be tens of thousands of randomized controlled trials concerned with mental health care is a major challenge.

The most important thing to keep in mind is that it is no longer acceptable to try and guess what the evidence says about particular forms of care. As Tom Chalmers and others have shown that is just too high risk a strategy. You get the answer wrong too often. And when you compare the amount of resources needed to assemble the evidence—the evidence that is already available and should be informing our physicians—with the amount of resources going into primary research and into health care services themselves, you see that systematic reviews of RCTs are a rather important investment. But it will take time to sensitize funding organizations to that insight, but we really can't afford *not* to do the work. The interesting thing about the proposal for the Cochrane Collaboration is that no one is coming up with strong arguments *against* doing what is being proposed.

PETER SANDERCOCK (*University of Edinburgh*): The key point about the cost of any systematic review is that it is completely trivial compared to the cost of the primary research. And the second thing is the Cochrane Collaboration itself, which has wider implications because in many fields competition is encouraged and competition impedes collaboration. These overviews do not need to be very expensive provided they're collaborative, and they are certainly not expensive in terms of the cost of the primary research or the health care costs associated with the disease in question. The health care costs for stroke in the U.K. consume about 5 percent of the total NHS budget.

CHALMERS: We're moving quite fast nevertheless. When you recall that Cynthia Mulrow's article was published in 1987, and it only took 5 years after publication to be regarded as a classic, we see just how rapid progress has been. This article drew attention to the unscientific nature of most review articles. And while progress has been phenomenal since then, I certainly hope that it will always seem too slow for those of us who are interested in trying to make even faster progress. The organization of this meeting is in itself an expression of the need for this sort of work. Let us fumble our way into the future, keeping in mind the image of what's required to make better decisions for patients.

JOHN WENNBERG: (*Dartmouth Medical School, Hanover, N.H.*): I want to ask Iain Chalmers to say more about the issue of priorities. One of the problems that I see with this advance is that constituencies become organized on a particular front such as cardiovascular disease and questions of anticoagulation therapy. But for some diseases, and one that we've been particularly interested in is prostate disease, there simply aren't any randomized trials. Consequently no one is doing meta-analyses for this disease because there is nothing to work on. So the question arises on how we are going to organize across a broad spectrum of conditions where some conditions, for reasons that have more to do with historical accident, are neglected and others are, by comparison, overinvestigated. I'm sure that people who are interested in breast cancer would not agree with that statement, yet there are hundreds of randomized clinical trials for breast cancer and none for prostate cancer, just to give an example.

So priority-setting needs to be carried out at a very high level of oversight, and it seems to me ultimately has to be a governmental function.

CHALMERS: As far as the governmental function is concerned, we have both a white paper called "Health of the Nation," which has identified priorities, and also priorities identified within the NHS Research and Development Programme (on the advice of a working party of the Central Research and Development Committee). Most of the priorities that have been identified are uncontentious, such as cardiovascular disease and stroke, mental illness, physical disability, maternal and child health, and respiratory disease.

In terms of getting the Cochrane Collaboration going we have to take these priorities into account as well as what is already available within the U.K. in terms of systematic, periodically updated overviews. For that reason I'm very glad that the UK Cochrane Centre is closely affiliated with the Clinical Trial Service Unit at Oxford—and thus with Richard Peto, Rory Collins, Richard Gray and their colleagues—because they have been a central part of that movement.

All of us involved in trying to help the Collaboration to succeed have had to put ourselves where people are already. For example, if someone has already done work comparing fluoxetine and related antidepressant preparations with the tricyclic antidepressants, and they are interested in continuing to investigate that question, then we need to build on that interest and enthusiasm. Gradually the gaps in coverage will be filled in and we will have a better map of the epidemiology of controlled trials throughout health care. We will often see that the research agenda is quite substantially distorted by particular vested interests. For example, it's very difficult to get anyone within the pregnancy and childbirth field to look at all of the trials of how to stop women breast-feeding. There are about 200 or 300 trials on lactation suppression, but only about 20 on how to help women who want to breast feed do it more successfully. There are distortions in the research agenda which can be described more clearly once we know where the trials have been done.

There are going to be some areas where not only are there *no* trials, but where it is very unlikely that there will *ever* be any randomized trials. In these circumstances, it will be necessary to rely on systematic, scientifically defensible reviews of nonrandomized studies.

Panel Discussion 1

Suzanne Fletcher (Annals of Internal Medicine, *Philadelphia, Pa.*): Because Dr. Jerome Kassirer, editor of the *New England Journal of Medicine*, has been caught in a snow storm in Boston, we are going to have an impromptu panel of editors of several journals whose task will be to discuss the problems of dissemination of information from their particular vantage point. Our panelists include Dr. Jerold Lucey, editor of *Pediatrics*, Dr. Maria Lebrón, Managing Editor of the *Online Journal of Current Clinical Trials*, Dr. Charles Hennekens, editor of the *American Journal of Preventive Medicine* and the *Annals of Epidemiology*, Dr. John Clarke, editor of *The Journal of Theoretical Surgery*, and myself as editor of the *Annals of Internal Medicine*.

I'll start by bringing up two topics. One is a continuation of a theme that Dr. Dickersin discussed most directly. I'd like to suggest from the perspective of an editor of a large medical journal that we have a new kind of possibility for publication bias and that is financial conflict of interest. This is something of ever-increasing concern for editors of journals.

In the United States support of studies by pharmaceutical houses now rivals that given by the federal government and may even surpass it. As a result it is time to think carefully about developing standards to reveal any possible conflict of interest and to ensure that it is minimized in the conduct and reporting of these trials. The potential reach of this bias extends beyond the authors—it goes to the level of reviewers as well. Recently the *Annals of Internal Medicine* published a paper investigating how independent viewers assessed the validity of advertisements in medical journals. The authors of this paper wanted reviewers who had no financial ties with any pharmaceutical companies. When they selected reviewers for the advertisements they discovered that a large percentage of these persons—about three-quarters—*did* have financial ties. So the authors had to adjust their criterion to be a *large* financial tie rather then just any financial tie. Financial conflict of interest may be getting into the peer-review system as well as into the production of research.

Finally, some have suggested that it's actually gone all the way to the editorial office, saying that editors themselves may have financial ties that would skew their judgment of the manuscripts coming in. This has become such an item of concern that the International Committee of Medical Journal Editors that is sometimes called the Vancouver Group—which comprises an *ad hoc* group of the editors of the *Lancet*, the *British Medical Journal*, the *New England Journal of Medicine*, *JAMA*, the *Annals of Internal Medicine*, and several other major medical journals—issued a statement about it that is going to be published in the *Lancet* next month as well as in the *Annals of Internal Medicine*.[a] The issue of financial conflict of interest has an impact on what this meeting is all about, and it is time for scientists to figure out the ground rules in this new world of financing the medical research that we're involved in.

The second topic I want to mention is related to the question of how journals disseminate evidence in the first place. We've become increasingly impressed at how little we know about how and what and to what degree journals disseminate anything at all. The only groups routinely studying whether physicians even open up medical journals are the pharmaceutical companies themselves—the editors know little about their readers. We have to rely on the studies that the drug companies do to learn how our readers are reading our medical journals. We've

---

[a] International Committee of Medical Journal Editors. 1993. Conflict of interest. Ann. Intern. Med. **118:** 646–647.

discovered some brand new approaches to research, including a check study, in which checks are blown into the journal at random pages so that the marketers know exactly which pages readers look at. At the *Annals of Internal Medicine*, when we discovered this technique, we contemplated blowing checks into the editorial pages of the journal to see whether any of the articles are being read. We learned a great deal. However, editors don't know how well they are communicating to the readers, and some of these readers, by the way, are the reviewers who don't seem to know the studies that Tom Chalmers mentioned.

Many journals are trying to help to teach the readers about some of the concepts that are being discussed here at this conference, and most major medical journals now use a structured abstract. Brian Haynes and Ed Huth deserve the credit for starting this practice, which has now spread to many journals. Still, we find that not only do readers often not know all the components of the structured abstract, but that the authors don't know either. More journals are setting up abstracting services, and we like to think that the ACP Journal Club, a bimonthly supplement to the *Annals of Internal Medicine* that is edited by Brian Haynes, is the flagship of that kind of service because it not only picks out articles from all over the medical literature that are important to clinical medicine, but picks those that are methodologically sound.

We're trying to figure out ways to get readers to just open up the journal so we've started to include departments that are not necessarily scientific such as personal anecdotes in "On Being a Doctor," which retails the human experiences of a physician; we hope that they will then go to the meta-analyses and reports of clinical trials. We're trying to entice them into the journal!

Lastly, I just want to say that an underlying theme for disseminating evidence is how little we know about it and it's time that medical journal editors themselves started doing research to determine whether they're doing more good than harm.

CHARLES HENNEKENS (Annals of Epidemiology, *Boston, Mass.*): The *Annals of Epidemiology* was established by Julie Buring and myself in 1989, partly in response to the ever-increasing numbers of high-quality papers being submitted in the field. The *American Journal of Epidemiology*, the standard bearer in the United States and sponsored by the Society of Epidemiologic Research, then had a lag time of over 15 months from acceptance to publication. In addition, the American College of Epidemiology wished to sponsor a new journal since it was a relatively new society. I also became editor-in-chief of the *American Journal of Preventive Medicine* in 1991. The *AJPM* is the official journal of the American College of Preventive Medicine as well as of the American Teachers of Preventive Medicine and encompasses a wide range of health promotion and disease prevention initiatives. The journal was actually in some disarray after the untimely death of Joe Stokes; our predecessor, Bob Lawrence, became editor-in-chief and did a lot to improve the quality of the journal.

In general, advances in knowledge proceed on several fronts, optimally simultaneously, because each discipline provides importantly relevant and complementary information to a totality of evidence upon which rational clinical decisions for individual patients as well as policy for the health of the general public can be based reliably. In such circumstances, I believe we can be assured that we are far more likely to be doing good rather than harm. Yet I should point out that having trained at a medical school I've been impressed by the enormous strength and breadth of basic and clinical research, but noticed occasional disdain for epidemiology and preventive medicine. On the other hand, having trained at a school of public health, I've also been impressed by the depth and breadth of research in epidemiology and prevention, but was aware of an occasional disdain for basic and clinical investigation! So our goal is to encourage high-quality submissions in epidemiology and preventive medicine which will allow an equal partnership of these disciplines with basic and clinical research to advance knowledge. We emphasize the principles not as ends in themselves, but rather as means to answer important questions, and we insist on a clear explanation of the strengths and limitations of various approaches, including descriptive, observational analytic studies and randomized trials to advance knowledge and understand how each contributes to the totality of evidence. We wish to thank many of you here today, including Sir Richard Doll from Oxford, Suzanne Fletcher from Philadelphia, Elisheva Simchen from Jerusalem, and others for doing an outstanding job on our editorial boards and we also wish to thank the leaders like yourselves in the audience who are making important contributions to these journals.

JEROLD LUCEY (Pediatrics, *Burlington, Vt.*): We survey our readers every few years and we pay a good deal of money to do it. Part of my job is trying to find out what's really read in the journal and what's of interest to the readers. The last survey, which was just done last year, revealed the discouraging information that young doctors are not buying textbooks anymore—any textbook company will tell you that. And young doctors are not reading long articles. We're probably dealing with a Nintendo generation that wants short sound bites and quick communication. Most physicians who read our journal do not read the whole article, but they do read the structured abstract, which may be a mixed blessing. Randomized control trials are particularly unread *in toto*. Very few of our readers ever claim that they read the total trial information. That is not representative, I know, of this audience, who would, of course, read the whole trial. We love randomized trials—we'd like to have more of them. But it takes a very long time to generate a trial—a couple of years of planning, three years of doing, one year of analyzing; then it is submitted to a journal and it is dithered about for nearly a year. We've tried to do something about this by letting it be known that we're willing to accept the trial based on the protocol, if we can be assured that the protocol has been adhered to. That would save some time in publication.

Meta-analyses present a puzzling problem for me. I never know how to regard these articles—are they new articles or review articles?—and we don't necessarily publish many review articles. You must realize something about the readership that we stumbled onto, and that is that a reader who's 10 years out of medical school has not even heard of meta-analysis. He may have seen it in the newspapers, but he's never had any course in which this is discussed. The readers find such studies boring and usually make comments like "the authors waffle," "I can't understand what they're trying to say to me," or "it doesn't seem to apply to my practice." And the careful language which is used to construct the meta-analysis often isn't conducive to encouraging readership. People want clear conclusions, which is not always possible in analyses of such complexity.

I'm probably making a mistake in having meta-analyses reviewed, and probably pick the wrong persons to do it. The old-fashioned authorities routinely find the meta-analyses to be uninspiring. I'm also confused about what to do when somebody sends me a meta-analysis based on 10 studies and then another comes along that's based on 34 studies. I know if I swap the reviewers between the two that one will say that they eliminated many studies and the one with 34 took everything and the one with 10 was a better study and then I'd get the reverse opinion and back and forth it would go and would probably never get published until I used a third reviewer to break the tie.

Somebody mentioned something about team writing. That's a horror and usually results in a very bland, legalistic kind of language, like the kind used in guidelines, which have a very low readership. So our current methods of communication are ineffectual in influencing physician behavior after a trial. We're not able to convey the good points of the trial and the practical value of the trial. The issue of communication has to be borne in mind in planning a trial. I know that the PORTs are being planned in a different way. You have to plan on how to get the information diffused. Unfortunately there is a lot of useless duplication of information through the small special mailings of newsletters and newspapers, and publishing in double journals. We've had several requests over the last few years for simultaneous publications of new guidelines based on re-examination of the evidence. However, it should be published in two places, say for the ophthalmologists and the pediatricians because they don't read the same journal. Again that is one of our major problems.

In *Pediatrics* we're plagued with too many small trials. Tom Chalmers sounded like he was encouraging 115 trials on magnesium, for instance, but that's a terrible thought to me. The time that's been spent on republishing 115 trials—are they that different?—is staggering. Do we want to encourage small trials? I don't think so. I think it's really unethical to keep exposing people, especially children, to small trials leading nowhere, unless you do a meta-analysis on the trials, and then you have to wait for 20 or 30 such studies to accumulate.

MARIA LEBRÓN (The Online Journal of Clinical Trials, *Washington, DC*): The *Online Journal* is a new publication that started on the first of July 1992 and our editor-in-chief is Ed Huth. And, although we're not a print journal, we will undoubtedly experience the same trials and tribulations noted by the other editors on this panel. I would like to focus on some of the things that we're trying to do with the journal and touch on the issues raised by the new electronic publishing technology. There are a lot of questions about it that still remain unanswered and many questions still to be formulated regarding its promise, its limitations, and what it augers for the future of scientific communication.

We are a peer-review journal that publishes studies on trials, therapies, procedures, and anything that is relevant to patient care. The primary difference that we have is that once an article has gone through peer review and been accepted for publication we can release that document within 48 hours after acceptance throughout the electronic networks. The electronic medium is the primary medium that we use for publication; we do not exist as a hard-copy publication. The classic peer-review process that you have in your quality medical journals is observed in our publication too, and we publish a variety of kinds of papers including research reports, meta-analytic reviews, and methodologic papers. One thing that the electronic environment can provide is facilitation in searching, which is much easier when there is access to all documents published simultaneously. So if you have a specific subject that you wish to look at, say gastroenterology, you can keyboard that term and anywhere that term appears all those documents are automatically searched and prepared as a list for you.

We are trying to address one aspect of the subject of publication bias by allowing the publication of quality small trials or trials that report negative results. We do not have page limitations, and can therefore offer this option for publication. And although we have no manuscript page limitations, there's a fairly strong warning in the letter that goes to reviewers that this does not mean that verbosity is accepted. We want quality materials—the fact that the technology is open-ended does not mean that anything goes. A number of other items that are important are that we are able to link follow-up reports, corrections, rebuttals, and retractions to the original document, and in the case of meta-analyses we will be able to link the original document that we published with subsequent versions of it. Thus you would have an electronic "paper trail" of that particular document.

It is important to keep in mind about electronic publishing, *vis-à-vis* any subject matter, that what we're embarking on is a highly educational process for everyone concerned—a process that involves the authors, the editors, the publishers, and the readers. We can, or at least my colleagues at OCLC can likely tell you—if the privacy laws were not to forbid them from doing so—what articles were being read, how many times, and by whom. That information is not disclosed, however, because it is protected by privacy laws. But the online environment allows a number of these things to be studied and who knows whether things may change in the future. One thing is certain: the fact that online or electronic publishing can be, or may be, or will be more frequent in the future will demand that we re-examine the tenets and practices in publishing today.

JOHN CLARKE (The Journal of Theoretical Surgery, *Philadelphia, Pa.*): The *Journal of Theoretical Surgery* is a small new journal with a special interest in applying meta-analyses and other methodologic processes to surgery. It was founded by Wilfred Lorenz about 4 or 5 years ago. In contrast to more established journals such as the *New England Journal,* we're trying to build interest in the field and therefore taking a more active editorial role in terms of soliciting and working with authors rather then just reviewing manuscripts that come over the transom. We try to maintain the quality, but in a new field such as ours we need to take a much more active role.

Our objectives remain the same, however, and we too must ask: Is the work valid? Is the work new? And as a specialty journal we also must ask whether it is within the domain of our mission and our readership. Finally, as a practical issue, we're also concerned about whether an article will interest the readers and whether it is of interest to the journal—specifically we have to ask whether we want to be associated or identified with a methodology and its results since we're trying to establish a reputation. We then ask whether the article contributes to the field and helps the growth of the field. As with any journal there's competition for space and, as a result, depending on the time of year and the size of our backlog good articles might not be accepted when there's a limit in space, while marginal articles might be accepted if there's a gap. Again, we're trying to both get good-quality work and also promote the field. Like our authors, we have a particular position, and we must particularly guard ourself against the bias that inheres in an advocacy of the discipline.

ROBERT BROOK (*The RAND Corporation, Santa Monica, California*): Let me put three notions on the table. First, the purpose of journals is not to disseminate information, but to promote faculty—this is the sole reason and justification for the journals' existence. Second, the major conflict of interest of clinical researchers is that they don't follow through on whether their results are ever used. They do care about whether they are published and promoted, for they would behave very differently if they cared whether their results are used. Third, we *do* know about the readership of journals and the news isn't great. We did a major study of physician's reading habits as part of our evaluation of the NIH consensus development process, trying to determine whether physicians had read the conference statements. We did a detailed, random survey of doctors in this country, and I can tell you that they don't read much. Doctors read virtually nothing in journals—they don't even read the abstracts whether they're structured or not, though I do thank Brian Haynes for making them structured. The doctors basically want guidelines or short statements available to them at the point in time when they need them. That's what they told us over and over in the surveys we did.

So the question becomes one of how we preserve the promotion philosophy of academics and yet produce a service component to doctors who need to use some of the information that's published in a way that affects patient care. And that balancing act has not yet been brought off. I propose that what is really needed is a "talking wall" that a doctor can ask a question of while examining a patient. The wall would respond with an answer, the question then becoming: How is all the information that you publish going to produce that answer? How are we going to get to that point where all the different approaches to information including meta-analysis, decision analysis, and large and small randomized trials are going to come together to say to the doctor "this is the answer."

FLETCHER: To address the issue of journals' existing to promote faculty: usually journals get started by groups of physicians or associations, and they're probably started in order for the associations to have some sense of identity. They may move on to help the researcher, and in fact some journals are primarily for that. But there's a growing sense among editors, at least of major journals, that they have a duty to help the readers as well. I agree that looking out for the readers' interests has not always been a high priority historically, but I think that it may be growing.

BROOK: Let me challenge you with this question: If the ideal is really to do service to the reader, why don't you let the author get up in front of the press as soon as the article is accepted and announce the results? The journal could then use its editorial function to comment on the original article. All the policies we've implemented up to now preserve the function of the journal as a way of making money, of expanding its circulation, of getting it read, and of getting more advertisements as opposed to servicing the field. Editorial embargoes pose a huge conflict of interest here that needs to be addressed.

ALAN MORRIS (*University of Utah, Salt Lake City, Utah*): I'd like to follow up on Dr. Brook's remark, and would just ask a rhetorical question. Why should the financial conflict of interest be the only one which focuses our attention? Other major conflicts of interest involved in the reading process are not being brought to the table for discussion. In that regard I want to discuss the methods section of a paper and the issue of guidelines, which was discussed recently by Dr. Chalmers, because I think the guidelines issue—the rules provided to physicians get directly at whether or not we'll help practitioners make decisions—is very important. Among the purposes of a methods section are two extremely important goals: One is to provide enough detail to let an interested reviewer critically review the results and discussion sections. The second is to provide enough detail to let an interested investigator duplicate the work. My experience in reading the medical literature is that it's almost always impossible to attempt to duplicate the work from a reading of the paper. When we set up a clinical trial of extracorporeal CO_2 removal for ARDS patients in 1985, I had to go to Italy to speak with the author of a paper that appeared in *JAMA* to find out what was done because it was literally impossible from reading the paper to determine the method. Now that has a couple of implications, one of which is that the journals don't require in the methods section that medical researchers articulate the rules, the protocols, the recipes, that are used to carry out a particular work. This has the unfortunate effect of fostering a very diffuse approach to the management of medical research which precludes an articulation of rules for the practitioner. How much more useful it would be to read a paper that has a precise delineation of the methods used so that they could perhaps even be programmed; such information would then be more readily transferable to the practicing physician. But editorial policy, as I have experienced it, precludes the publication of adequate detail. For example, if you were all editors of a gastronomic journal and someone was doing a randomized control trial with a technique for making a flan or a chocolate mousse or a cake, and you were comparing the results, say, of two ways to make a cake, would you be willing to accept statements like those that are common in medical protocols such as "maximize antibiotic therapy," "optimize positive pressure application," "optimize hemodynamic support," or "control anticoagulation according to standard techniques"?

LEBRÓN: In our particular journal we do not limit the methods section, or indeed any other section, so if the author wishes to put a very detailed protocol we would welcome that. That is one option that you have in the online environment, but I am very sympathetic with your point because I come from the hard-copy environment where you sometimes do not have all the space that you need to be able to provide detailed information.

HENNEKENS: To address the concerns of both Dr. Brook and Dr. Morris, whether it relates rapid communication to promote the faculty or to the clear exposition of methods so that the practicing clinician can understand them, I think we should all be proactive towards achieving these goals.

Dissemination of Medical Information: A Journal's Role

JEROME P. KASSIRER

Editor-in-Chief, New England Journal of Medicine
10 Shattuck Street
Boston, Massachusetts 02115

Results of biomedical research reach the scientific community and the public through medical meetings, scientific publications, textbooks, and media reports. Just where do journals fit in this process? Should journals be merely a conduit between one investigator and another; between the investigator and the clinician; or between the research laboratory and the textbook? What is the responsibility of editors for the material published in their journals? Can they guarantee its validity? Can they assure that the conclusions are unbiased? Do they have a role in disseminating the information beyond their printed pages? To whom? And finally, what can we predict about the journal of the future?

Journals carry the permanent record of the advances of science. Without such a record, it is difficult to imagine how science could progress. To many, the medical journal is the most critical and most important stage in the process of dissemination of the results of medical research. Critical, because it is here that the work is subjected to a detailed quality assessment by individuals independent of the investigators. Optimizing the quality of a journal's published papers is one of the most important responsibilities of an editor.

I examine here how journals acquire their manuscripts, how they judge the material, the extent to which they can eliminate bias and assure validity in the papers they publish, the responsibility of others that participate in decision making, and the mode of transmission of a journal's information.

MANUSCRIPT SUBMISSION

Because progress in science is unpredictable, the results of research projects become available at irregular intervals. Experiments cannot be speeded up or slowed down simply to meet a publication deadline. Spontaneous, unsolicited submission of manuscripts parallels the unpredictable completion of scientific studies, and this timetable drives publication. Although some claim that a call by a journal for scientific papers in a certain subject for a "theme issue" drives research, this claim is unsubstantiated. I believe, quite the contrary, that research should drive publication. Calls for papers and the holding of symposia may attract superb studies that, by happenstance, are ready for publication on a given date of publication, but theme issues and symposia are unlikely to attract uniformly high-quality work. And the pressure to fill a theme issue or a symposium issue provides a strong incentive to shave on the quality of the material that is accepted for publication. For these reasons, except for extremely rare circumstances, I believe that journal editors are wise to eschew the practice of soliciting scientific studies for theme issues.

173

ASSESSMENT OF VALIDITY

Throughout the entire process of handling of submitted manuscripts by authors, reviewers, and editors, two closely related themes are dominant: evaluating (as much as possible) the validity of a study and reducing the possibility of bias, including that arising from financial conflicts of interest.

The process of evaluating a manuscript differs widely among journals. At the *New England Journal of Medicine,* all papers are first screened by the Editor-in-Chief, and some are immediately rejected as clearly unsuitable or inappropriate for publication. All scientific papers that are eventually published and most of the other papers submitted are sent out for peer review, typically to two expert reviewers.[1] Authors are expected to describe their work accurately, clearly, and concisely, and to make the editors aware of any published or submitted material that might overlap with the study they are submitting. All authors are asked to sign a statement that certifies that they have approved the manuscript and have taken due diligence to ensure the integrity of the work.[2] Any financial conflict of interest must be disclosed: in research involving pharmaceuticals or medical devices, for example, the holding of equity interests in a company, membership on the scientific advisory committee, engagement as an ongoing consultant, and employment by a company making a product or a competing product must be disclosed. This information is not provided to reviewers, but if the paper is published, it may be provided to readers on the title page of the article. Finally, we ask authors not to make public disclosures of their work until the date of publication: at that time the peer review process has been completed and other physician subscribers will have had an opportunity to review the study.

Reviewers are expected to act as consultants to the editors, providing expert opinion about the quality of the manuscript.[3] They are expected to provide their technical critiques as objectively, fairly, and constructively as possible. At the *New England Journal of Medicine,* when we send manuscripts to potential reviewers, we ask them to return them if their interests conflict with those of the author or if they have a close relationship with the author. We do not ask them to divulge any financial conflict of interest in part because the editor, not the reviewer, makes the final decision about the suitability of a given paper for publication. We ask reviewers to treat the manuscripts as privileged documents and not to share them with others or to copy them. Reviewers provide not only technical critiques, but also make recommendations to the editor about the appropriateness of a given paper for the journal.

At the *New England Journal of Medicine,* we make no attempt to hide the authors' identity from the reviewers.[3] Blinding may not be effective; there are usually ample clues as to the identity of the authors in the subject, style, and references. We give reviewers the choice of whether to sign their critiques, but only a minority choose to do so. We believe that requiring signatures on reviews encourages less critical, less rigorous, and thus less helpful assessments, though this point is arguable.[4] Needless to say, anonymity of reviewers opens the door to irresponsible or intemperate criticisms, but such commentaries usually can be identified by the editorial staff.

The editor must carefully weigh the reviewers' opinions, which may be discrepant, decide whether the reviewers' opinions on the experimental design and methods are sound, judge whether the paper is appropriate and relevant for the journal's readers, and ensure that the peer review process is as objective as possible. Editors are bound to have personal prejudices about certain kinds of research, but they must do their best to avoid personal, professional, or financial conflicts of interest and judge each manuscript on its merits. In making judgments about manuscripts, it is essential that the editor is independent and free of external constraints from journal owners, advertisers, politicians, government, or others.

The process of peer review is admittedly imperfect. Some have attacked it as secretive, lacking in objectivity, and insufficiently quantitative.[5] Certainly it is true that peer review cannot ensure that research results are accurately reported and it cannot root out fraud. Most of the time it cannot even identify all the honest errors in a manuscript. But properly supervised by an editor, the peer review process does assess and criticize the appropriateness of experimental design, methods, and analysis of results.[6] It weighs the quality of the evidence presented and provides a measure of the soundness of the authors' interpretations of their own data. Because of these features, the nature of an individual journal's peer review process sets a standard for quality to which authors measure their work: journals with a reputation for their rigorous peer review process are likely to receive better manuscripts than those whose peer review process is more lax.[6] Authors learn which journals are willing to accept papers without the often tedious and sometimes lengthy process of peer review and choose which of their studies to send to such journals. By the same token, many readers realize which of the journals shortcut the process of peer review, and they rely less on the studies in such journals. Peer review improves the scientific quality of individual manuscripts by the recommendations it offers authors for different kinds of data analysis, and sometimes even for additional data.[6]

Peer review also offers substantial protection against dissemination of invalid information. Though peer review cannot guarantee that a study is valid, it does increase the chance that it is valid. In some instances, the disclosure to the media of the results of a study prior to peer review has been followed by the revelation that the information released was invalid. We have only to recall the excitement over cold fusion, and the claims in press conferences (subsequently disproved) that ribavirin and cyclosporin were of value in the treatment of HIV infection.[7] The public is already skeptical and confused about the claims of medical science, and the release of incomplete or invalid conclusions only increases their cynicism or bewilderment.

JOURNALS, COURTS, AND THE QUALITY OF INFORMATION

Considerable ambiguity exists about the quality of evidence presented in court by expert witnesses. Many courts, which rely on decades-old standards imposed by the Supreme Court, insist that scientific testimony be based on generally accepted principles, a tacit proxy for peer-reviewed, published data. Other courts, which rely on rules of evidence enacted by Congress nearly 20 years ago, specify the qualifications of witnesses, but do not specify the nature of the evidence they can present. In recent months the Supreme Court agreed to hear a case in which expert testimony based on unpublished data was used to support a scientific argument in a lower court. The decision in this case (*Daubert et al.* vs. *Merrell Dow Pharmaceuticals, Inc.*) could have a profound effect on the quality of evidence presented to juries.

Those who assert that courts should admit evidence from experts that has not been published argue that scientific evidence need not be supported by consensus and need not be published in any particular form to be considered. Many of these proponents also criticize the peer review process as biased and flawed. They believe that judges and juries should be capable of weighing all the evidence and coming to their own conclusions. Those on the other side of the argument believe that reliable testimony should be defined as meeting an accepted standard, and that a decisive criterion for such a standard is publication preceded by critical review of data and hypotheses by a scientist's peers.

Journals, scientists, and scientific organizations have weighed in on both sides of this complex issue. The *New England Journal of Medicine,* the *Annals of Internal Medicine,* and the *Journal of the American Medical Association* have filed a joint brief in support of courts' reliance on published, peer-reviewed material. The decision by the Supreme Court probably will be rendered soon, and the decision is likely to influence not only how the courts set standards of evidence, but also the integrity of the peer review process. At issue is whether on the scale of scientific validity we will give greater strength to independently assessed scientific material than to unpublished data.

THE PUBLIC AND A JOURNAL'S MESSAGE

Medical journals do not direct their information message to the public. Instead, the public receives news of medical research from newspapers, magazines, and television. Much of the focus in the popular media has been on medical ethics, social issues, legal aspects of medicine, and health policy, but complex medical science has also become of great interest to the public. Each week news of medical "breakthroughs" abound in the news and on television. Though the general public has exhibited increasing interest in such information, segments of the public have a special appetite for medical news. Activists on behalf of patients with HIV infection, Alzheimer's disease, and other conditions regularly scour the news, searching for new hope. These groups have become sentinels over the scientific establishment in an effort to ensure that information on new advances is released and implemented as rapidly as possible.

The financial world is equally alert to medical advances. Many people invest in the pharmaceutical and biotechnology industries, and the publication of a study of a new agent in a journal such as the *New England Journal of Medicine* can have enormous implications on the price of a company's stocks. Brokers who translate such published information into financial advice watch medical journals in a timely fashion and sometimes even get their advice "from the network" before the date of publication.

It is the responsibility of journal editors, in agreement with authors and the printed and electronic media, to avoid disclosure of scientific information before the peer review process is complete. A study should not be considered complete until it has passed peer review and has been revised according to the recommendations of the journal's editors. To assure that authors do not disclose the results of their studies prematurely, most journals impose rules that preclude considering papers that have been largely published elsewhere, including the popular press, and they also impose an embargo on release of a study until the date of publication. In the case of the *New England Journal of Medicine,* those journalists who agree to abide by these restrictions may receive an advance copy of the journal several days before the publication date, a lead that allows them to research their stories, interview authors, and gather opinions from experts. Though some journalists object to the embargo, claiming that they have the capacity and expertise to interpret medical science to the public, most reporters agree with the embargo policy, and prefer having a few days to formulate their stories before the publication date.

Most material published in medical journals does not have immediate clinical applications; most studies need to be verified before applying their results to patients. Nevertheless, journal editors have a responsibility not to keep medical information critical to the health of the public under wraps as it goes through the routine mechanisms of publication, a process that can take months. Thus, the *New England Journal of Medicine* exempts from its policies on duplicate publication and its embargo any presentation of material at medical meetings, any material that the National Institutes of Health or the Centers for Disease Control and Prevention or other governmental agencies decide has immediate implications for the health of the public, and material that is released in the course of governmental deliberations.[7] In addition, at an author's request, we will consider a rapid review of a paper that might have immediate implications for the health of the public.[7] Such reviews can be expedited or even short-circuited when appropriate. For example, we often expedite reviews of studies of patients with HIV infection that have therapeutic implications. By observing such policies, journals do not hold up information that could save lives or alleviate suffering.[7]

Should journals address the public directly? Some journal editors provide press releases and some hold press conferences in an effort to publicize their messages. Contrary to the belief of many, the *New England Journal of Medicine* never holds press conferences and never provides press releases on its contents: many of our papers (2–3 per week) are accompanied by editorials which consider the significance of studies and place papers in context for both our readers and for reporters. In turn, the media interpret these studies and our editorials for the public. Should medical journals take a more active role in direct education of the public? We think they should, and we are exploring ways in which to carry out such a mission.

THE FORM OF THE MESSAGE

Until very recently, journal editors have focused entirely on the quality of the contents in their paper edition. Other forms of communication were simply not available, or if available, were unsuitable for direct transmission of medical science. Two advances in information transfer have broadened an editor's concerns to include media other than the printed page.[8] First, the capacity to transform virtually all scientific information into digital form makes it possible to transmit text, figures, and tables by phone line or cable. Second, the development of media with which physicians have familiarity and ready access has facilitated such transmission. In 1992 the *New England Journal of Medicine* inaugurated a weekly cable television presentation in collaboration with Lifetime Medical Television called "This Week in the New England Journal of Medicine."[9] This half-hour show, which airs on the cable network oriented to physicians, is shown two to three times on the Sunday following the *Journal*'s publication date. It is intended as a complement, not a substitute for the paper issue of the *Journal*. It expands on the contents of one or more original or review articles and offers special advantages when visual images are helpful in clarifying the material. For some time the contents of the *New England Journal of Medicine* have been available on a variety of electronic media, including Medline and CD-ROM disks. Simulations of the front cover containing the table of contents, as well as abstracts, are published each week in a disk version of *Current Contents,* a feature that allows a reader to browse though the *Journal*'s contents. The *Journal* has yet to be published fully online, though it would be possible with the technology under development in our offices.

THE JOURNAL OF THE FUTURE

The capacity to convert information of all kinds (print, audio, video) into a digitized form and to send digitized data out over an expanding number of networks has the potential of completely revolutionizing our definition of a journal.[8] Considering only the technology available today, it is easy to imagine the journal of tomorrow. It might be fully electronic without any printed version. Though it would be accessible from today's desktop terminals, equipment for using the data probably will be sufficiently portable to take to the patient's bedside, the conference room, or the doctor's office or bedside table. This electronic journal could contain audio or video segments. It would be capable of carrying out searches in innumerable medical and nonmedical databases. The electronic journal of the future could be individualized and tailored to a reader's interests, or it might be in a familiar form with a table of contents or series of abstracts that a reader could scan. If it were personalized, a physician could opt for certain kinds of review articles, certain kinds of original scientific studies, meta-analyses or cumulative meta-analyses. The "journal" could form a basis for a physician's continuing education or even for his or her continuing certification.

Developments of this kind are accompanied by many unsolved problems.[8] We should be concerned about whether authors will be tempted to send their data out over such networks without peer review, and how the process of peer review would be carried out. Many other concerns have been raised: how would authors get credit for their work; what would happen to the archival function of journals; how would such journals be funded? Finally, will physicians be willing to give up their paper journals for an electronic form? If so, when?

No matter what form information takes in the journal of the future, I believe the hurdle of editorial peer review should be preserved. Judging the validity of a study and assessing authors' interpretations of their papers is as important to the advance of science as the observations themselves.

REFERENCES

1. RELMAN, A. S. & M. ANGELL. 1989. The *Journal*'s peer-review process. N. Engl. J. Med. **321:** 837–839.
2. KASSIRER, J. P. & M. ANGELL. 1991. On authorship and acknowledgments. N. Engl. J. Med. **325:** 1510–1512.
3. RELMAN, A. S. 1990. Publishing biomedical research: Roles and responsibilities. Hastings Center Rep. May/June: 23–27.
4. McNUTT, R. A., A. T. EVANS, R. H. FLETCHER & S. W. FLETCHER. 1990. The effects of blinding on the quality of peer review. JAMA **263:** 1371–1376.
5. LOCK, S. 1992. Journalology: evolution of medical journals and some current problems. J. Int. Med. **232:** 199–205.
6. RELMAN, A. S. & M. ANGELL. 1989. How good is peer review? N. Engl. J. Med. **321:** 827–829.

7. ANGELL, M. & J. P. KASSIRER. 1991. The Ingelfinger Rule revisited. N. Engl. J. Med. **325:** 1371–1373.
8. KASSIRER, J. P. 1992. Journals in bits and bytes. N. Engl. J. Med. **326:** 195–197.
9. KASSIRER, J. P. 1992. This week in the *New England Journal of Medicine*. N. Engl. J. Med. **327:** 1754.

NIH Consensus Conferences:
Dissemination and Impact

JOHN H. FERGUSON

Office of Medical Applications of Research
National Institutes of Health
Bethesda, Maryland 20892

INTRODUCTION

The history of medicine is replete with the record of treatments, practices, and procedures to which patients have been subjected for which there was no medically sound basis. For example, bleeding and purging were performed for many illnesses, including stroke, which was treated by applying leeches to the anus.[1] Neurosyphilis was treated by the direct injection of malarial parasites,[2] and frontal lobotomy was performed for the treatment of various mental disorders.[3] It is instructive to bear in mind that Nobel prizes were awarded for these latter two invasive therapies.[3] Some now discarded surgical procedures for such things as constipation and descended abdominal organs ("ptosis") achieved popularity earlier in this century without adequate assessment.[4] More recent examples include such invasive procedures as portacaval shunt for esophageal varices, gastric freezing for peptic ulcer, radical mastectomy for breast cancer, and internal mammary artery ligation for angina.[5]

By contrast, in the last century some treatments were quite reasonably studied and their results published but not accepted. James Lind's clinical trial for the treatment of scurvy showed the efficacy of citrus fruit in 2 of the 12 patients who received it.[6] It took 40 years for these published results to be adopted as practice by the British Navy for its sailors. Pierre Louis published findings that early bleeding for pneumonia decreased survival in some 70 personally treated patients, yet bleeding continued to be a common treatment for many conditions.[7] It was known and published as early as 1831 that intravenous fluids for the treatment of cholera could be life-saving, but this information was not used. Instead, and this was worse than no treatment, fluids were *removed* by blood-letting and cathartics.[8]

On the other hand, treatments and procedures were evaluated without the benefit of randomized controlled trials and found to be effective and safe. These include the treatment of pernicious anemia with vitamin B_{12}, and the use of X rays to guide the setting of fractures, cortisone for adrenal insufficiency, penicillin for subacute bacterial endocarditis and for syphilis, and insulin for severe diabetes.[7]

HEALTH TECHNOLOGY ASSESSMENT

Health technology assessment is necessary to evaluate treatments and procedures, to inform providers, improve health care, and ultimately to improve health.[9,10] Appropriately influencing our increasing health care costs is an expected benefit. In an ideal world, no new procedure, treatment, diagnostic test, or other innovative health technology would be used routinely or paid for on a general basis until it had been fully assessed.[11]

Evaluation or health technology assessment is a continuous process which may follow a complex path along a continuum. For this continuum, it is useful to consider four categories of medical technologies: therapeutic procedures (both medical and surgical), diagnostic procedures, preventive techniques, and adjunctive technologies. The adjunctive category might include various devices such as hospital beds, braces, or intravenous tubing and the like. Assessments in each category may follow a distinct path along the continuum. Assessment has generally been for safety and efficacy but more recently, cost-effectiveness, cost–benefit ratio, and patient outcomes have been rightly added to assessment protocols adding to the complexity, time, and cost of any assessment.[12]

For discussion, some *theoretical* steps in this continuum have been proposed.[13] *Inception*—the technology is untested; *innovation*—preliminary testing; *investigation*—confined largely to research protocols in humans; *promising*—appropriate for some indications in certain patient populations; *established*—fully evaluated for given indications; *guidelines*—routine and standard of care. A schema that more closely resembles the real path taken by many technologies as they become part of practice has been discussed by McKinlay. The lack of proper assessment along this *actual* path emphasizes the need for evaluation.[11]

Once reimbursed by a large or major payer, perhaps not before the "established" step above, the use of a technology will spread.[14,15] It behooves those responsible for the health and safety of our citizens and for those allocating the use of health resources to make reimbursement decisions based on carefully done evaluations, judging the *quality of the evidence* upon which the assessment is based.[16–19]

Therapeutic technologies for life-threatening disorders should follow a different path of assessment for general use than that used for less serious diseases. What is generally deemed experimental may be the only available therapy for certain serious disorders and require reimbursement during the "investigational" step.[13,20] Surgical therapies require innovative assessments for obvious reasons (e.g., blinding). Too frequently they have not been subjected to proper evaluation.[4,11] Preventive technologies, especially primary preventive technologies (e.g., vaccine development), deserve a separate, and perhaps accelerated path. It is clear that preventive medicine has historically been, and continues to be, relatively ignored by the U.S. medical profession and certainly by the third-party payers, to the disadvantage of society and health.

Other factors to consider for any of these continua—whether diagnostic, therapeutic, or preventive—are: the nature of the illness; the number of patients or people involved; that prevention is more achievable than cure; cost; expected benefit; and quality of life. Is an adequate alternative available? Additionally, one should ask: will reimbursement spread the use of the technology, prevent a clinical trial from taking place, prevent patients from entering a trial, or prevent patients from being randomized? Once a technique is reimbursed and being performed, can it be studied in controlled trials? Is it ethical to do so?

The gathering of assessment information for any given technology for synthesis is complex and dynamic, with feedback from many time points in the continuum. This may come from varied groups such as clinical trials researchers, government and academic programs, hospitals, insurers, health care providers, patient groups, the media, medical journals, and governing bodies like the Congress. The point at which a technology can be termed "fully evaluated" and therefore "established," put into broad general use, and paid for by the appropriate parties may be fuzzy and extend over time. The information is not usually being funneled into or being gathered by just one source. Meta-analysis and group judgement processes like consensus conferences are attempts to bring these diverse elements of information together for synthesis. Various methods of technology assessment are discussed in recent reviews.[5,21]

THE CHANGING CLIMATE OF THE 1970s

In the late 1960s and '70s, expenditures for health care began to increase markedly. Technology development was more rapid and expensive for both drugs and devices such as computerized tomography scanners. With the more acute and infectious disorders under control by prevention or antibiotic treatment, and with the aging of the population, more-chronic conditions such as cancer, heart disease, diabetes, and arthritis became the targets for research and treatment. In these conditions, where the margin of success of any treatment is smaller, larger and more expensive trials became necessary. The United States was spending much more for health care than previously and proportionately more than other countries in the world, and yet statistics did not show a necessarily healthier population. It was clear that there were, and still are, wide disparities in health care both in quality and availability, and some began to ask whether the health care community knew about the results of research that were applicable to practicing physicians and their patients.

In 1975 the Congress asked its Office of Technology Assessment (OTA) "to examine current Federal policies and existing medical practices to determine whether a reasonable amount of justification should be provided before costly new medical technologies and procedures are put into general use." In 1976, in response to Congress' request, the OTA published *The Development of Medical Technology: Opportunities for Assessment.*[22] In 1975, Senator Kennedy's Health Subcommittee asked the question, "What should the role of the National Institutes of Health (NIH) be in assuring effective introduction into the health care system of new knowledge pertinent to disease prevention, detection, diagnosis, treatment, and rehabilitation: [and] what new organizational approaches are needed to discharge this role?" In 1976, the Director of the NIH, Dr. Donald Fredrickson, stated before a Senate Labor and Public Welfare Subcommittee on Health that "It seems clear that in the future, the NIH and the rest of the scientific community must assume greater responsibility for the effect of research on the quality and cost of health care. The need for assuring effective transfer of useful new knowledge across the interface between biomedical research and the health care community and systems is a major issue."[23,24] In May 1977, the Director of the NIH requested the Department of HEW to established OMAR, the Office of Medical Applications of Research. In September 1977, the first Consensus Development Conference (CDC) was held entitled "Breast Cancer Screening."[25-27] In October 1978, the OMAR was officially established by the Assistant Secretary of Management and Budget.[23]

The OMAR's mandate as published in the October 13 *Federal Register* in 1978 states that the office:

a. advises the NIH Director on medical applications of research;
b. promotes systematic identification and evaluation of clinically relevant NIH research information;
c. promotes effective transfer of this information to the health care community and other agencies;

d. provides a link between the technology assessment activities of the NIH and the Office for Health Technology Assessment (OHTA) (now in the Agency of Health Care Policy and Research [AHCPR]); and

e. monitors the effectiveness and progress of the assessment and transfer activities of the NIH.

Item *e* indicates that the OMAR is charged with evaluating how well it does.

In this report I will present some of the past and present studies and discuss some of the difficulties in gathering hard data to measure the effectiveness of these exercises.

NIH CONSENSUS CONFERENCES

The consensus conference format evolved with great care so that the NIH would not be perceived as attempting to regulate health care. The three essential ingredients of the consensus conference are (1) that it is a public meeting, (2) that it is a scientific meeting appropriate for the NIH, and should include scientific viewpoints on all sides of the issues, and (3), most importantly, that the panel (the "jury") weighing the issues is not biased. By including ample discussion time in a public forum, the OMAR hopes to include critical viewpoints from the audience. The scientists who present expert testimony are chosen to include scientific viewpoints on all sides of the issues to the extent possible.[28]

The panel, the key ingredient to the process, is chosen from scientists, clinicians, biometricians, and a public representative who are all experts in the general area. If their published research and viewpoints can be used to answer the questions of the conference they are not chosen to be on the panel. They may not be government employees and they are screened for both scientific and commercial conflicts of interest. Consensus panels are convened by the NIH but they are not advisory to the NIH.[29] The OMAR encourages the panels to be critical and adhere as much as possible to data so that their statement represents a fair evaluation of the information presented. Because the statements address controversial issues, departmental review (Department of Health and Human Services) has occasionally been suggested, but thus far successfully resisted. The statements are in a sense peer-reviewed by members of the panel, the audience, and the speakers. Therefore the OMAR resists further substantive editing during the journal publication process. Consensus panels work hard on these statements and the OMAR tries to keep them intact.

Topic Selection

Topics are generally selected by one of the NIH Institutes. Major criteria for topic selection include importance to public health, controversial or unresolved problems, and data upon which to resolve the issues. Of additional importance are perceived inappropriate or widespread use before adequate testing, wide variations in practice, unawareness of a safe and effective measure, and political concerns. Potential for prevention, public interest, and the timing of an evaluation are also considered.[29] Generally a form of technology must have been tested in humans in order to be evaluated in the consensus conference format. In the previously presented schema of "inception" to "guidelines," the consensus process probably best fits in during or after "investigation." If it is too early, there are not enough data. If it is too late, there may be no chance for a conference to effect appropriate change. The NIH consensus statements would logically become a part of the database for certain guidelines and thus precede guidelines development. Some forms of technology may be in need of re-evaluation as they are replaced by newer procedures or because other issues such as safety have emerged that could not be determined except by longer use.[30] We have readdressed several topics in the NIH consensus program, such as dental implants, endoscopy in ulcer disease, treatment for breast cancer, and surgery for obesity.

For the past five years, we have reviewed consensus statements that are five years old or older with the co-sponsoring institute to identify those statements that may no longer be current. To date, (November 1993) 31 statements have been thus identified. When one of these is requested, the OMAR indicates to the requester that the statement is not current and sends the more recent statement from an appropriate conference, sends the requested statement with updated material, or sends newer material as recommended by the co-sponsoring institute. Of the 10 conferences held through 1979, the one on lung cancer screening is still current,[31] while the others are not.[32–39] Of the 11 conferences held in 1979, 4 are considered current—the statements on pain, consumer blood pressure devices, postmenopausal estrogen use, and removal of third molars.[40–43] Substitution, as above, has been made for the others.[44–50] Of the 8 held in 1980, the ones on febrile seizures and CEA are current.[51,52] Substitution is made for the others.[53–58] Of the 11 held in 1981 through 1983, the conferences on diets and hyperactivity, hip joint replacement, critical care medicine, drugs and insomnia, and dental sealants are still current.[59–63] Substitutions are made for the others for those years.[64–69] Additionally, three other statements from conferences on routine HTLV-III testing, neurofibromatosis, and MRI held in 1986 and 1987 are no longer considered current.[70–72] All others are considered to be up-to-date.

As a rough overview of topics in 93 CDCs held to date, we have had 17 on cancer topics, 12 on heart and blood topics, 12 on neurologic topics (some of these were sponsored by the National Institute of Child Health and Human Development or by the National Institute on Aging), and 11 on gastrointestinal or urologic subjects. We have had 5 conferences on mental disorders, 5 on dental disorders, 6 on maternal child health problems, 4 on aging disorders other than dementia, and 14 on surgical topics.

Assessment Criteria

The major assessment criteria that the OMAR has used has been whether a treatment, procedure, device, or drug was safe and effective. There was initial concern, and continues to be, about whether or not economic, social, ethical, and legal aspects of these medical issues are appropriate for an NIH pane.[73] The concern was that if NIH strayed too far from its basic mission of biomedical research, this mission would be undermined. While recognizing the clear importance of these issues in the total picture of technology assessment, it was felt perhaps best for the NIH to evaluate safety and efficacy based on medical science, so called "technical consensus," and let other groups, institutes, or agencies address the other aspects in what was termed "interface consensus."[23,26]

Because the OMAR has been criticized for not addressing some of these issues in consensus conferences (see Refs. 104, 108 and 109), we were interested to find out just how often these topics had actually been discussed. All 93 consensus statements plus 8 technology assessment statements, including a list of the panel members, speakers, and titles of speaker presentations, are now on floppy disks in a consistent format and are being transformed into a searchable full-text online database by the National Library of Medicine. They possibly will be put onto CD-ROMs. Additionally, all are available and searchable on the Internet using the "Gopher" interface. All can presently be easily installed into one directory on a computer hard disk. We therefore have been able to readily search past consensus statements and answer some of these questions.

Cost issues have been discussed in 53 conferences. The word "cost effectiveness" was used in 16 conference statements and used as a question in 3 conferences in 1979, 1980, and 1990. (A planning committee a year or so before the conference frames the conference issues in the form of 4–6 questions. After hearing scientific testimony at the conference, the panel uses that information to answer the questions. Therefore, issues that are directly raised in one of the conference questions assume greater importance.) The phrase "cost effectiveness" was used in the title of a presentation for 3 conferences in 1990, 1991 and 1993. One can conclude that cost issues have certainly not been neglected in well over half of the NIH consensus conferences. It is clear that economic issues are playing an increasingly important role in the consensus process. Given the present state of the U.S. health care system, in which costs are seen to be out of control, this is indeed appropriate.

On somewhat more slippery ground for the NIH consensus process are legal and ethical issues, although they have recently gotten a lot of attention from the NIH regarding gene therapy, gene patenting, and genetic screening, and patenting issues in general. Legal issues have been discussed in 14 consensus conferences and ethical issues in 17 conferences. Legal and ethical questions were posed in 2 conferences in the early years of the OMAR in 1979 and 1980. The words "legal" and "ethical" appeared in the titles of talks for 3 conferences (in 1982, 1984, and 1987).

Dissemination

Every effort is made to disseminate the statements emerging from these conferences as widely as possible. The entire statement is read in public on the last day of the conference and critiqued by the expert speakers and the public. Changes are made as necessary and a press conference is held. Often the conference results make television and radio news and are summarized nationwide in the major newspapers. The statement is printed by the government and a mass mailing of anywhere from 20,000 to 100,000 statements will take place, about 4 to 6 months after the conference. The OMAR maintains a booth at several medical meetings each year to distribute statements and inform participants about NIH and the consensus program. Since 1988, 54% of the statements have been published in the *Journal of the American Medical Association*. Others are generally published in various specialty journals. Besides the mass mailing, statements are mailed on request to individuals and groups. Occasionally, as many as 500 are requested by one group. The OMAR maintains a database to track these requests and is analyzing what triggers them and where they come from. We also maintain a news clipping service to determine how widespread the newspaper reporting is and we are comparing this with news retrieval from electronic databases.

The database of requests was started in August of 1989. The average number of requests for all statements from all conferences is about 400 per month. The conferences on urinary incontinence, sunlight and ultraviolet light, destructive behaviors, noise-induced hearing loss, sleep disorders in older people, and breast cancer[74–79] have all been more popular than average. The requests for the statement on urinary incontinence of about 2,000 in one month, mostly from non-physicians, resulted from a special marketing effort.

A videotape was made of this conference and marketed one year after the conference. A brochure announcing the videotape was direct-mailed to nursing homes, hospitals, and medical libraries. Availability notices of the videotape were sent to a variety of medical, geriatric and media organizations such as syndicated television and radio health shows, satellite TV networks, health sections of newspapers and others. A panel member who was the director of an organization for incontinent people participated in media interviews in the Chicago area announcing a toll-free number. An article about this videotape and the conference appeared in the *Chicago Tribune,* which directed readers to request the CDC statement from the OMAR. Other newspapers around the country also picked up the story. This marketing effort indicates that the public can be made aware of health messages and will seek information. Targeting the mailing of the consensus statement on osteoporosis[80] to a given city also increased physician awareness of this statement compared to a non-targeted similar metropolitan area.[81] The effect on actual health or on health care–provider behavior is less certain.

We have tried to analyze various aspects of the dissemination process using this database of requests for statements, data on conference attendance, number of pre-conference announcement brochures mailed and date of mailing, the number of statements mass-mailed after the conference and when they were mailed, and the publication date in *JAMA.*

There has been a rise in typical conference attendance over the past five years from about 280 to 580. Regression analysis shows a slight positive relationship between requests for a statement and conference attendance. Thus, the more persons who attend, the more requests for the statement we receive. There does not seem to be a clear relationship between the number of announcements mailed, or when they were mailed, to the number of attenders. For some conferences, the mass mailing of the statement appears to trigger requests for the statement.[77–79,82] For some, the publication in *JAMA* seems to provoke requests.[77,82,83] But for other conferences, there appears to be no relationship.[84]

TECHNOLOGY ASSESSMENT CONFERENCES

The criteria for a consensus conference are lacking for some topics, mostly because of insufficient data to resolve controversy. To address these issues, we have held a number of conferences that have been termed "technology assessment conferences" in order to remain true to our consensus conference guidelines.[29] These conferences follow the NIH consensus conference process, which is well established and perceived as a credible method of publicly addressing controversial issues. The impetus for these conferences comes from a variety of sources and is often political. One can argue appropriately that the NIH has an obligation to address health issues of concern to society where the application of science and scientific principles are necessary in the evaluation process.

Three technology assessment conferences were held before I became director of the OMAR.[85–87] The conference entitled "Modeling in Biomedical Research"[88] was prompted by the perceived need for the NIH to make a statement on the necessity for the use of animals in biomedical research to counteract the negative attention directed at the NIH by the animal rights activists.

The OMAR held a conference on bovine somatotropin (BST)[89] in December 1990 to address political concerns of some members of Congress regarding small-dairy farmers, and concerns in the dairy industry and others, that BST might hurt cows and therefore the people that drink the milk and eat the meat. BST, made by recombinant techniques by several pharmaceutical companies, makes cows give more milk without eating proportionately more. The panel determined that available evidence indicated meat and milk from treated cows was as safe as that from untreated cows, and that BST does increase milk production without affecting the cow's general health.

The conference on dental restorative materials in August 1991 occurred mostly because of the concerns of various groups that mercury amalgam fillings were responsible for absorption of mercury, leading to such diseases as epilepsy, depression, and multiple sclerosis, and that these fillings are best removed and replaced with substitute materials.[90] The NIH technology assessment panel found these concerns to be scientifically unfounded, as did a panel previously convened by the FDA.

In March 1992, a technology assessment conference on voluntary weight loss was held to address congressional concern that this $34 billion-a-year industry was selling weight-loss diets and supplements to the public that were ineffective and/or perhaps unsafe.[91] The panel concluded that these methods were generally safe and effective in the short term, but less clearly so in the long term. Unfortunately, most people regain the lost weight.

Besides these conferences, we have held a number of other workshops to address other kinds of issues. Because it appeared that hospital-based centers for extracorporeal membrane oxygenation (ECMO) were diffusing rapidly throughout the country, the OMAR and the National Institute of Child Health and Human Development and several other institutes held a 2-day workshop to study this issue.[92]

A workshop was convened with AHCPR and the FDA to examine the evidence for the presumed superior safety of low osmolar contrast agents (LOCA) over the high osmolar agents (HOCA), given the extremely high cost of the former. Literature used was graded for quality after the method of the Canadian Task Force.[16] Unless patients were at high risk, the panel found no clear evidence to support the use of LOCA over the less expensive HOCA.[93,94]

Impressed that there was a great need for sound medical information on many treatments and procedures and other aspects of health care that could not be studied by large multi-center clinical trials, the OMAR hosted a workshop on an innovative method of performing randomized trials relatively cheaply. This Metro Firm method was pioneered at the Cleveland Metropolitan General Hospital. The workshop resulted in a supplement to *Medical Care*.[95,96–98]

A number of problems arose when the results of some clinical trials, deemed too important to await publication ("clinical alerts"), were announced early. To address these issues, the OMAR and the NLM convened a workshop with a panel composed of journal editors, media representatives, principal investigators from six different trials representing different clinical alert problems, and NIH clinical trials and communications representatives. The public was invited. Much useful, and occasionally heated, discussion of the six examples resulted in some understanding among the groups represented.[99,100] Journal editorial policies were reexamined.[101,102] NIH guidelines on clinical alerts or early announcements of clinical trials have been formulated as a result.[102a] Additionally, the NLM has made these alerts available immediately as an opening message upon dialing into Medline.

Because of increasing interest in nonlinear dynamic phenomena in biology, a workshop on chaos theory as applied in heart and brain was convened by the OMAR with several other institutes. An effort was made to bring the mathematical theorists and biologists together for cross fertilization, with some success.[103]

PAST STUDIES OF THE OMAR IN THE CONSENSUS PROCESS

The NIH consensus development program has been studied extensively. These studies have primarily focused on the earlier years of the program. The Rand Corporation published a study in 1989 of the NIH consensus process and its information dissemination and impact, but only covered the first 24 conferences, those held through 1980.[104-107] A University of Michigan study was also based on the very early conferences covering process and to some extent, dissemination.[108] A review of the NIH consensus process by the Institute of Medicine with suggestions for improvement was published in 1990.[109] The OMAR has adopted a number of the recommendations from these studies and believes that the NIH consensus development program has benefitted considerably as a result.

CRITIQUES OR EVALUATIONS OF SELECTED CONFERENCES FROM THE LITERATURE

The 1980 conference on cesarean childbirth[57] addressed the problem of the increasing rate of cesarean sections in the U.S. and made a strong recommendation for a trial of labor in appropriate circumstances for women who had had a previous C-section. This statement was published in two journals[110,111] and a larger conference report was published a year later.[112] The American College of Obstetrics and Gynecology adopted guidelines for vaginal birth after cesarean (VBACS) based in large part on this CDC.[113] The RAND study considered that this conference was one of the more successful of the 24 they studied.[104] However, the effect of this conference on physician behavior has been questioned as rates of C-section continue to rise.[114] An extensive review of VBACS in 1988 suggests that there is hope for ending the rule of routine repeat abdominal delivery,[115] and data indicate that VBACS has increased from 3.4% to 12.6% between 1980 and 1988.[116] The leveling off and stability of C-section rate, and increase of VBACS, could be viewed as appropriate effects of the CDC on physician behavior.[117] However, some have judged the effect, if any, to be disappointing.[118]

The NIH consensus conference entitled "Lowering Blood Cholesterol to Prevent Heart Disease" held in December 1984[119] spawned much discussion and criticism.[120-123] Studies of physicians' practices in 1983 and again in 1986 suggested changes in behavior and knowledge commensurate with the panel's recommendations.[124] Eighty-seven percent agreed with the treatment levels of cholesterol suggested by the panel. However, only 55% of physicians surveyed in 1986 were aware that a consensus statement had been released and 50% had not heard of the Lipid Research Clinics Coronary Primary Prevention Trial (see Ref. 125) published in 1984, which was an important piece of data for the consensus conference. This would suggest that dissemination of the CDC recommendations was incomplete or ineffective and/or that knowledge was gained through other channels. Additionally, a public survey of non-physicians was done, comparing knowledge and habits in 1983 and 1986.[126] These data showed gains in public awareness of the risks relating cholesterol to heart disease, but less of a change than in the physicians' survey.

A recent study of physician practice in transfusion decision making[127] would indicate that the recommendations of the 1988 CDC on perioperative red blood cell transfusion[128] were not being followed. This study did not discern knowledge of the conference recommendations *per se*, but did base its survey questions in part on the CDC statement. In a related area of medical practice, a French study concluded that a consensus conference on the use of albumen in hypovolemia organized by the French Society of Intensive Care Medicine did have an appropriate impact.[129]

An editorial accompanying the printing of the complete NIH consensus statement on cochlear implants[129a] in the *British Journal of Audiology* implies that the consensus statement was fundamental to the decision of the British National Health Service to make funds available for these devices. Other comments on the statement are included in this citation.

An editorial in the *Lancet* criticized the statement on intravenous immunoglobulin (IVIG),[84] saying that some data were perversely ignored, that serious account was not taken of work that did not include a U.S. investigator, and that issues of the variety and side effects of products were sidestepped. The panel was criticized for complacency in failing to address what the editorial writer considers to be some danger to the recipients of IVIG of non-A non-B hepatitis.[130]

A recent report on endoscopic hemostasis for bleeding ulcer using meta-analysis[131] compared their results with the 1989 consensus conference on that subject.[132] The authors, not convinced there was a paucity of controlled trials in this area as the NIH consensus panel stated, found 25 studies appropriate for analysis, 5 of which were in abstract form. The study confirmed the conclusions of the NIH consensus panel on the safety and efficacy of this treatment and agreed with the panel that questions remain about which mode of therapy is best. This study also agreed with the panel on the need for standardization of terms such as "rebleeding."

The consensus conference on liver transplantation occurred in 1983, concluding that it was ". . . a therapeutic modality for end-stage liver disease that deserves broader application. . . . but must be the object of comprehensive, coordinated, and ongoing evaluation in the years ahead."[67] A recent economic analysis of liver transplantation indicates that the NIH consensus conference had a profound effect in moving this procedure from "investigational" toward more general acceptance in the health care system. The study states that the sentence regarding broader application of liver transplantation quoted in part above was the major reason that public and private insurers began covering the procedure.[132a] A colorfully critical review of this conference discussed some of the politics surrounding this issue and argued that the CDC acted as a "mechanism to contain rather than to resolve controversy" and that the conference results were "formal and predictable."[133] Often the planners of any given consensus conference are aware of a likely outcome and use the conference as a mechanism to inform the health care community. This was one of the original reasons for the establishment of the OMAR at the NIH. On the other hand, as an example of the independence that panels may exhibit by not always recommending what the planners had envisioned, a recent consensus panel on adjuvant chemotherapy for early-stage breast cancer[79] were cautious in their statement on the use of adjuvant chemotherapy in this disease and were accused of a "totally wimpy" statement by some of the planners.[134]

One of the problems of the NIH consensus program has been that although the program's intent has been to inform the health care givers, primarily practicing physicians, the conferences are organized by and largely constituted from members of the academic community. The difficulties in communication between these two groups was analyzed using the audiotapes of discussion at the 1980 conference[58] on adjuvant chemotherapy for breast cancer.[135] This problem, also discussed by Greer,[136] and in the Institute of Medicine report,[109] has been at least in part addressed by the OMAR by including members of the practicing community on the planning committees of most conferences and on all the panels.

Recent studies of the consensus process, including the NIH consensus program, conclude that these exercises rarely have an effect on physician behavior even when physicians are aware that such conferences have occurred and produced recommendations.[105,137,138] There has been the suggestion that these conferences may influence policymakers,[139] perhaps more so from abroad, as mentioned above for cochlear implants. I recently learned that the consensus conference on mammography, the very first consensus conference held in 1977,[25] had an effect in Quebec, Canada.[140] The conference concluded that breast cancer screening using thermography was not effective. The number of thermograms in Quebec had gone up from 4,000 in 1972 to a peak of 84,000 in 1976. Between 1975 and 1976, information regarding breast thermography had also been produced by the American Cancer Society and negotiations begun in 1976 on breast thermography between physician specialty groups and the government of Quebec. The consensus conference took place in September of 1977 and its conclusions regarding screening thermography immediately adopted by the Quebec government. Reimbursement ceased. The number of procedures, which had begun to drop before the conference, fell to zero in 1978.

In the last several years the OMAR has received calls from various insurance programs or companies asking whether or not it recommended reimbursement for a particular procedure. In Illinois, a statute exists indicating that organ transplant will be a "covered expense" unless deemed "experimental or investigational" by the NIH Office of Medical Applications of Research.[141] The statute further states that failure of the OMAR to respond to the request for information within 90 days may be understood as "a determination the procedure is deemed to be experimental or investigational." Several companies have said that similar clauses are in the coverage policies of their employees. We have been unable to ascertain how this language got into this law or these policies. Several past directors have requested its withdrawal. Although the OMAR is pleased that the NIH consensus statements are being used by payers and other health policy formulators as a reliable source of information regarding the safety and effectiveness of various medical procedures, we acknowledge that we cannot—and will not—be the arbiters of reimbursement policy.

THE OMAR'S EVALUATION AND IMPACT STUDIES

The OMAR has conducted four focus groups consisting of 34 practicing physicians in two cities, Chicago and Tucson. Twenty-six of the 34 doctors were in solo practice. The Chicago groups consisted of 9 and 11 physicians and the Tucson groups of 6 and 8, respectively. Most of them had heard of the NIH. None knew of the OMAR. There was only minimal and vague recollection of the consensus development program or consensus conferences. When told about the process and shown some of the statements, the Chicago group was not very receptive of the concept, especially regarding the government's role, but in Tucson the groups appeared more enthusiastic about the OMAR's attempts to inform physicians.

The OMAR has generic approval from the Office of Management and Budget for a "Quick Launch" survey of physicians' knowledge and behavior before and after nine different conferences. The first survey on a recently held conference on hearing loss in infants and children[142] is under way. Physicians, dentists, and others also come to our conferences and get continuing medical education (CME) credit. We are analyzing these questionnaires as part of our ongoing studies. Each panel member after a conference also fills out a questionnaire and we are in the process of analyzing these.

We have studied physician use of two therapies before and after the prostate cancer conference, which occurred in 1987[143] using the SEER and Medicare databases.[144] This conference concluded that radical prostatectomy or radiation therapy were effective for nonmetastatic prostate cancer. When the number of patients who had radical prostatectomies, radiation therapy only, or both surgery and radiation, was tabulated for a period of several years before the conference to several years after, there did not appear to be a change in the number of these procedures or an inflection point in the year 1987. There possibly was a flattening of the curve just before the conference with an upward slope after, but this was questionable. We could not conclude from this study that there was a change in behavior as a result of this conference.

A major impact of the NIH program has been the spawning of consensus conferences throughout the world. Programs have started in Canada, Denmark, Finland, the Netherlands, Norway, Sweden, Switzerland, United Kingdom, France, and Israel.[145]

The following are preliminary data from a physician survey conducted with the National Cancer Institute (NCI). The Breast Cancer and Colon Cancer conferences occurred in the spring and early summer of 1990.[79,82] This survey was taken in the summer and fall of 1991, one year after the conferences. Physicians who had patients diagnosed with Stage I or II breast cancer within the past 12 months, were asked the question "Are you familiar with the NIH Consensus Conference on this subject?" About 8% were very familiar, 40% somewhat familiar, and 50% not at all familiar with this conference. Those who were "very" or "somewhat" familiar with the conference were asked "Are you recommending breast conservation therapy for more, the same, or fewer Stage I patients?" The conference strongly recommended breast conservation therapy for patients with Stage I and Stage II disease. It is disappointing to note that although 45% said more, about the same number said it was just the same. One would have hoped that if the message of the conference was received and acted upon, a much larger percentage of those physicians who were familiar with the conference would have recommended breast conservation therapy for more of their patients. Similar conclusions about the underutilization of breast conservation therapy for patients with Stage I or II breast cancer were found in a recently published survey of 8,095 patients in Washington state using the SEER database.[146] The authors comment that although the study was terminated before the NIH consensus conference, the results of the randomized clinical trials were available a decade earlier.

A similar set of questions was asked regarding colon and rectal cancer. Physicians who had taken care of patients with Duke's Stage B2 or C colon or rectal cancer in the past 12 months were asked whether they were familiar with the NIH consensus conference. The response was similar to that of the breast cancer conference: about 5% were very familiar, some 40% were somewhat familiar, and about 55% not at all familiar. Those who were somewhat or very familiar, were asked "Are you recommending surgery followed by adjuvant therapy for more, the same, or fewer Duke's Stage C patients?" (The conference strongly recommended adjuvant therapy for Duke's Stage C patients following surgery.) Here the results are a little more encouraging in that some 68% said they were recommending more adjuvant therapy for this group of patients and only 30% said they were recommending it for the same number of patients. Perhaps for this conference and for those physicians who were very or somewhat familiar with it, there was a behavior change. One should bear in mind, however, that physicians may not actually do what they report that they do.[137]

CONCLUSIONS

The NIH consensus program has spawned consensus programs worldwide and in effect has been a model for such programs.[145] The NIH CDC is perceived as a creditable way to evaluate controversial subjects in a public forum. The NIH has been requested to convene consensus conferences by various groups, including the Congress. These conferences are perceived as scientifically credible landmarks, anchors, or summaries of current knowledge, especially by the academic health care community, but also by the government and by some insurers, including those outside the United States. The conferences focus attention on some health problems for future research and for improvements in health care.

It is, however, very difficult to measure changes in physician behavior as a result of these conferences. This may be because the U.S. health care system is fragmented and not centrally administered. A national health care system is threatening for some who espouse a free enterprise approach to health care. When the buyer and seller need not be concerned with cost which is borne by a third party, free enterprise will not work. The U.S. health care system is an example. Additionally, there are a lot of nonmedical influences on physician behavior in the U.S. The NIH consensus program has had more of a general impact and less of an effect on physician behavior. As our marketing studies indicate, the program could have more effect on physicians by reaching patients and the public.

It is important to emphasize that technologies need to be assessed before they are routinely paid for and widely disseminated. Public deliberative assessments by independent groups such as the NIH consensus conferences provide a needed gathering of information for some technologies as the technologies evolve from "experimental" through "promising" to "established." Information on completely evaluated or "established" technologies then becomes part of the database that groups developing guidelines, such as the forum at AHCPR, may use.

REFERENCES

1. GUBLER, A. 1971. Alternating hemiplegia, a sign of pontine lesion, and documentation of the proof of the facial decussation. *In* The Classical Brainstem Syndromes. J. K. Wolf, Ed.: 9–30. Charles C Thomas. Springfield, IL.
2. AUSTIN, S. C., P. D. STOLLEY & T. LASKY. 1992. The history of malariotherapy for neurosyphilis. J. Am. Med. Assoc. **268**(4): 516–519.
3. VALENSTEIN, E. S. 1986. Great and Desperate Cures: The Rise and Decline of Psychosurgery and Other Radical Treatments for Mental Illness.: 338. Basic Books. New York.
4. BARNES, B. A. 1977. Discarded operations: Surgical innovation by trial and error. *In* Cost, Risks, and Benefits of Surgery. J. P. Bunker, B. A. Barnes & F. Mosteller, Eds.: 109–123. Oxford University Press. New York.
5. MOSTELLER, F. 1985. Assessing Medical Technologies.: 573. National Academy Press. Washington, DC.
6. LIND, J. 1753. A Treatise of The Scurvy in Three Parts, Containing an Inquiry into the Nature, Causes and Cure of That Disease, together with a Critical and Chronological View of What has been Published on the Subject. Sands, Murray, and Cochran. Edinburgh.
7. MOSES, L. E. 1992. The series of consecutive cases as a device for assessing outcomes of interventions. *In* Medical Uses of Statistics. J. C. Bailar III & F. Mosteller, Eds.: 125–140. New England Journal of Medicine Books. Boston, MA.
8. CARPENTER, C. C. J. 1992. The treatise of cholera: Clinical science at the bedside. J. Infect. Dis. **166**(1): 2–14.

9. FINEBERG, H. & H. HIATT. 1979. Evaluation of medical practices: The case for technology assessment. N. Engl. J. Med. **301:** 1086–1091.

10. RELMAN, A. S. 1988. Assessment and accountability: The third revolution in medical care. N. Engl. J. Med. **319**(18): 1220–1222.

11. MCKINLAY, J. B. 1981. From 'promising report' to 'standard procedure': Seven stages in the career of medical innovation. Milbank Mem. Fund Quart. **59:** 374–411.

12. FUCHS, F. R. & A. M. GARBER. 1990. The new technology assessment. N. Engl. J. Med. **323**(10): 673–677.

13. FERGUSON, J. H. 1992. Perspective from the National Institutes of Health. *In* New Medical Technology: Experimental or State-of-the-Art? M. L. Grady, Ed.: 19–22. Agency for Health Care Policy and Research. Publication No. 92-0057. Rockville, MD.

14. BUNKER, J. P., J. FOWLES & R. SCHAFFARZICK. 1982. Evaluation of medical-technology strategies: Effects of coverage and reimbursement (first of two parts). N. Engl. J. Med. **306**(10): 620–624.

15. LARSON, E. B. & D. L. KENT. 1989. The relevance of socioeconomic and health policy issues to clinical research, the case of MRI and neuroradiology. Int. J. Technol. Assess. Health Care **5:** 195–206.

16. CANADIAN TASK FORCE ON THE PERIODIC HEALTH EXAMINATION. 1979. The periodic health examination. Canad. Med. Assoc. J. **121:** 1193–1254.

17. 1989. Guide to Clinical Preventive Services: An Assessment of Effectiveness of 169 Interventions. Williams and Wilkins. Baltimore, MD.

18. ENKIN, M., M. J. N. C. KEIRSE & I. CHALMERS. 1989. A Guide to Effective Care in Pregnancy and Childbirth.: 376. Oxford University Press. New York.

19. SACKETT, D. L. 1989. Rules of evidence and clinical recommendations on the use of antithrombotic agents. Chest **95**(Suppl.)(2): 2s–4s.

20. ANTMAN, K., L. E. SCHNIPPER & E. FREI, III. 1988. The crisis in clinical cancer research: Third-party insurance and investigational therapy. N. Engl. J. Med. **319**(1): 46–48.

21. SOX, H., S. STERN, D. OWENS & H. L. ABRAMS. 1989. Assessment of diagnostic technology in health care.: 143. National Academy Press. Washington, DC.

22. U.S. CONGRESS, OFFICE OF TECHNOLOGY ASSESSMENT. 1976. Development of Medical Technology: Opportunities for Assessment. U.S. Government Printing Office. Washington, DC.

23. PERRY, S. & J. T. KALBERER, JR. 1980. The NIH Consensus-Development Program and the assessment of health-care technologies: The first two years. N. Engl. J. Med. **303**(3): 169–172.

24. OFFICE OF THE DIRECTOR, NATIONAL INSTITUTES OF HEALTH. 1977. The Responsibilities of the NIH at the Health Research/Health Care Interface. Bethesda, MD.

25. 1978. National Institutes of Health/National Cancer Institute consensus development meeting on breast cancer screening: Issues and recommendations. J. Natl. Cancer Inst. **60**(6): 1519—1521.

26. FREDRICKSON, D. 1978. Seeking technical consensus on medical interventions. Clin. Res. **26**(3): 116–117.

27. PERRY, S. 1978. The biomedical research community: Its place in consensus development. JAMA **239**(6): 485–488.

28. MULLAN, F. & I. JACOBY. 1985. The town meeting for technology: The maturation of consensus conferences. JAMA **254**(8): 1068–1072.

29. NATIONAL INSTITUTES OF HEALTH, OFFICE OF MEDICAL APPLICATIONS OF RESEARCH. 1988. Guidelines for the Selection and Management of Consensus Development Conferences. U.S. Government Printing Office. Bethesda, MD.

30. BANTA, H. D. & S. B. THACKER. 1990. The case for reassessment of health care technology: Once is not enough. JAMA **264**(2): 235–240.

31. Mass Screening for Lung Cancer. 1978. NIH Consensus Statement, September 18–20; **1**(8).

32. Breast Cancer Screening. 1977. NIH Consensus Statement, September 14–16; **1**(1).

33. Educational Needs of Physicians and Public Regarding Asbestos Exposure. 1978. NIH Consensus Statement, May 22; **1**(2).

34. Dental Implants: Benefits and Risk. 1978. NIH Consensus Statement, June 13–14; **1**(3).
35. Mass Screening for Colo-Rectal Cancer. 1978. NIH Consensus Statement, June 26–28; **1**(4).
36. Treatable Brain Diseases in the Elderly. 1978. NIH Consensus Statement, July 10–11; **1**(5).
37. Availability of Insect Sting Kits to Non-physicians. 1978. NIH Consensus Statement, September 14; **1**(7).
38. Supportive Therapy in Burn Care. 1978. NIH Consensus Statement, November 10–11; **1**(9).
39. Surgical Treatment of Morbid Obesity. 1978. NIH Consensus Statement, December 4–5; **1**(10).
40. Pain, Discomfort, and Humanitarian Care. 1979. NIH Consensus Statement, February 16; **2**(1).
41. Improving Clinical and Consumer Use of Blood Pressure Measuring Devices. 1979. NIH Consensus Statement, April 26–27; **2**(4).
42. Removal of Third Molars. 1979. NIH Consensus Statement, November 28–30; **2**(11).
43. Estrogen Use and Postmenopausal Women. 1979. NIH Consensus Statement, September 13–14; **2**(8).
44. Antenatal Diagnosis. 1979. NIH Consensus Statement, March 5–7; **2**(2).
45. Transfusion Therapy in Pregnant Sickle Cell Disease Patients. 1979. NIH Consensus Statement, April 23–24; **2**(3).
46. The Treatment of Primary Breast Cancer: Management of Local Disease. 1979. NIH Consensus Statement, June 5; **2**(5).
47. Steroid Receptors in Breast Cancer. 1979. NIH Consensus Statement, June 27–29; **2**(6).
48. Intraocular Lens Implantation. 1979. NIH Consensus Statement, September 10–11; **2**(7).
49. Amantadine: Does It Have a Role in the Prevention and Treatment of Influenza. 1979. NIH Consensus Statement, October 15–16; **2**(9).
50. Microprocessor-Based "Intelligent" Machines in Patient Care. 1979. NIH Consensus Statement, October 17–19; **2**(10).
51. Febrile Seizures. 1980. NIH Consensus Statement, May 19–21; **3**(2).
52. CEA (Carcinoembryonic Antigen): Its Role as a Marker in the Management of Cancer. 1980. NIH Consensus Statement, October 1; **3**(7).
53. Thrombolytic Therapy in Thrombosis. 1980. NIH Consensus Statement, April 10–12; **3**(1).
54. Cervical Cancer Screening: The Pap Smear. 1980. NIH Consensus Statement, July 23–25; **3**(4).
55. Endoscopy in Upper GI Bleeding. 1980. NIH Consensus Statement, August 20–22; **3**(5).
56. Coronary Artery Bypass Surgery: Scientific and Clinical Aspects. 1980. NIH Consensus Statement, December 3–5; **3**(8).
57. Cesarean Childbirth. 1980. NIH Consensus Statement, September 22–24; **3**(6).
58. Adjuvant Chemotherapy for Breast Cancer. 1980. NIH Consensus Statement, July 14–16; **3**(3).
59. Dental Sealants in the Prevention of Tooth Decay. 1983. NIH Consensus Statement, December 5–7; **4**(11).
60. Defined Diets and Childhood Hyperactivity. 1982. NIH Consensus Statement, January 13–15; **4**(3).
61. Total Hip Joint Replacement. 1982. NIH Consensus Statement, March 1–3; **4**(4).
62. Critical Care Medicine. 1983. NIH Consensus Statement, March 7–9; **4**(6).
63. Drugs and Insomnia: The Use of Medications to Promote Sleep. 1983. NIH Consensus Statement, November 15–17; **4**(10).
64. The Diagnosis and Treatment of Reye's Syndrome. 1981. NIH Consensus Statement, March 2–4; **4**(1).

65. Computed Tomographic Scanning of the Brain. 1981. NIH Consensus Statement, November 4–6; **4**(2).
66. Clinical Applications of Biomaterials. 1982. NIH Consensus Statement, November 1–3; **4**(5).
67. Liver Transplantation. 1983. NIH Consensus Statement, June 20–23; **4**(7).
68. Treatment of Hypertriglyceridemia. 1983. NIH Consensus Statement, September 27–29; **4**(8).
69. Precursors to Malignant Melanoma. 1983. NIH Consensus Statement, October 24–26; **4**(9).
70. The Impact of Routine HTLV-III Antibody Testing on Public Health. 1986. NIH Consensus Statement, July 7–9; **6**(5).
71. Neurofibromatosis. 1987. NIH Consensus Statement, July 13–15; **6**(12).
72. Magnetic Resonance Imaging. 1987. NIH Consensus Statement, October 26–28; **6**(14).
73. PERRY, S. 1987. The NIH Consensus Development Program: A decade later. N. Engl. J. Med. **317**: 485–488.
74. 1989. Consensus Conference. Urinary incontinence in adults. JAMA **261**(18): 2685–2690.
75. Sunlight, ultraviolet radiation, and the skin. 1989. NIH Consensus Statement, May 8–10; **7**(8).
76. Treatment of Destructive Behaviors in Persons with Developmental Disabilities. 1989. NIH Consensus Statement, September 11–13; **7**(9).
77. 1990. Consensus Conference. Noise and hearing loss. JAMA **263**(23): 3185–3190.
78. The Treatment of Sleep Disorders of Older People. 1990. NIH Consensus Statement, March 26–28; **8**(3).
79. 1991. NIH Consensus Conference. Treatment of early-stage breast cancer. JAMA **265**(3): 391–395.
80. 1984. Consensus Conference: Osteoporosis. JAMA **252**(6): 799–802.
81. JACOBY, I. & S. M. CLARK. 1986. Direct mailing as a means of disseminating NIH consensus statements: A comparison with current techniques. JAMA **255**(10): 1328–1330.
82. 1990. NIH Consensus Conference. Adjuvant therapy for patients with colon and rectal cancer. JAMA **264**(11): 1444–1450.
83. 1990. National Institutes of Health Consensus Conference. Surgery for epilepsy. JAMA **264**(6): 729–733.
84. 1990. NIH Consensus Conference. Intravenous immunoglobulin. Prevention and treatment of disease. JAMA **264**(24): 3189–3193.
85. 1983. Evaluating the Elderly Patient: The Case for Assessment Technology. NIH Technology Assessment Statement, June 29–30.
86. 1985. Donor Registries for Bone Marrow Transplantation. NIH Technology Assessment Statement, May 13–15.
87. 1987. Health Benefits of Pets. NIH Technology Assessment Statement, September 10–11.
88. 1989. Modeling in Biomedical Research: An Assessment of Current and Potential Approaches. NIH Technology Assessment Statement, May 1–3.
89. 1991. NIH Technology Assessment Conference statement on bovine somatotropin. JAMA **265**(11): 1423–1425.
90. 1992. Statement: Effects and side-effects of dental restorative materials. Advan. Dental Res. **6**(September): 139–144.
91. 1992. Methods for voluntary weight loss and control. NIH technology assessment conference panel. Ann. Intern. Med. **116**(11): 942–949.
92. WRIGHT, L. L., ED. 1993. Report of the Workshop on Diffusion of ECMO Technology: Extracorporeal Membrane Oxygenation. Publ. No. 93-3399. 93. NIH/PHS/DHHS. Rockville, MD.
93. LAWRENCE, V., W. MATTHAI & S. HARTMAIER. 1992. Comparative safety of high-osmolality and low-osmolality radiographic contrast agents: Report of a multidisciplinary working group. J. Invest. Radiol. **27**(1): 2–28.
94. HILLMAN, B. J. 1992. The consensus of committees. J. Invest. Radiol. **27**(1): 1.

95. FERGUSON, J. H. 1991. Foreward: Research on the delivery of medical care using hospital firms. Med. Care **29**(7 Suppl.): JS1–JS2.

96. MOSTELLER, F. 1991. The contributions of firms: A fresh movement in medicine. Med. Care **29**(7 Suppl.): JS3–JS4.

97. NEUHAUSER, D. 1991. Parallel providers, ongoing randomization, and continuous improvement. Med. Care. **29**(7 Suppl.): JS5–JS8.

98. CEBUL, R. D. 1991. Randomized, controlled trials using the Metro firm system. Med. Care **29**(7 Suppl.): JS9–JS18.

99. PALCA, J. 1991. Conflict over release of clinical research data. Science **251**(25 Jan.): 374–375.

100. SCHWAB, L. E. 1991. Clinical announcements: Where do we go from here? J. Natl. Cancer Inst. **83**(4): 237–238.

101. ANGELL, M. & J. P. KASSIRER. 1991. The Ingelfinger rule revisited. N. Engl. J. Med. **325**(19): 1371–1373.

102. LUNDBERG, G. D., R. M. GLASS & L. E. JOYCE. 1991. Policy of AMA journals regarding release of information to the public. JAMA **265**(3): 400.

102a. HEALY, B. 1993. From the National Institutes of Health: Issuing clinical alerts. JAMA **269**(24): 3096.

103. AMATO, I. 1992. Chaos breaks out at NIH, but order may come of it. Science **256**(26 June): 65–66.

104. KANOUSE, D. E., *et al.* 1989. Changing Medical Practice through Technology Assessment: An Evaluation of the National Institutes of Health Consensus Development Program. The Rand Corp. Santa Monica, CA.

105. KOSECOFF, J. *et al.* 1987. Effects of the National Institutes of Health consensus development program on physician practice. JAMA **258**(19): 2708–2713.

106. FINK, A., J. KOSECOFF, M. CHASSIN & R. H. BROOK. 1984. Consensus methods: Characteristics and guidelines for use. Am. J. Public Health **74**(9): 979–983.

107. WINKLER, J. D., D. E. KANOUSE, L. BRODSLEY & R. H. BROOK. 1986. Popular press coverage of eight National Institutes of Health consensus development topics. JAMA **255**(10): 1323–1327.

108. WORTMAN, P. M., A. VINOKUR & L. SECHREST. 1988. Do consensus conferences work? A process evaluation of the NIH consensus development program. J. Health Politics, Policy & Law **13**(3): 469–497.

109. 1990. Consensus Development at the NIH: Improving the Program.: 81. National Academy Press. Washington, DC.

110. ROSEN, M. G. 1981. Introduction and NIH consensus development statement on cesarean childbirth. Am. J. Obstet. Gynecol. **139**: 901–909.

111. ROSEN, M. G. 1981. Introduction and NIH consensus development statement on cesarean childbirth. Obstet. Gynecol. **57**: 537–545.

112. 1981. Cesarean Childbirth. Report of a Consensus Development Conference sponsored by the National Institute of Child Health and Human Development. NIH Publication No. 82-2067. National Institutes of Health. Bethesda, MD.

113. 1982. Guidelines for Vaginal Delivery after a Cesarean Childbirth. American College of Obstetricians and Gynecologists Committee on Obstetrics: Maternal and Fetal Medicine. Washington, DC.

114. GLEICHER, N. 1984. Cesarean section rates in the United States: The short-term failure of the National Consensus Development Conference in 1980. JAMA **252**(23): 3273–3276.

115. MARTIN, J. N., J. C. MORRISON & W. L. WISER. 1988. Vaginal birth after cesarean section: The demise of routine repeat abdominal delivery. Obstet. Gynecol. Clin. N. Am. **15**(4): 719–736.

116. TAFFEL, S. M. 1989. Cesarean section in America: dramatic trends, 1970 to 1987. Bull. Metropolitan Insurance Company **70**: 2–11.

117. TAFFEL, S. M., P. J. PLACEK & M. MOIEN. 1990. 1988 U.S. cesarean-section rate at 24.7 per 100 births—A plateau? N. Engl. J. Med. **323**(3): 199–200.

118. MYERS, S. A. & N. GLEICHER. 1990. 1988 U.S. cesarean-section rage: Good news or bad? N. Engl. J. Med. **323**(3): 200.

119. 1985. Consensus conference. Lowering blood cholesterol to prevent heart disease. JAMA **253**(14): 2080–2086.

120. AHRENS, E. H., JR. 1985. The diet-heart question in 1985: Has it really been settled? Lancet **i**(May 11): 1085–1087.

121. OLIVER, M. F. 1985. Consensus or nonsensus conferences on coronary heart disease. Lancet **i**(May 11): 1087–1089.

122. STEINBERG, D. 1985. Consensus conference on cholesterol and heart disease. Lancet **ii**(27 July): 205–207.

123. JACOBY, I. & M. ROSE. 1985. Consensus conference on cholesterol and heart disease. Lancet **ii**: 205.

124. SCHUCKER, B. *et al.* 1987. Change in physician perspective on cholesterol and heart disease. JAMA **258**(24): 3521–3526.

125. KRONMAL, R. A. 1985. Commentary on the published results of the lipid research clinics coronary primary prevention trial. JAMA **253**(14): 2091–2093.

126. SCHUCKER, B. *et al.* 1987. Change in public perspective on cholesterol and heart disease: Results from two national surveys. JAMA **258**(24): 3527–3531.

127. SALEM-SCHATZ, S. R., J. AVORN & S. B. SOUMERAI. 1990. Influence of clinical knowledge, organizational context, and practice style on transfusion decision making: Implications for practice change strategies. JAMA **264**(4): 471–475.

128. 1988. Consensus conference. Perioperative red blood cell transfusion. JAMA **260**(18): 2700–2703.

129. DURAND-ZALESKI, I. *et al.* 1992. Usefulness of consensus conferences: The case of albumin. Lancet **340**(5 Dec.): 1388–1390.

129a. ROSEN, S. 1990. Cochlear implants: Some consensus at last? Br. J. Audiol. **24**: 361–373.

130. 1990. Consensus on IVIG. Lancet **336**(25 Aug.): 470–472.

131. SACKS, H. S. *et al.* 1990. Endoscopic hemostasis: An effective therapy for bleeding peptic ulcers. JAMA **264**(4): 494–499.

132. 1989. Consensus conference: Therapeutic endoscopy and bleeding ulcers. JAMA **262**(10): 1369–1372.

132a. EVANS, R. W., D. L. MANNINEN & F. B. DONG. 1993. An economic analysis of liver transplantation. Gastroenterol. Clin. N. Amer. **22**(2): 451–473.

133. MARKLE, G. E. & D. E. CHUBIN. 1987. Consensus development in biomedicine: The liver transplant controversy. Milbank Quart. **65**(1–24).

134. OKIE, S. & S. ROVNER. 1990. Drug treatments for early breast cancer: Panel of experts offers little guidance for women. Washington Post (*Health*), June 26. :9. Washington, DC.

135. MONTINI, T. & K. SLOBIN. 1991. Tensions between good science and good practice: Lagging behind and leapfrogging ahead along the cancer care continuum. Res. Soc. Health Care **9**: 127–140.

136. GREER, A. L. 1987. The Two Cultures of Biomedicine: Can There Be Consensus? JAMA **258**(19): 2739–2740.

137. LOMAS, J. *et al.* 1989. Do practice guidelines guide practice? The effect of a consensus statement on the practice of physicians. N. Engl. J. Med. **321**(19): 1306–1311.

138. LOMAS, J. 1991. Words without action? The production, dissemination, and impact of consensus recommendations. Annu. Rev. Public Health. **12**: 41–65.

139. 1992. Guidelines for doctors in the new world. Lancet **339**(May 16): 1197–1198.

140. JACOB, R. 1992. Diffusion of mammary thermography in Quebec. Personal communication.

141. 1984. The Voluntary Health Services Plan Act of the State of Illinois. State of Illinois. Public Act 83-1274, Chapt. 32, Sect. 609.14, §15.14.

142. Early Identification of Hearing Impairment in Infants and Young Children. 1993. NIH Consensus Statement, March 1–3; **11**(1).

143. 1987. Consensus conference. The management of clinically localized prostate cancer. JAMA **258**(19): 2727–2730.

144. SHERMAN, C. R., A. L. POTOSKY, K. A. WEIS & J. H. FERGUSON. 1992. The consensus development program: Detecting changes in medical practice following a consensus

conference on the treatment of prostate cancer. Int. J. Technol. Assessment Health Care **8**(4): 683–693.

145. GOODMAN, C. & S. R. BARATZ, Ed. 1990. Improving Consensus Development for Health Technology Assessment: An International Perspective.: 163. National Academy Press, Washington, DC.

146. LAZOVICH, D., E. WHITE, D. B. THOMAS, & R. E. MOE. 1991. Underutilization of breast-conserving surgery and radiation therapy among women with stage I or II breast cancer. JAMA **266**(24): 3433–3438.

DISCUSSION

ALAN MORRIS *(Latter-Day Saints Hospital, Salt Lake City, Utah)*: Is there any plan to accumulate data that will ultimately enable you to draw conclusions about the impact of these conferences on physician behavior? For example, would you entertain the idea of putting the results out to selected institutions in an effort to look at pre- and post-conference behavior?

JOHN FERGUSON *(National Institutes of Health, Bethesda, Md.)*: We'd consider that, although it's very difficult to actually measure what the physicians do. As has been pointed out, claims data aren't always the best indication. With our OMB approval we have plans to survey physicians, even though as Jonathan Lomas and others have pointed out, what physicians *say* they do and what they actually do are not always the same. We're open to suggestions—I would very much like to know how much good we're doing.

SUZANNE FLETCHER (Annals of Internal Medicine, *Philadelphia, Pa.*): Having participated in one of these conferences, I was struck by the fact that the rules for participation have been developed in such a way that you don't want anybody with a conflict of interest, which is good. But I wonder whether maybe you've carried that stricture too far. When I was called and asked to participate in a particular conference I agreed but said that I didn't know anything about that field. The persons inviting my input said that's why we want you. But in that 3-day session, in which a great deal of information was presented, I felt very uncomfortable about the fact that I didn't feel like I could evaluate such a great amount of data in 3 days and, moreover, I didn't even know what other data were out there that should have been included because I was not an expert in the field. Do you have thoughts about that?

FERGUSON: You're right—it's very difficult to get the ideal participant. If we get people who have published on it and are very knowledgeable, then we're shooting ourselves. But if we get people who come in with a *tabula rasa*, that's not good either. Our job is to try to educate you beforehand with information that normally takes busy people a month to assimilate, and that is closer to our goal. But you're right—we have been criticized for having panelists who don't know enough about the subject, especially in the area of cholesterol. But I think that smart participants can evaluate what they hear and come to conclusions a little bit more dispassionately than those that are involved in the subject.

DAVID SACKETT *(McMaster University, Hamilton, Ontario, Canada)*: An alternative approach, used both here in the United States by the American College of Chest Physicians and in Canada, is to have the experts there, but to force them to categorize the evidence that they're presenting by its level of scientific validity. We have found that experts, even though they hold strong views, do rapidly achieve consensus on whether they're basing their conclusions and recommendations on results from large randomized trials, overviews, too-small trials, or cohort case series, and they reach rapid consensus on this. We then permit them to make recommendations, but force them to give the grade of evidence that's associated with those recommendations. By this means it seems that we can have the best of both worlds. Having been in a consensus conference here on thromboembolism, I can say that it was very difficult to become sufficiently expert in 3 days to be able to assess the evidence and come up with a coherent statement.

FERGUSON: I'm familiar with that work. It costs money to have somebody evaluate all the literature and I know we all have a limit on that. Your suggestion is very good, Dr. Sackett, and is one of the reasons why we want to start a database of trials with the National Library of Medicine.

Bringing the News to the Public:
The Role of the Media

LAWRENCE K. ALTMAN

The New York Times
229 West 43rd Street
New York, New York 10036

We are here about 90 years too late, but better late than never.

Early in this century a Boston surgeon, Dr. Ernest A. Codman, proposed what he called the "end result card,"[1-3] an evaluation based on a follow-up examination exactly 1 year after surgery or discharge from a hospital. Dr. Codman urged that all hospitals standardize pertinent data and then publish them. He contended that such analyses would substantially reduce the time it took doctors to learn whether certain operations were worth doing or whether they were a waste of time, or even hazardous. For its day, it was a radical suggestion. Today, of course, it's common practice, showing how far we've come.

Dr. Codman also urged that such evaluations be used to assess the types of errors doctors made and to help determine promotions in hospitals and medical schools. Additionally, he believed that patients could use the data in "end result cards" to choose where to obtain medical care.

Where was the Health Care Financing Administration when Dr. Codman needed it? To help patients determine what might be worthwhile, Dr. Codman advocated that they pay consultants, which was not a routine practice at the time. In advocating such consultations, Dr. Codman became an architect of the modern second-opinion programs.

Dr. Codman was a flamboyant, wealthy Boston Brahmin who worked at the Massachusetts General Hospital and taught at Harvard Medical School. After he began practicing medicine in 1895, he learned a lot about "doing more good than harm" and the obstacles that the medical profession created to block his efforts to reach that goal. He was an unrelenting advocate of accountability, efficiency, competition, and even advertising. He strongly promoted the use of statistics to reduce costs and improve quality of medical care.

Dr. Codman knew how hard it is to distinguish between operations that are done to save lives and those to relieve suffering. He also understood the complexities of developing and analyzing statistics relevant to such assessments.

He pointed out that the analyses must account for such variables as the attending doctors, the medical facility where the treatment was carried out, the disease and condition of the patient, and the personal and social conditions influencing the patient's cooperation.

Remember, this was in the early 1900s. We can only imagine how this went over with his colleagues at Harvard and the Massachusetts General Hospital!

In his work, Dr. Codman asked such fundamental questions as:

- What was the patient's problem?
- Did the doctors diagnose it in time?
- Did the patient get entirely well? If not, why not?

• Was it the fault of the surgeon, the disease, or the patient?
• What could be done to prevent similar failures in the future?

Dr. Codman studied the annual reports of many large hospitals elsewhere in the United States, thereby identifying a major obstacle to the compilation of "end result cards": Hospital annual reports scarcely mentioned facts critical for the evaluation of medical care.

It is clear that Dr. Codman's views were unpopular among his colleagues at Harvard and the Massachusetts General Hospital for many reasons. One is that the outcomes of the evaluations might not be complimentary to certain doctors on the staff and to hospital administrators. So he resigned from both positions to open his own private hospital, where he proposed to challenge the underlying beliefs of long-established medical institutions. Dr. Codman lowered the prices to compete with Massachusetts General. He set a maximum surgical fee. The hospital offered the essentials, but no luxuries.

But competing against the Massachusetts General Hospital and other Boston medical centers was difficult, and Dr. Codman lost money. He complained that his competitors, as charitable institutions, received subsidies and did not pay taxes.

He tried to practice what he preached. As part of his plan to develop "end result cards," Dr. Codman petitioned and won permission from the Massachusetts General Hospital to review 2,000 operations he had performed before leaving there. But the Massachusetts General Hospital refused Dr. Codman permission to examine the patients at his new hospital. The fear was that the venerable Massachusetts General Hospital might lose the patients to the upstart Codman Hospital. Because Dr. Codman said he could not afford to leave his new hospital to go to Massachusetts General to carry out the follow-up examinations they were not done. And, eventually, Dr. Codman's hospital closed.

So here we are today, and how pleased Dr. Codman would be, not the least that we are also dealing with far more than surgery in trying to determine how much more good than harm is done in medicine.

Dr. Codman's was a lonely voice, though he did have his followers. One was Dr. William J. Mayo, a founder of the Clinic bearing his name. But Dr. Codman attracted little attention in medical journals or the lay press. In retrospect, that's easy to understand: in those days, medicine was almost entirely a private entrepreneurial business, and nothing like the public institution that it is today. Furthermore, unlike today, medical journals in Dr. Codman's era generally defended vested interests. In those days journalists had little opportunity to expose problems in health care partly because the crucial medical data that critics like Dr. Codman needed were entirely in private hands.

Now the public pays for most medical care through Medicare and Medicaid programs and through third-party insurance plans that are subject to government regulation. And one dividend of the transformation of American medicine from a private entrepreneurial system to a public institution is that the public has gained control over the collection, analysis, and dissemination of medical data. Also, that revolution, making medicine more of a public institution, has given new reason for journalism to cover medicine and to hold medicine's feet to the fire. Just as our Founding Fathers wanted a strong press to challenge the awesome—some might say awful—power of government, journalism has a responsibility to challenge the life-and-death action of doctors, particularly when so much of medical education and research comes from the public purse.

∾

American journalism has an old tradition of reporting on public health. In 1799, for example, when Dr. Benjamin Waterhouse learned about Dr. Edward Jenner's smallpox vaccination technique, Dr. Waterhouse said he "was struck with the unspeakable advantages" that smallpox vaccination could offer.[4] Dr. Waterhouse then proposed its routine use for his fellow Americans through the usual channel of communications—a newspaper article. Dr. Waterhouse said, "As the ordinary mode of communicating even medical discoveries in this country is by newspapers, I drew up the following account of the cow pox, which was printed in the "Columbian Centinal" March 12, 1799." American journalism has continued in that tradition. Many times it has performed extremely well, even though at other times it was deserving of criticism.

At the core of the current journalistic and health policy debate is the charge that the public is paying too much for what it gets in health care. In response, federal and state agencies have begun to evaluate the performance of hospitals and doctors. Each year, for several years, the Health Care Financing Administration has tried to evaluate the performance of hospitals that have received Medicare funds—and that means most hospitals in the United States.[5-7] Independently, the New York State Health Department has developed score cards for heart surgery and other cardiological procedures.[8] Leaders in cardiology and cardiac surgery helped establish the criteria for such evaluations, and several papers describing this work have already been published in medical journals.[9-13]

The current efforts of the Health Care Financing Administration and the New York State Health Department have sparked no less controversy than Dr. Codman did when he was given the cold shoulder by his medical colleagues. In a variant of Dr. Codman's "end result cards," newspapers in New York have published the rank listing of hospitals and doctors performing cardiac surgery. But even in the 1990s, nearly a century after Dr. Codman's pioneering efforts, publishing this information did not come easily. Newspapers had to appeal to the rights upheld in the Freedom of Information Act in order to obtain the information. In the case of the Health Care Financing Administration, it was *The New York Times*, through my colleague Joel Brinkley, that made this effort. In the case of the New York State Health Department, *Newsday* went to court to have the data released. But the debate continues over whether the dissemination of such information does more good than harm[14]—the new head of HCFA, Dr. Bruce Vladeck, for instance, has announced his intention of preventing the public release of such data.[15]

There are valid concerns over using such data as score cards. One reason is the uncertainty about how accurately current methodology can measure the severity of illness in the first place, so that outcomes attributable to the nature of a disease itself may be wrongly blamed on the treatment. Another reason is that surgeons, mindful of their batting averages, might tackle only the easiest cases and avoid operating on the sickest patients.

To be sure, Dr. Codman was not a statistician, and he was hardly on his way to developing meta-analyses, case-control studies, and other tools to measure the effectiveness of interventions. But if the medical journals and newspapers of Dr. Codman's time had supported his position, Richard Peto and Iain Chalmers most likely would not be our honorees at this meeting. Assuredly, others would have come along sooner to do what they have done. Increased discussion and reporting of Dr. Codman's efforts would have encouraged wider acceptance of his proposals, and there would have been many more attempts to develop new modes of statistical analysis. All of these steps would have sped up research into accountability, evaluations, outcomes, and effectiveness of therapies.

I have spoken about Dr. Codman for several reasons. One reason is that his story is not as well known as it should be. In the second place, the nature and importance of journalism's role in disseminating medical information has changed since Dr. Codman's era because of medicine's increasingly public complexion. A third reason is that Dr. Codman's story illustrates some points about doing more good than harm in disseminating information about interventions in medicine.

The public needs information to improve its health and to establish sound health policy. Individuals may need information about conditions that affect them directly. Doctors need information to keep up to date with developments in medicine, even—or particularly—when the news affects events far afield from their specialities. The media disseminate huge amounts of data and report on many types of studies. The reporting of medical data may seem new to many of you, but the phenomenon is not new. What *is* new is the sheer volume of such reporting. This volume reflects not only vast increases in public funding, but also the larger number of scientific advances. Yet, even today, there is little agreement on the best way to disseminate medical information. There may never be agreement between the news media and medicine. But there may one day be a better understanding of one another's special aims and responsibilities.

Scientific journals and the lay press are concerned with new data—both the journals and the lay press deal with news. News can be either entirely new information, or new information about an old subject. It is not repetition of old information (although that may be brought in as background). The trouble is that, for a journalist, what is new may not be true, and what is true may not be new. And by "journalist" I include editors of medical journals who, I believe, are acting as journalists during the hours they edit their journals. So I was delighted to hear Dr. Suzanne Fletcher's remarks at this meeting, and to learn that the editors of medical journals are belatedly discovering that they *are* journalists—a fact that most editors have long denied.

News varies in its importance, both to society and to the readership of a publication, and what is important to each news organization is a matter of judgment. Journalism's role is not limited to reporting the latest advances in medicine and public health, critically important as that function may be. The dissemination of medical information is a decidely more complex task, involving economics, politics, ethics, and many other factors. Journalism prods and probes. Journalism seeks greater accountability, in part by uncovering waste and dishonesty. Journalism also aims at pointing to the need for new ideas. Journalism explores what does and does not make sense. Another journalistic function is to be a provocateur, and one way of doing that is by identifying trends in science and medicine as reported in the professional journals.

Dr. Lucey noted that newspapers have reported on meta-analysis, making the information available to the public, but that many doctors do not even know what meta-analysis is. Dr. Ken Warren, in inviting me to speak at this meeting, specifically cited an article I wrote on meta-analysis in 1990.[16]

One problem in disseminating scientific information is the difference between the way in which scientists and journalists view public controversies. Controversy is the lifeblood of journalism, but most scientists abhor it. Yet, reporting controversy can be educational—but there is an important distinction in what scientists and journalists tend to mean by the word "education".

Scientists tend to think of education in the formal sense, as the kind of schooling in which students are a captive audience, absorbing prescribed material in a predigested course. They go to lectures, no matter how exciting or boring. They may very well gripe about them, but they know they have to listen to them in order to pass examinations and to earn a degree. The captive-audience idea extends to the relation of scientists to scientific journals. The overwhelming majority of scientific journals are aimed at members of the professional society that owns or publishes the journal.

But for laypeople, media journalism is the main form of continuing education after they finish their formal schooling. However, journalism does not grant degrees. Journalism has to compete for the public's attention and time. Thus, journalism must find the quickest and most interesting way to entice readers into a story—no matter how important or trivial the science might be. The journalist must keep the reader in mind, and cannot feel free to "talk to the wall." When I write an article, I try to think of the reader as a patient, as personally concerned with information important to some acknowledged need. I try to anticipate what the patient/reader wants to know and what questions he or she might ask. But I cannot think of all these questions. And if I did, there would not be enough space to publish all the material in an article.

I was also happy to hear Dr. Brook speak out in discussion as a researcher–author to criticize the embargo policy that journal editors enforce, and that I among other journalists have long criticized. In the same discussion Dr. Suzanne Fletcher spoke of financial conflicts of interests on the part of authors, reviewers, and editors. We should also give a thought to the interests of the organizations that own the scientific journals. They refuse to tell you how much money they make or lose, and what they do with the profits. The point is important because much of the research they publish is paid for by the American taxpayer through the National Institutes of Health and other agencies that support the medical centers where the scientists do their work.

At times, there *is* an element of entertainment and drama in journalism. But so too is there one in formal education. Think back on your best teachers. Wasn't it a flair for the theatrical that helped make them so successful? Though there is an educational component in news, reporters think of themselves as informers rather than educators. It's the difference between a scientific lecture session and a continuing medical education course.

When it comes to the dissemination of new information, the professional journals seem to have the upper hand. The journals, for example, exert strong controls on the types of studies that are published. And, in recent years, journals have assumed the primary responsibility for determining the character of most of the scientific information that is disseminated to the public. Endorsing this state of affairs, many scientists and doctors believe that media journalism should play a secretarial role, spoon-feeding to the public only what appears in peer-reviewed journals after the data are published, and not before—not even reporting news from scientific meetings, since about only one-half of the presentations eventually get published.[17,18]

The wisdom of this approach can be debated endlessly, particularly as regards the restriction that information must first be published in a peer-reviewed journal as a means of ensuring the quality of the data disseminated to the public.

But let me say at once that the press—given the nature of its mission—will forever regard such a restriction as unacceptable. In the second place, consider an editorial in the March 1993 issue of the *Archives of Ophthalmology* that implies a challenge to that restriction. The editorial, in effect, says that editors of peer-reviewed journals have published too many articles of poor statistical and methodological design. The editorial focused on the problems that a panel appointed by the U.S. Public Health Service encountered in developing a new guideline for the treatment of cataracts.[19] The panel began its work by evaluating for content and methods 8,000 articles published in peer-reviewed journals in the 15-year period from 1975 through 1990. In the editorial, Dr. Denis M. O'Day wrote: "Despite the large data base, the amount of usable and valid data in the literature proved to be meager since many of the articles were too weak methodologically to be useful. They, therefore, could not provide much information to answer the important questions." If this is true, editors of medical journals—at least in this area—may have been doing less good than they believed in disseminating information to doctors as well as to patients. (Perhaps editors of medical and scientific journals might follow Dr. Codman's example and try to find a way to evaluate their publications periodically.)

In disseminating information, a news organization's primary obligation is to its readers or listeners or viewers. It goes without saying that the news organization should strive above all to report the facts accurately. When circumstances warrant, journalism should also strive to be provocative, to raise questions, and to be skeptical. In fulfilling its responsibilities to report on new advances in medicine, journalism explores many avenues. One is the interview—with doctors, scientists, and patients. Another is the meeting, whatever form this may take. A third is the journal. I doubt that anyone knows what proportion of the information that journalism disseminates about interventions comes from meetings, journals, or interviews. (My impresson is that journalists covered meetings much more in the past than they do now.)

In many ways, journalism is the first draft of history. The dissemination of information about medical advances also proceeds in drafts, and that includes scientific journals. Rarely can a medical story be told in full in one study or one scientific report. News organizations often follow the progress of a line of research. The path usually is winding and often leads to dead ends. Yet the accounts published in medical and scientific journals do not always provide an accurate and complete picture of the complicated process, so that it is unlikely that news organizations serving general audiences will be able to publish all the ins and outs of a research project. But news organizations should nevertheless be free to disseminate information at any step of the process, to report the steps involved, the results of preliminary trials, the caveats, and the follow-ups.

To be fully informative, scientific and medical journals have an obligation to follow up on what they report as preliminary results. Follow-up has been a theme through this meeting, But all too often, early reports are left standing without follow-up—as Dr. Chalmers, our honoree, has reported.[20,21] When a failure to follow up on an initial report is criticized, scientists and doctors typically respond by saying that the failure itself is significant enough. It tells you all you need to know, namely, that the research or therapies or whatever failed along the way. But such silence is too subtle. It smacks of evasion. Doesn't it amount to a different form of publication bias, a bias against reporting failure? The authors of a scientific report and the editors who published their reports should be diligent in following up, particularly when the initial promise fails to hold. When journalists try to follow up many initial reports, they often are handicapped because the authors have not published a follow-up or have not even sought to do so.

We should also take account of disagreement within the scientific community about the relative merits of the different methods for conducting studies. The gold standard today is the double-blind randomized controlled trial. We hear that new therapies should not be approved unless they have been tested in a randomized controlled trial. But it probably is not realistic to believe that everything can be tested in a randomized controlled trial. So in disseminating new medical information, it is unrealistic to think that journalists should be limited to reporting only the results of a randomized controlled trial, or of any single type of study. If news organizations did do that, they would be losing perspective and overlooking the value of anecdotal information. Obviously, the type of study and its statistical reliability are important factors in evaluating the importance of a study. Yet in our zeal for randomized controlled trials, there is a tendency to forget how we got to the point of needing a randomized controlled trial.

Rare indeed must be the research endeavor that started out directly as a randomized controlled trial. The public should be told about the steps leading up to it, about the process of discovery and how new therapies and diagnostic methods are evaluated—sometimes these stories are fascinating. Generally, things get started with an observation or a thesis. In human experiments, scientists generally do not line up hundreds of subjects in military style. They usually start by testing the thesis on one human. Then the researcher moves on to a pilot study. If the results seem favorable, eventually the researcher moves into a larger, randomized controlled trial.

In other words, most research starts out with an original idea and a situation in which, to use statistical jargon, "N equals one". Yet researchers are prone to reflexively scoff at N-equals-one situations, dismissing outright any observation or intervention that involves a small number. True enough, they are generally correct to do so. However, let me remind you that sometimes an N-equals-one fact can have tremendous value. Arguably, medicine's most significant accomplishment resulted from a study in which N equalled one—Jenner's smallpox vaccine. The original report of the study was rejected by a peer-reviewed journal. But Jenner persisted. He published the rejected account of his own as a book. And ultimately, Jenner's technique wiped out smallpox, making it the only natural disease that has been eradicated from the world. It began with an N-equals-one situation, and it went on from there.

I do not want to leave the impression that I advocate making the N-equals-one case the standard for trials in contemporary research, however valuable it may have been to the science of a different era. Nevertheless, we have talked about what can be learned from small trials. The N-equals-one case seems as small a sample as one can get. Yet, as we have heard in this meeting, many common therapies seem to have been based on N equaling zero! And so, lessons from history often can serve us well.

In discussing interventions that do more good than harm, we cannot limit ourselves to therapies. Scientists also intervene in trying to identify and control health hazards, and disseminating the news of both sorts of intervention is one journalistic function.

For example, consider the circumstances surrounding the recognition in 1989 of the relationship between a dietary supplement, L-tryptophan, and eosinophilia myalgia syndrome. A few bright doctors in New Mexico diagnosed the condition in a small number of patients. A reporter for the *Albuquerque Journal*, Tamar Stieber, learned about the cases. She asked the Health Department for further information. However, the New Mexico health officials scolded her for contemplating reporting the cases. The health officials insisted that premature publicity would hamper the investigation they were starting and that making public any suggestion of a link would be irresponsible and unethical.

But the reporter rejected the warning. She reported the cases immediately. The news allowed many primary-care doctors to learn much more precisely—and in timely fashion—about the condition that they were dealing with, a fact that in turn led to the savings of thousands of dollars of unnecessary tests by clinicians and public health researchers. Also, the news allowed readers to identify themselves as victims. Further, Ms. Stieber's reporting led to the quick discovery of a much larger, nation-wide outbreak of the syndrome and to a national recall of L-tryptophan.

Later, when I interviewed doctors and health officials in New Mexico for a follow-up story, they reluctantly conceded that the journalist's reporting had sped up the investigation and aided it in other ways.[12]

And Ms. Stieber won a well-deserved Pulitzer Prize.

Dr. Codman died in 1940, having realized, he said, that "the patients and the public do not yet understand the problem" of professional accountability. Let us hope that the time for that understanding has arrived.

REFERENCES

1. ALTMAN, L. K. The doctor's world: A reformer's battle. New York Times. June 12, 1984: C-5.
2. CODMAN, E. A. 1914. The product of a hospital. Surg. Gynecol. Obstet. **18:** 491–496.
3. CODMAN, E. A. 1916. A Study in Hospital Efficiency: As Demonstrated by the Case Report of the First Five Years of a Private Hospital. Thomas Todd. Boston.
4. WATERHOUSE, B. The history of the kine-pox commonly called the cow-pox. *In* Great Adventures in Medicine. S. Rapport & H. Wright, Eds.
5. BRINKLEY, J. Hospital death rate: At least one plus. New York Times. March 13, 1986.
6. BRINKLEY, J. U.S. releasing lists of hospitals with abnormal mortality rates. New York Times. March 12, 1986.
7. ALTMAN, L. K. Report on mortality: Guarded praise. New York Times. December 18, 1987: B-5.
8. ALTMAN, L. K. Heart-surgery death rates decline in New York. New York Times. December 5, 1990: B-10.
9. HANNAN, E. L., H. KILBURN, J. F. O'DONNELL, G. LUKACIK & E. P. SHIELDS. 1990. Adult open heart surgery in New York State. J. Am. Med. Assoc. **264:** 2768–2774.
10. HANNAN, E. L., H. KILBURN, H. BERNARD, J. F. O'DONNELL, G. LUKACIK & E. P. SHIELDS. 1991. Coronary artery bypass surgery. Medical Care **29:** 1094–1107.
11. HANNAN, E. L., H. R. BERNARD, H. C. KILBURN & J. F. O'DONNELL. 1992. Am. Heart J. **123:** 866–872.
12. HANNAN, E. L., H. KILBURN, M. L. LINDSEY & R. LEWIS. 1992. Clinical versus administrative data bases for CABG surgery. Medical Care **30:** 892–907.
13. HANNAN, E. L., D. T. ARANI, L. W. JOHNSON, H. G. KEMP & G. LUKACIK. 1992. Percutaneous transluminal coronary angioplasty in New York State. **268:** 3092–3097.
14. ALTMAN, L. K. The doctor's world. Surgical scorecards: Can doctors be rated just like ballplayers? New York Times. Jan. 14, 1992: C-3.
15. Associated Press. Rating of hospitals is delayed on ground of flaws in data. New York Times. June 23, 1993: A-19.
16. ALTMAN, L. K. New method of analyzing health data stirs debate. New York Times. August 21, 1990: C-1.
17. RELMAN, A. S. 1979. An open letter to the news media. N. Engl. J. Med. **300:** 554–555.

18. RELMAN, A. S. 1980. News reports of medical meetings: How reliable are abstracts? N. Engl. J. Med. **303:** 277–278.
19. O'DAY, D. M. 1993. A new guideline for patients with cataract. Arch Ophthalmol. **111:** 317–318.
20. CHALMERS, I., M. ADAMS, K. DICKERSIN, J. HETHERINGTON, W. TARNOW-MORDI, C. MEINERT, S. TONASCIA & T. C. CHALMERS. 1990. A cohort study of summary reports of controlled trials. J. Am. Med. Assoc. **263:** 1401–1405.
21. CHALMERS, I. 1990. Underreporting research is scientific misconduct. J. Am. Med. Assoc. **263:** 1405–1408.
22. ALTMAN, L. K. The doctor's world: How medical detectives identified the culprit behind a rare disorder. New York Times. Nov. 28, 1989: C-3.

DISCUSSION

UNIDENTIFIED SPEAKER: Four or five years ago Elizabeth Whalen published an article showing that magazines that took cigarette advertising seldom ran stories about the hazards of cigarettes. Would you comment on the influence of advertising on the selection of topics for stories?

LAWRENCE ALTMAN (The New York Times, *New York, N.Y.*): This is an important issue. My reporting has not been influenced by advertising. To get a broader perspective on the issue, studies could be done as they are in medicine. It would be useful to look at the policies of newspapers, magazines, and television and radio stations. As I view it, the *New York Times*'s extensive reporting on smoking and health outweighs the impact of cigarette advertising. The point we are discussing applies to any publication that becomes too heavily dependent on any type of advertising revenue. Newspapers, for example, once were said to rely too heavily on department store advertising. Now newspapers are hurting because they have lost a lot of department store advertising resulting from the demise of many stores, at least in New York City. As for the influence of advertising on the selection of articles, we should strive harder to learn about how the point applies to the drug industry and publications in the scientific literature. Some journals that eked out a small profit measured in thousands of dollars 25 years ago more recently have become accustomed to profits in the millions of dollars, chiefly due to increased revenues from drug company advertising and reprint fees. For many reasons, drug companies are now cutting back on advertising, and representatives of these journals are complaining about the loss of advertising income.

UNIDENTIFIED SPEAKER: I'm a freelance medical writer and I teach medical writing at NYU. You said that when you are writing your articles you imagine yourself talking to a patient, which provides a good perspective to your work. I've been working with a group called the International Medical Benefit Risk Foundation in Geneva and we're trying to come up with ways of improving the reporting of risk in the media. This work is still very preliminary, but one of the things that is coming up in discussion is that everybody uses relative risk. Relative risk makes a better story, both for the journals and for the newspapers, although they usually give a poor idea of that person's absolute risk. Preliminary talks with some journalists showed that it was difficult to find discussions of absolute risk in the papers they read, and while I don't believe journalists should be spoon-fed, they should ask these questions and the information should be available. It would help if investigators were able to tell us other measures of both risk and benefits of treatment, things like numbers needed to treat and absolute risk. I want to repeat these concerns in a company of epidemiologists because this sort of information would help us put the things we report into perspective.

ALTMAN: I agree with you and I can think of a couple of times in recent weeks where I put in this information when it was not reported by the authors.

RICHARD DOLL (*Radcliffe Infirmary, Oxford, England*): Obviously the journalist has his ordinary responsibility in reporting any event to check that the report is reliable and to attempt to make some assessment of the character of the source of the information before reporting it. But I don't think that's any different for so-called medical discoveries and for anything else that the journalist is concerned with. To me it seems that the principal responsibility lies with the scientist in releasing the information, and if the scientist releases information it's fair game. And he mustn't complain if it is reported. I don't think that there should be reports until after papers have been published in peer-reviewed journals, but if the scientist releases the information beforehand then he has no justifiable complaint if someone takes that up. So to my mind the responsibility is equally shared and as often as not when there are complaints, when things go wrong, it is because the scientist has released the information without checking his results and seeing that they are repeatable.

ALTMAN: Thank you; I'm glad to hear you say that.

Some Problems in Applying Evidence in Clinical Practice[a]

R. BRIAN HAYNES

Health Information Research Unit
McMaster University
Faculty of Health Sciences
1200 Main Street West
Hamilton, Ontario, Canada L8N 3Z5

INTRODUCTION

The increased public and private investment in biomedical and health care research since the Second World War has led to a burgeoning flow of accurate diagnostic tests and efficacious treatments. This presages a new era in which there is an evidential basis for health care, but there remain at least two fundamental barriers blocking the way to this goal. First, the evidence that is generated from most applied research in health care and services provides incomplete coverage of the clinical situations that confront practitioners, so that application of evidence in practice is far from straightforward. Second, the health care system and its practitioners have difficulty implementing changes even when the evidence clearly supports those changes. Thus, there is a large gap between what sound evidence shows will work or not work, and what patients and the public receive in the name of health care, even when care is not restrained by resources.

There are numerous ways of characterizing barriers to the successful application of health care evidence[1] and at least 50 randomized trials of interventions designed to overcome them.[2] Nevertheless, our understanding of the barriers remains incomplete and the effects of interventions to date are not impressive, with studies showing that practitioner performance can be changed at most by a modest amount, with even less effect on patient outcomes. Furthermore, the interventions that have some impact on performance or outcome have not been tested for durability and also would be very expensive to implement on a broad scale. It is clear that we do not understand the problems of improving practitioner performance well enough to overcome them efficiently. While empirical research should continue, we may profit by exploring why interventions have not been more successful.

The purpose of this paper is to seek better understanding of the barriers to dissemination and application of validated health care knowledge, mainly by juxtaposing the steps that must be taken to apply sound health care evidence with the problems that practitioners face in engaging fully in this process. I will dwell on the problems of translating evidence into action without delving into ways to overcome them. (This would be a morose task if it were not for the following paper, by Jonathan Lomas,[3] which deals in part with solutions.)

[a] This work was supported in part by the B. C. Decker Health Informatics Research Fund. Dr. Haynes is supported in part by a National Health Scientist Award from the National Health Research and Development Program of Canada.

As a point of departure, I will address only those situations in which sound evidence fails to have the impact on health care practice that it merits, not those in which faulty or incomplete evidence penetrates practice, receiving greater application than it merits, or situations in which practitioner performance changes in the absence of evidence. This focus on faulty application of validated interventions is rather narrow. No one knows exactly the proportion of all clinical interventions for which there is sound evidence for or against clinical application, but it is likely less than half. For example, in their comprehensive review of randomized controlled trials of interventions in obstetrics and childbirth, Iain Chalmers, Murray Enkin, and Marc Keirse[4] list 43 forms of care that improved outcomes, 36 that appeared promising but required further evaluation, 86 with unknown effects, and 61 forms of care that should be abandoned in the light of available evidence. Thus, sound evidence of value could be found for only 19% of clinical procedures, and sound evidence of lack of value for a slightly higher percentage, 27%. It is these two groups that provide the starting point for the paper.

Furthermore, my perspective mainly will be that of the health care practitioner in a decision-making role, rather than that of co-providers, the patient, administrators, or third-party payers. In taking the perspective of the providers of services, I am aware of the models of "continuous quality improvement" and "total quality management," which attribute problems in the quality of health care to faults in the system rather than in individuals.[5,6] For the most part I agree with this model as an attractive approach to the solutions for the problems—but I will focus on the problems and not the solutions.

THE MAGNITUDE OF THE PROBLEM

Numerous studies have documented the extent to which implementation of evidence from sound health care research has fallen short of the ideal, and the following reports illustrate this over the past three decades. Stross and Harlan demonstrated substantial delays in the awareness of family physicians and internists about the value of photocoagulation for diabetic retinopathy.[7] These investigators later showed delays in awareness of new information about the management of hypertension.[8] More recently, Williamson and his colleagues found that primary care practitioners lacked awareness of several common and recommended procedures for patient management.[9] Anderson and colleagues[10] recently reported that less than a third of patients at high risk for venous thrombosis and pulmonary embolism in 16 hospitals received prophylaxis, with variation in implementation in the hospitals ranging from 9% to 56%. For thrombolytic therapy during acute myocardial infarction, life-sparing benefits consistently have been shown in trials since the early 1970s,[11] but in two hospitals in Southern Ontario, streptokinase was used appropriately in just 36% of patients in 1990, with a decrease to 29% in 1991[12] after publication of consensus guidelines by the Canadian Cardiovascular Society.[13] This finding is perplexing since both hospitals had participated in international trials of streptokinase during the 1980s, which formed the basis for the guidelines.

Despite increasing numbers of new, effective treatments and increasing research in continuing education[2] and quality improvement, there is little evidence that we are improving the speed and fidelity with which validated health care evidence is deployed. This begs the question of what is wrong.

TABLE 1. Barriers to Dissemination and Application of Health Care Evidence from the Perspective of the Practitioner

Steps	Major Barriers	
Getting the evidence straight	Difficulties in finding sound evidence	Time pressures
Developing clinical policy	Unclear standards of evidence and interpretation	Time pressures
Applying clinical policy	Mismatch between evidence and clinical situations	Time pressures

A SIMPLE MODEL OF THE STEPS FROM EVIDENCE TO APPLICATION

Simplistically, one can characterize the transformation of evidence into action as requiring three steps (TABLE 1). The first of these steps is getting the evidence straight; the second, developing the evidence into clinical practice guidelines; and the third is applying clinical practice guidelines to the right person at the right time, and in the right way (the "three Rs of application"). Each step is at least partly dependent on the successful negotiation of the preceding step, so that problems in the first and second steps can accumulate and multiply their effects on the third and final step. Furthermore, failures in one of the higher steps can nullify successes in preceding steps. Each step has its own unique problems, but one problem runs through all: time pressures. I will use this framework to identify and describe some of the obstacles that block the path from evidence to application.

Getting the Evidence Straight

Recalling that the departure for this essay was studies providing convincing evidence of the value of specific clinical procedures, we see that there are a number of problems in "getting the evidence straight." Two groups of these problems include the difficulties of finding of sound evidence and time pressures in assembling, evaluating, and interpreting evidence.

Difficulties of finding sound evidence. Practitioners face many frustrations in attempting, themselves, to retrieve evidence to support clinical decisions. First, practitioners seeking evidence that they do not already know about often will not know in advance whether there is any good evidence or where or how to find it. The odds are that a blind search will not be productive. As the work of Chalmers, Enkin, and Keirse shows,[4] there are many clinical interventions for which there is inadequate evidence of efficacy. The majority of searches are ill-fated at the outset for lack of adequate evidence, and practitioners may need to do searches on several different topics to find one piece of solid evidence. For example, in a recent study of MEDLINE use in clinical settings, less than 1% of citations retrieved on questions of clinical management contributed to a new or changed decision.[14] This appears to be a key reason why practitioners do not turn to the medical literature when questions arise in clinical practice.[15]

Second, for most clinical topics there is no practical way to invoke closure on an unproductive search for evidence. Most information sources are not well organized for clinical practice[16] so that it is not possible to determine for an unproductive search whether there is no adequate evidence or the search simply failed to uncover the evidence. A resource such as the Oxford Database of Perinatal Trials[17] can overcome this, and the Cochrane Collaboration will rapidly extend this service for topics in other clinical disciplines.

Third, most health care practitioners are not well versed in the handling of research evidence. Thus, when definitive evidence is uncovered, its value may remain opaque to the seeker. It is to be hoped that the principles of evidence-based medicine will quickly take hold,[18] but this is not the case now.

Fourth, even if there were adequate evidence for clinical decisions and clinicians had the skills (or the staff) to assemble the evidence, it is likely to be buried in a plethora of evidence of lesser ilk, much of it conflicting, and much of it claiming to be adequate. Thus, a considerable amount of sorting is required to retrieve applicable and acceptable evidence from all reports even with the advantage of electronic access.

Time pressures. It can take considerable time and resources to assemble and evaluate evidence. Most health professionals pace themselves quickly, allowing little time for each problem they confront, with no scheduled time for seeking answers to questions that arise. Of interest, when Covell and colleagues observed how internists dealt with questions that arose in clinical practice, 70% of the questions went unanswered and internists gave lack of time and out-of-date textbooks as reasons.[15]

Electronic information services can provide access to current medical research evidence in clinical settings. Many libraries have modern information tools, but these tools usually are not situated in clinical settings, and are not used much even when they are available.[14] Furthermore, for whatever reason, most clinicians do not provide themselves with personal access to electronic information services. For example, when the American College of Physicians (ACP, Philadelphia, PA) and the National Library of Medicine (NLM, Bethesda, MD) offered unlimited use of MEDLINE to ACP members in 1992 for an annual flat fee of $200, including software, only 850 of the 77,483 members signed up.[19] Even when MEDLINE access was made available at no charge in clinical settings in a teaching hospital, average use was less than twice a week,[14] even though a study in a similar setting had shown that MEDLINE was among the best potential sources of information for about one question per patient.[20] Although it would be easy to label physicians as Luddites, they are no strangers to adopting new technology, and at least part of the problem is with the state of electronic information services. As a manifestation of the relatively low yield from a general bibliographic database such as MEDLINE, the average time to complete a MEDLINE search on a clinical problem was over 20 minutes in one study,[21] and then the search provided the searcher with only a set of citations and abstracts to sort through.

An alternative to electronic access is a textbook such as *Scientific American Medicine*,[22] which comes in subscription form with regular updates, usually driven by new evidence. While this is an important advance on traditional textbooks, it lacks a systematic and explicit policy for the collection and interpretation of evidence, and there is a considerable logistical burden to replacing obsolete text with new. The CD-ROM version of *Scientific American Medicine* can overcome this problem, but not many clinicians have equipped themselves with CD-ROM access.

The usual alternative to looking up the answers for clinical questions is to refer the patient to a specialist,[15] but this cannot easily occur in isolated communities. Even when specialists are available, referral does not occur if the physician is unaware of his own ignorance, particularly if the problem falls within the scope of problems for which the practitioner is expected to be expert. Referring to an expert also increases the time and cost for the patient to get an answer for his or her problem.

Finally, even if practitioners do take the time and trouble to assemble, sort, and synthesize evidence, they are confronted by the perishability of evidence, so that evidence forays must be repeated periodically. For example, studies of the efficacy of digoxin in patients with congestive heart failure in sinus rhythm show a benefit,[23] but these studies were all done before the advent of angiotensin-converting enzyme (ACE) inhibitor therapy, and it is not known whether digoxin now has any incremental value for patients for whom ACE inhibition is appropriate. Unfortunately, there can be no "best before . . ." time dating on evidence and it doesn't smell when it is overripe. Thus, practitioners lack reliable warnings of when new evidence should be considered, and efficiency in doing so is problematic. Current information resources are certainly not adequate for decision support at the usual breathless pace of health care. It is worthwhile noting here that one of the most important and attractive features of the ***Oxford Database of Perinatal Trials***[17] and the promised progeny of the Cochrane Collaboration is continuous updating of the trials database and regular updating of the reviews.

Developing Evidence into Clinical Practice Guidelines

While attention to appropriate research evidence can reduce the uncertainty in making a clinical decision, evidence from research can be only one element in the decision process. Other elements include the severity of the patient's condition, co-morbidity and other treatments, the patient's personal preferences and situation, and so on. How the evidence is to be combined with the other elements is often problematic, and may be one of the most important barriers to application of new knowledge. Although there are many organizations now involved in developing clinical practice guidelines to assist practitioners, they do not currently cover more than a fraction of health care and thus most of clinical practice continues to be based on the knowledge, beliefs, and actions of individual practitioners.

Of interest, there is a considerable difference between what doctors say their clinical policy is, what expert groups recommend, and what actually happens. For example, Woo and colleagues[24] studied the screening practices of internists and found for a sample of patients that published guidelines recommended mammography for 185 patients, internists recommended mammography for 59, and that the procedure was actually performed for only 9 patients. It would be easy in this situation to blame the practitioners for being lazy, forgetful, or disorganized, but it is fairer to say that we do not understand the reasons for the discrepancies between evidence, policy, intentions, and practice. Ironically, the clinicians' actions for mammography may have been more appropriate than their words or those of the expert groups in light of new evidence concerning the lack of efficacy of mammography.[25,26] One wonders how the disparity among recommendations, intentions, and actions can be resolved and in this case, even whether it should be.

During the past decade, professional organizations and scientific bodies have attempted to help practitioners bridge the gap between evidence and practice by investing increasing resources in developing clinical practice guidelines. In 1990, the Institute of Medicine (Washington, DC) defined guidelines as "systematically developed statements to assist practitioner and patient decisions about appropriate health care for specific clinical circumstances."[27] (Products of attempts to develop rules for clinical practice go by many names, including parameters, guidelines, standards, and algorithms, of which guidelines is the commonest and will be used generically here.) Ideally, clinical practice guidelines are the product of available evidence, clinical experience, and collective wisdom, and provide guidance for clinical actions that is true both to the strengths and limitations of evidence, and to the circumstances of clinical practice.

At their best, clinical practice guidelines are formulated in an explicit way that permits users and observers to follow and verify the process as being an accurate reflection of evidence and responsive to the circumstances of clinical practice. The pitfalls in attempting to achieve this balance are plentiful. In addition to problems in "getting the evidence straight," difficulties include unclear standards for evidence assessment and interpretation, and time pressures in the consensus process. The net result of these problems can be disagreement among the recommendations from different groups about the same clinical problems, leading to confusion and rejection by intended users.

In illustrating the problems, I will pay particular attention to the National Institutes of Health (NIH, Bethesda, MD) consensus process since this is highly visible, prolific, and well described.[28-31] It has many robust features, including broad representation of experts and stakeholders, extensive advanced preparation, public participation when appropriate, detailed evidence review, and widespread dissemination of the recommendations of the conference. It is important to bear these strengths in mind when considering what I believe to be some weaknesses from the perspective of improving the linkage between evidence and clinical practice.

Unclear evidence standards. Standards for assembling, evaluating, analyzing, and interpreting evidence have been developing rapidly,[32,33] but there is no general agreement on whether or how these standards should be applied in making clinical practice recommendations. The Canadian Task Force on the Periodic Health Examination,[34] the U.S. Preventive Services Task Force,[35] and the American College of Chest Physicians[36,37] (ACCP, Northbrook, IL) have pioneered the approach of "levels of evidence" based on scientific merit, and "grades of recommendation" based on the level of evidence supporting a recommendation, but other organizations are just beginning to follow suit. Even when there is an extensive literature review in support of clinical recommendations, consensus committees may not connect items of evidence with specific recommendations, making it difficult for users to verify the process and, at least as important, to determine when new evidence might supersede the recommendation. For example, as of early February, 1993, the 1990–1993 current MEDLINE file listed 120 citations under the term "consensus development conference, NIH (pt)", which reported on consensus conferences on 25 unique topics, 22 of which provided no references for their recommendations. In discussing this with John Ferguson, the Director of the Office of Medical Applications of Research (OMAR, Bethesda, MD), which organizes the NIH consensus conferences, consensus committees are given the option of citing references in their publications, but this option is seldom exercised. Thus, only those who attended the consensus conference will know what and how evidence has been considered.

Even if groups attempting to formulate clinical policy conduct a thorough review of evidence and have adequate time to formulate recommendations, and attempt to cite evidence in support of their recommendations, uncertainties remain in how far to generalize the evidence, how far to go in making recommendations when there are gaps in the evidence, and what other factors should be taken into account. The result of these uncertainties is that different expert bodies take different approaches to handling evidence in formulating recommendations, and may issue conflicting statements, all claiming to be based on the "best scientific evidence."

Comparison of the current recommendations from two expert bodies about the screening and treatment of elevated cholesterol illustrates this problem.[38] Although the guidelines for the two groups are based on much of the same evidence, the U.S. National Cholesterol Education Program (NCEP) recommends screening all people over 20 years of age,[39] whereas the Canadian Task Force (CTF) recommends screening males between 35 and 59 years and others at high risk.[40] The level for diet intervention is set much lower by the NCEP. The result for men aged 35 to 59 years is that intervention would be prescribed for 54% in the U.S. but only 19% in Canada. The implications of the two policies for practitioners are profoundly different. Which one is "correct"? How can the practitioner or patient decide? Whether one or neither of the sets of recommendations is correct, their disagreement undermines the credibility of the consensus process. Attempts to document and overcome "missed opportunities"[41] by physicians, based on the more aggressive NCEP recommendations, appear to be premature. The fallout will be worse still if practitioners actually follow recommendations that are eventually shown to do more harm than good.

How could this have happened if the consensus groups started with the same evidence? Clearly, there must be disagreement about the strengths and limitations of the evidence or the role of evidence in making recommendations for health care practice. There may also be a host of distorting influences, including the quest for simplification so that practitioners will find recommendations easier to apply; vested interests, both personal and financial; the imperative to "do something"; group and interpersonal dynamics in the consensus process so that the views of the strongest or most persistent prevail; the mistaking of expertise, experience, and logic for generalizable knowledge; and overly optimistic notions (such as that diet recommendations can do no harm even if we cannot be sure that they will be of benefit). Unless there is agreement on, and acceptance of, standards for the assembly, synthesis, interpretation, extrapolation, and application of evidence in developing clinical practice guidelines, and how far guidelines should go in the absence of conclusive evidence, the guideline movement risks undermining its credibility. Fortunately, there are efforts to improve the consensus process.[31,42]

Time pressures in the consensus process. It takes time and resources to assemble evidence and time to publish and disseminate recommendations based on evidence, both of which make it demanding to accomplish the tasks satisfactorily while the evidence is still current. For practical reasons, most meetings to formulate clinical practice guidelines convene for two or three days at most, which may—or may not—provide for full consideration of the evidence and achievement of meaningful consensus on its interpretation. For example, the NIH has a formula for consensus conferences that provides just over two days for evidence presentation and discussion, development of recommendations, and presentation to a press conference. Even with the considerable background work that takes place before each meeting, it seems unlikely that a fixed meeting time would be appropriate for all topics. The requirement for reaching recommendations and reporting them to the press in just over two days is administratively tidy, but may undermine the final product. Presumably, this is one of the reasons why NIH consensus conference committees choose not to include references in their final reports. If the fixed duration also undercuts systematic and comprehensive review of the evidence, then the recommendations may also suffer.

Once recommendations are made, there is often an unpredictable delay until publication, during which time new evidence may become available. Even if there is no new evidence in the interval to publication, there is seldom provision for regular review of recommendations. Although there have been attempts to warn users about the need for updating after a period of time,[13] such predictions are bound to be speculative. It would take considerable resources and monumental organizational efforts to ensure regular review of practice guidelines. It is conceivable that this could occur with international collaboration, but the professional societies that often take on this type of activity are mainly organized within national boundaries and may even see similar organizations in other countries as rivals, competing for whose current round of recommendations is published first.

Despite the problems with practice guidelines, progress is being made in developing a rigorous process that will do justice to both evidence and clinical realities.[43]

Applying Evidence and Clinical Practice Guidelines

As mentioned, for most clinical situations practitioners remain responsible for whatever attention is paid to evidence in clinical practice. Even when strong evidence is faithfully embedded in clinical practice guidelines from an authoritative source, there are numerous impediments to delivering evidence to the patient in the right way at the right place and at the right time. Two groups of these impediments include mismatches between evidence or guidelines and clinical situations, and time pressures in health care practice.

Mismatches between evidence or guidelines and clinical situations. Most clinical trials are quite narrow in their scope and attempt to answer a question for patients who are carefully selected to maximize risk for adverse outcomes and responsiveness to the intervention that is being tested. Combining the results of multiple trials on the same type of clinical problem can help to "fill in the blanks" for different types and severity of clinical presentations, but the process of addressing all clinical issues that relate to even a single clinical disorder is daunting. Take, for example, thrombolytic therapy for acute myocardial infarction, one of the most important and well-documented breakthroughs in modern therapeutics. According to the current evidence-based clinical practice guidelines,[44] based on a multitude of trials, patients should receive streptokinase for acute myocardial infarction only if they have chest pain typical of myocardial infarction and at least 1-millimeter ST-segment elevation in at least two adjacent-limb electrocardiographic leads or at least 1–2 millimeter ST-segment elevations in at least two adjacent precordial leads. They should not receive thrombolysis if they have had a cerebrovascular hemorrhage, a recent nonhemorrhagic stroke, peptic ulcer, surgical wound, or previous use of streptokinase, or diabetic proliferative retinopathy, or if they are pregnant, or have a bleeding disorder, hepatic dysfunction, pancreatitis, or severe hypertension, or if they might have aortic dissection, or if they are more than 6 hours' beyond the time of onset of their myocardial infarction (or 24 hours, depending on which evidence one goes by[45]). If one uses the entry criteria of the trials as the basis for deciding who should receive thrombolytic therapy, it has been reported that the overwhelming majority of patients presenting with myocardial infarctions—as many as 90%—are ineligible.[46] But many of the "ineligible" patients are likely to have "relative" contraindications, leaving the practitioner in a situation of having to process a considerable amount of information about the patient only to find that clear evidence is lacking to support a decision for them.

Two consecutive patients who recently were cared for on my clinical service illustrate the problem:

A 78-year-old woman presented to the emergency room of our hospital with dyspnea, discovered on examination to be due to congestive heart failure. She denied any history of myocardial infarction or prolonged chest pain, but had deep Q-waves in four precordial leads of her electrocardiogram, indicating that she had had an anterior myocardial infarction at some undetermined time. Further, her electrocardiogram showed 1.5-mm ST-segment elevation in two adjacent precordial leads.

Minutes later a 50-year-old man arrived with crushing retrosternal chest pain radiating down his left arm, following 2 weeks of chest tightness on exertion. His electrocardiogram showed ST segment elevation of less than 1 mm in two limb leads and three lateral chest leads.

The first patient met the electrocardiographic criterion for thrombolytic therapy, but she did not have chest pain, and so did not meet the second essential criterion.[44] Cardiac enzyme tests subsequently showed a rise indicating acute myocardial damage, but the lack of chest pain meant she lacked a reference time for judging whether thrombolytic therapy might be beneficial since this must be given within the first 24 hours of an infarct to be effective. Judging by the changes in her electrocardiogram and the enzyme rise, however, she likely developed her congestive heart failure because of acute myocardial ischemia. Furthermore, even though silent myocardial ischemia and infarction are well recognized, it is unlikely that there will ever be evidence concerning whether she should be given thrombolysis, because she does not meet the entry criteria that are currently used for trials or likely to be used in the future.

The second patient had classical chest pain for acute myocardial infarction, but did not quite meet electrocardiographic criteria for this and so was not given streptokinase. Subsequently, his cardiac enzymes showed that he had indeed suffered an acute myocardial infarction, but these results were not available until about 20 hours after the onset of chest pain and it was decided to forego streptokinase therapy at that late time.

If one can extrapolate from the status of evidence in obstetrics to that in cardiology, even for the 20% or so of clinical interventions for which there is unequivocal evidence of benefit, only some patients with the specific clinical problem for which an intervention has been found beneficial will have the features regarded as appropriate for the intervention's application. Attempting to sort out which patients should have what validated procedure and providing this validated procedure at the right place in the right way at the right time is not a straightforward task. At present there is incomplete evidence concerning most clinical procedures, even for those procedures for which the evidence is strongest, and in most clinical situations the evidence is too slim for clinicians to apply it easily or well. To put this in perspective, almost all clear-cut evidence about the value of health care interventions has been generated in the past three decades and the coverage of clinical problems is rapidly expanding; thus, the current limitations of evidence will dissipate with time. Nevertheless, practitioners are very accustomed to making decisions in situations of uncertainty and the opportunities in which it is not necessary to do so may be so few at present that there is little impetus to shift from the current "experiential" and "qualitative" modes of conducting practice to a quantitative or "evidence-based" mode.

Even when there is strong evidence concerning specific interventions, the decision to intervene must be tempered by consideration of other aspects of the patient's clinical situation (including the severity of the patient's condition, comorbidity, treatment allergies and intolerances and so on) and by the patient's personal wishes (including his aversiveness to risk, and his desire to live or die). These additional considerations may explain much of the apparent discrepancy between practice guidelines, clinician's general policies, and the clinician's decisions for individual patients.[47]

The situation for thrombolytic therapy for acute myocardial infarction is typical, not unique. For example, trials of antihypertensive therapy have been producing results for almost three decades now and there is still not conclusive evidence that pharmacologic intervention for individuals with uncomplicated mild hypertension does more good than harm.[48,49] Thus, the current recommendations of the Canadian Hypertension Society call for "clinical judgment" in dealing with such patients, "taking into account" other risk factors (gender, race, age, family history, cholesterol, diabetes and so on) in deciding whether to initiate therapy.[50]

Given the complexity of clinical situations that arise for the same disorder, and the difficulty and cost of doing clinical trials, it will be a very long time before we generate answers to most of the questions that confront practitioners. Thus, bridges from evidence to clinical practice are bound to be fragile for the foreseeable future. There is a real risk during this period that bridge builders will discredit themselves if they succumb to the "imperative" to build bridges on quicksand either by failing to do justice to good evidence or by making recommendations when there is no good evidence. Unfortunately, they may also paint themselves into ivory towers, so to speak, from the perspective of full-time clinicians, if they do not provide "grade C" recommendations when no "grade A" recommendations can be made because of lack of solid evidence. There is a difficult balance here that needs to be addressed at "consensus conferences on consensus conferences" such as that held recently by a partnership of professional medical bodies in Canada.[42]

Time pressures. It takes time to learn new procedures and ways of delivering care. The forms of continuing education that have been tested and found effective include such methods as supervised practice or preceptorships that are labor-intensive for both the practitioner and the CME provider.[2] Unfortunately, practitioners prefer to spend their learning time discussing patients with their colleagues, reading, or attending rounds or conferences,[51] activities for which there have been no studies of effectiveness. Even if journal-reading were an effective way to learn of new evidence, there is too much new evidence for individual practitioners to consume, journals are too poorly organized for clinical practitioners to use,[16] and practitioners readily admit that they are overwhelmed by the literature.[52] Much of the time that practitioners are willing to put into continuing education may be misspent.

Perhaps the most potent stimulus to learning is a patient's problems for which the practitioner is unsure of the answer. The style of medical practice, however, does not include time for effective continuing education when clinical opportunities arise for application of new procedures. As Covell and colleagues discovered,[15] practitioners have good intentions about looking up the answers to questions that arise when seeing patients, but seldom seek answers for these questions because of lack of time.

Some forms of health care must be delivered within a very brief time window to be effective, and for many patients there may not be enough time to deliver the treatment at the right time. Thrombolytic therapy must be given within a few hours to be fully effective, but patients often delay coming for care, and many hospitals are not properly organized to minimize the delay in administration of appropriate therapy.[53] It takes additional time to determine whether a patient is an appropriate candidate for thrombolysis. Although this time may be modest for each patient, if only one in ten qualifies according to current guidelines, the time burden may be excessive, discouraging attempts to be certain that every patient who could benefit receives this treatment.

DISCUSSION

Consideration of some of the problems of evidence about health care interventions and its diffusion, dissemination, and application provides ample reason for concern about the prospects for a tight linkage between evidence and practice in the near future. Health care trials that ask pragmatic questions are very expensive and seldom done, but we need more of these to provide practitioners with less fragmentary evidence concerning the value of tests and interventions in usual clinical circumstances. A source of funding for more pragmatic trials could be through elimination of unnecessary replications. Ongoing cumulative meta-analyses of clinical trials would permit earlier decisions about which questions no longer need to be studied, and the Oxford groups[4,54–56] and their colleagues in Boston[11,57] and around the world[58] have shown us how to go about this. Furthermore, pooling of trials permits examination of the effects of interventions in subgroups of patients who are not represented in enough numbers in individual trials. This is important and essential research itself and must be elevated in status and funding so that no evidence from trials is wasted. As new evidence accumulates, the waste becomes increasingly tragic.

The process of developing clinical practice guidelines that attempt to merge evidence with clinical practice circumstances is difficult, and more resources and work are needed to improve this process. A committee of the Institute of Medicine[31] reviewed the process for NIH consensus conferences and recommended a number of improvements including permitting a more flexible period of time for meeting, depending on the topic; grading evidence for quality; including experts in applied research evidence (epidemiologists and biostatisticians) in the guidelines process; preparing an overview and meta-analysis of existing evidence before the consensus conference; having speakers provide a standardized summary of their answers to the questions being addressed by the conference, including the specific evidence in support of these answers; not allowing speakers to make verbal presentations of unpublished evidence except in exceptional circumstances; and indicating in conference reports the degree of agreement for individual recommendations. Some of these recommendations have been adopted by the NIH, including preparation of meta-analyses for some meetings for which it is appropriate, and inclusion of an epidemiologist or biostatistician on committees dealing with applied research evidence. However, the recommendations on the grading of evidence and indicating the degree of dissent have not yet been adopted, and citing of evidence in consensus conference reports is a seldom-used option (J. Ferguson, Director of the Office of Medical Applications of Research, personal communication). More recently, a coalition of professional and medical education groups in Canada has produced a consensus on guidelines for developing clinical practice guidelines[42] that will provide a better link between evidence and practice if followed.

Of the many barriers to applying evidence at the bedside, perhaps the most important is that current methods of continuing education and quality improvement are expensive and inadequate. There is not enough research into the nature of the problems of continuous improvement of performance in the special situation of health care in which the evidence base keeps changing. A recent review of evidence concerning continuing education interventions[2] uncovered only 50 randomized controlled trials, spread thinly across a large variety of interventions, and showing modest effects on performance with inconsistent effects on the health of patients. The stimulus for more and better research for this orphan area may come from the realization that we can no longer afford a casual approach to the gap between evidence and practice. It is troubling to spend billions on health care research while neglecting the fact that most of the evidence generated from such studies is going to waste because we do not know how to overcome the problems of dissemination and application.

Nevertheless, there is considerable reason for hope. The process of dissemination of evidence is slow, but practice does improve with time, as shown by increases in the proportion of hypertensive patients who are successfully treated at the community level.[59] Eventually self-directed lifelong learning[60] and the teaching of evidence-based medicine[18] may take hold, so that practitioners learn during their training how to learn for the rest of their professional lives, becoming adept at keeping up with new evidence and applying it to the betterment of their patients' health. There are also additional measures that can be mobilized to improve the application of new knowledge, as the following paper by Jonathan Lomas describes.

SUMMARY

There is a considerable gap between sound evidence concerning health care interventions and the services that patients actually receive as health care. Practitioners and the health care system must overcome a number of barriers to narrow the gap. Viewed simplistically, there are three steps from evidence to practice: getting the evidence straight; developing clinical practice guidelines that are faithful to both the evidence and the clinical and personal situations of patients; and applying these guidelines to the right patient at the right time in the right way. Special problems in getting the evidence straight stem from difficulties in finding sound evidence. Lack of agreement on evidence standards undermine the effectiveness of authoritative practice guidelines. Applying evidence and practice guidelines effectively and efficiently is often thwarted by mismatches between evidence and usual practice circumstances. Time pressures undermine interpretation and application of evidence at every step. Understanding these problems may permit development of more effective strategies to bridge the gap between evidence and practice.

REFERENCES

1. LOMAS, J. & R. B. HAYNES. 1988. A taxonomy and critical review of tested strategies for the application of clinical practice recommendations: From "official" to "individual" clinical policy. Am. J. Preventive Med. 4(Suppl. 2): 77–94.
2. DAVIS, D. A., M. A. THOMSON, A. D. OXMAN & R. B. HAYNES. 1992. Evidence for

the effectiveness of CME. A review of 50 randomized controlled trials. JAMA **268:** 1111–1117.

3. LOMAS, J. 1993. Diffusion, dissemination and implementation: who should do what? Ann. N.Y. Acad. Sci. This volume.

4. CHALMERS, I., M. ENKIN & M. J. N. C. KEIRSE, EDS. 1989. Effective Care in Pregnancy and Childbirth. Vol. **2:** 1471–1476. Oxford University Press. Oxford, UK.

5. BERWICK, D. M., A. ENTHOVEN & J. P. BUNKER. 1992. Quality management in the NHS: The doctor's role—I. Br. Med. J. **304:** 235–239.

6. BERWICK, D. M., A. ENTHOVEN & J. P. BUNKER. 1992. Quality management in the NHS: the doctor's role—II. Br. Med. J. **304:** 304–308.

7. STROSS, J. K. & W. R. HARLAN. 1979. The dissemination of new medical information. JAMA **241:** 2622–2624.

8. STROSS, J. K. & W. R. HARLAN. 1981. Dissemination of relevant information on hypertension. JAMA **246:** 360–362.

9. WILLIAMSON, J. W., P. S. GERMAN, R. WEISS, E. A. SKINNER & F. BOWES, III. 1989. Health science information management and continuing education of physicians. Ann. Intern. Med. **110:** 151–160.

10. ANDERSON, F. A., JR., H. B. WHEELER & R. J. GOLDBERG. 1991. Physician practices in the prevention of thromboembolism. Ann. Intern. Med. **115:** 591–595.

11. ANTMAN, E. M., J. LAU, B. KUPELNICK, F. MOSTELLER & T. C. CHALMERS. 1992. A comparison of results of meta-analyses of randomized control trials and recommendations of experts. JAMA **268:** 240–248.

12. HOLBROOK, A., R. B. HAYNES & M. JOHNSTON. 1993. The quality of prescribing for myocardial infarction [abstract]. Clin. Invest. Med. **16**(Suppl.): B19.

13. FALLEN, E. L., P. ARMSTRONG, J. CAIRNS, W. DAFOE, N. FRASURE-SMITH, A. LANGER, D. MASSEL, N. OLDRIDGE, D. PERETZ, G. J. TREMBLAY *et al.* 1991. Report of the Canadian Cardiovascular Society's Consensus Conference on the Management of the Postmyocardial Infarction Patient. Can. Med. Assoc. J. **144**(8): 1015–1025.

14. HAYNES, R. B., M. E. JOHNSTON, K. A. McKIBBON & C. J. WALKER. 1993. A randomized controlled trial of a program to enhance clinical use of MEDLINE. Online J. Current Clin. Trials. Doc. No. 56.

15. COVELL, D. G., G. C. UMAN & P. R. MANNING. 1985. Information needs in office practice: Are they being met? Ann. Intern. Med. **103:** 596–599.

16. HAYNES, R. B. 1990. Loose connections between peer-reviewed clinical journals and clinical practice. Ann. Intern. Med. **113:** 724–728.

17. CHALMERS, I., ED. Oxford Database of Perinatal Trials. Oxford Electronic Publishing. Oxford University Press. Oxford, UK.

18. EVIDENCE-BASED MEDICINE WORKING GROUP. 1992. Evidence-based medicine: A new approach to teaching the practice of medicine. JAMA **268:** 2420–2425.

19. ACP Update. 1993. ACP renews flat fee program with NLM; enrollment open year round. ACP Observer **13:** 7.

20. OSHEROFF, J. A., D. E. FORSYTHE, B. G. BUCHANAN, R. A. BANKOWITZ, B. H. BLUMENFELD & R. A. MILLER. 1991. Physicians' information needs: Analysis of questions posed during clinical teaching. Ann. Intern. Med. **114:** 576–581.

21. HAYNES, R. B., K. A. McKIBBON, C. J. WALKER, N. C. RYAN, D. FITZGERALD & M. F. RAMSDEN. 1990. Online access to MEDLINE in clinical settings. A study of use and usefulness. Ann. Intern. Med. **112:** 78–84.

22. RUBENSTEIN, E. & D. D. FEDERMAN, EDS. Scientific American Medicine. Scientific American Inc., New York.

23. JAESCHKE, R. & G. H. GUYATT. 1989. To what extent do congestive heart failure patients in sinus rhythm benefit from digoxin therapy? A systematic overview and meta-analysis. Am. J. Med. **88:** 279–286.

24. WOO, B., B. WOO, E. F. COOK, M. WEISBERG & L. GOLDMAN. 1985. Screening procedures in the asymptomatic adult. Comparison of physicians' recommendations, patients' desires, published guidelines, and actual practice. JAMA **254:** 1480–1484.

25. MILLER, A. B., C. J. BAINES, T. TO & C. WALL. 1992. Canadian National Breast

Screening Study: 1. Breast cancer detection and death rates among women aged 40 to 49 years. Can. Med. Assoc. J. **147**: 1459–1476.

26. MILLER, A. B., C. J. BAINES, T. TO & C. WALL. 1992. Canadian National Breast Screening Study: 2. Breast cancer detection and death rates among women aged 50 to 59 years. Can. Med. Assoc. J. **147**: 1477–1488.

27. FIELD, M. J. & K. N. LOHR, EDS. 1990. Clinical Practice Guidelines: Directions for a New Program.: 38. Committee to Advise the Public Health Service on Clinical Practice Guidelines, Institute of Medicine. National Academy Press. Washington, DC.

28. OFFICE OF MEDICAL APPLICATIONS OF RESEARCH, NATIONAL INSTITUTES OF HEALTH. 1988. Guidelines for selection and management of consensus development conferences. OMAR. Bethesda, MD.

29. JACOBY, I. 1985. The consensus development program of the National Institutes of Health. Int. J. Technol. Assess. Health Care. **1**: 107–115.

30. KANOUSE, D. E., R. H. BROOK, J. D. WINKLER, *et al.* 1989. Changing Medical Practice through Technology Assessment. An Evaluation of the NIH Consensus Development Program. The Rand Corporation. Santa Monica, CA.

31. Consensus Development at the NIH: Improving the Program. 1990. Institute of Medicine. National Academy Press. Washington, DC.

32. LIGHT, R. J. & D. B. PILLEMAR. 1984. Summing Up: The Science of Reviewing Research. Harvard University Press. Cambridge, MA.

33. OXMAN, A. D. & G. H. GUYATT. 1988. Guidelines for reading literature reviews. Can. Med. Assoc. J. **138**: 697–703.

34. GOLDBLOOM, R., R. N. BATTISTA & J. HAGGERTY. 1989. The periodic health examination: 1. Introduction. Can. Med. Assoc. J. **141**: 205–208.

35. HARRIS, S. S., C. J. CASPERSEN, G. H. DEFRIESE & E. H. ESTES, JR. 1989. Physical activity counseling for healthy adults as a primary prevention intervention in the clinical setting. Report for the US Preventive Services Task Force. JAMA **261**: 3588–3589.

36. SACKETT, D. L. 1989. Rules of evidence and clinical recommendations on the use of antithrombotic agents. Chest **95**(Suppl.): 2S–4S.

37. COOK, D. J., G. H. GUYATT, A. LAUPACIS & D. L. SACKETT. 1992. Rules of evidence and clinical recommendations on the use of antithrombotic agents. Chest. **102**(Suppl.): 305S–311S.

38. KRAHN, M., C. D. NAYLOR, A. S. BASINSKI & A. S. DETSKY. 1991. Comparison of an aggressive (U.S.) and a less aggressive (Canadian) policy for cholesterol screening and treatment. Ann. Intern. Med. **115**: 248–255.

39. Report of the National Cholesterol Education Program Expert Panel on the Detection, Evaluation, and Treatment of High Blood Cholesterol. 1988. Arch. Intern. Med. **148**: 36–69.

40. CANADIAN TASK FORCE ON THE PERIODIC HEALTH EXAMINATION. 1993. Periodic health examination, 1993 update: 2. Lowering blood cholesterol to prevent coronary heart disease. Can. Med. Assoc. J. **148**: 521–538.

41. GILES, W. H., R. F. ANDA, D. H. JONES, M. K. SERDULA, R. K. MERRITT & F. DESTAFANO. 1993. Recent trends in the identification and treatment of high blood cholesterol by physicians. Progress and missed opportunities. JAMA **269**: 1133–1138.

42. CARTER, A. 1992. Clinical practice guidelines. Can. Med. Assoc. J. **147**: 1649–1650.

43. BATTISTA, R. N. & M. J. HODGE. 1993. Clinical practice guidelines: Between science and art. Can. Med. Assoc. J. **148**: 385–389.

44. CAIRNS, J. A., V. FUSTER & J. W. KENNEDY. 1992. Coronary thrombolysis. Chest. **102**(Suppl.): 483S–507S.

45. ISIS-2 (Second International Study of Infarct Survival) Collaborative Group. 1988. Randomised trial of intravenous streptokinase, oral aspirin, both or neither among 17,187 cases of suspected acute myocardial infarction. Lancet **2**: 349–360.

46. DOOREY, A. J., E. L. MICHELSON & E. J. TOPOL. 1992. Thrombolytic therapy of acute myocardial infarction. JAMA **268**: 3108–3114.

47. REDELMEIER, D. A. & A. TVERSKY. 1990. Discrepancy between medical decisions for individual patients and for groups. N. Engl. J. Med. **322**: 1162–1164.

48. MacMahon, S., R. Peto, J. Cutler, R. Collins, P. Sorlie & J. Neaton, *et al.* 1990. Blood pressure, stroke, and coronary heart disease. Part 1: Prolonged differences in blood pressure: Prospective observational studies corrected for the regression dilution bias. Lancet **335**: 765–774.
49. Collins, R., R. Peto, S. MacMahon, P. Hebert, N. H. Fiebach & K. A. Eberlein, *et al.* 1990. Blood pressure, stroke, and coronary heart disease. Part 2: Short-term reductions in blood pressure: Overview of randomised drug trials in their epidemiological context. Lancet **335**: 827–838.
50. Haynes, R. B., Y. Lacourciere, S. W. Rabkin, F. H. H. Leenen, A. G. Logan, N. Wright & C. E. Evans. 1993. Practice guidelines for the diagnosis of hypertension in adults. Report of the Canadian Hypertension Society Consensus Conference Committee on Diagnosis. Can. Med. Assoc. J. **149**: 409–418.
51. Fox, R. D., P. E. Mazmanian & R. W. Putnam. 1989. Changing and Learning in the Lives of Physicians. Praeger. New York.
52. Williamson, J.W., P. S. German, R. Weiss, E. A. Skinner & F. Bowes III. 1989. Health science information management and continuing education of physicians. Ann. Intern. Med. **110**: 151–160.
53. Doorey, A. J., E. L. Michelson & E. J. Topol. 1992. Thrombolytic therapy of acute myocardial infarction. Keeping the unfulfilled promises. JAMA **268**: 3108–3114.
54. Chalmers, I., K. Dickersin & T. C. Chalmers. 1992. Getting to grips with Archie Cochrane's agenda [editorial]. Br. Med. J. **305**: 786–788.
55. Peto, R. 1987. Why do we need systematic overviews of randomized trials? Stat. Med. **6**: 233–244.
56. Collins, R., R. Gray, J. Godwin & R. Peto. 1987. Avoidance of large biases and large random errors in the assessment of moderate treatment effects: the need for systematic overviews. Stat. Med. **6**: 245–254.
57. Lau, J., E. M. Antman, J. Jiminez-Silva, B. Kupelnick, F. Mosteller & T. C. Chalmers. 1992. Cumulative meta-analysis of therapeutic trials for myocardial infarction. N. Engl. J. Med. **327**: 248–254.
58. Oxman, A. D. & G. H. Guyatt. 1988. Guidelines for reading literature reviews. Can. Med. Assoc. J. **138**: 697–703.
59. Birkett, N. J., C. E. Evans, R. B. Haynes, D. W. Taylor, D. L. Sackett, J. R. Gilbert, M. E. Johnston, S. A. Hewson & L. A. Macdonald. 1986. Hypertension control in two Canadian communities: Evidence for better treatment and overlabelling. J. Hypertension **4**: 369–374.
60. Shin, J. H., R. B. Haynes & M. E. Johnston. 1993. The effect of problem-based, self-directed undergraduate education on life-long learning. Can. Med. Assoc. J. **148**: 969–976.

DISCUSSION

Henry Greenberg *(St. Luke's-Roosevelt Medical Center, New York, N.Y.):* I agree that the refinements of clinical trials, such as the entry data, sometimes skew the population so that applicability is a problem. But I think that the example you use is a poor one and creates a poor impression. The entry criteria for the streptokinase trials are no different from any clinician's entry criteria for any patient. Perhaps the only thing that the trials initially restricted that would not be restricted in practice is age, but all of the items you listed for not giving streptokinase are simply common-sense clinical reasons for not giving it unless you were against the wall thinking that you had an imminent death on your hands. The clinical trials are not restricting the population entry into the trial any more than a clinician would judge the patient eligible for the drug under virtually any circumstance.

BRIAN HAYNES *(McMaster University, Hamilton, Ontario, Canada)*: I disagree that it's a poor example. I have partly relied on anecdotal evidence and partly made my remarks on the basis of the evidence that we generated from looking at the appropriateness of care according to the guidelines in our own area. I don't know how generalizeable that is, but I don't believe that the self-reports of clinicians about their policy corresponds very closely to what actually happens in practice. In only about 30% of patients for whom the guidelines appear to apply was the care actually provided. I tried to get a sense of this when I was on the ward service in January, when several patients came through for whom the residents, who saw the patients first during the night, had not applied thrombolytic therapy. When we reviewed the guidelines we saw that there were good reasons for withholding streptokinase therapy. Yet in both cases we reviewed in our paper, it is arguable that the care should have been or could have been provided. But it fell outside the limits of what had been recommended in the American College of Chest Physicians' guidelines for practice.

So there is a disjunction between what the evidence covers and what actually occurs in practice. I endorse Bob Brook's opinion about the difference between clinical practice circumstances and the types of patients who end up in clinical trials. I think you're getting a very selective group of patients in the trials and when you try to apply the trial evidence to patient care, you find out that there are many reasons why you don't want to apply the recommendation.

GREENBERG: Your general statement is valid. As director of a coronary care unit, I see this sort of thing a lot—we administer thrombolysis to 50% or more of our patients using precisely those same criteria; in fact, we use more because our residents will call up an attending physician in the middle of the night to say, for example, that a patient has retinopathy but here is the clinical situation and here's the time frame. We will break the guidelines in the sense of balanced clinical risk, but I still insist that streptokinase is not a good example for the point that you want to make and that you weaken your own point by using that particular example.

UNIDENTIFIED SPEAKER: It occurred to me that medicine can't be the only field facing this problem of rapid dissemination and application of new technologies. Fields that come instantly to mind include agriculture and new cars, which have changed considerably so that mechanics have to be brought up to speed. Are there other models from other fields that we should be thinking about?

HAYNES: The original studies of dissemination were in agriculture, for example, where attempts were made to introduce new seed lines. That's where the idea of educational influentials came in, which was one of the prominent approaches. I'm suggesting that if you take a look at the studies that have tested those innovations that have been based on research in other fields and applied to medical care, you find only a modest effect on practitioners' behavior, which makes it very difficult to document a difference in patient outcomes. We're stuck at that plateau and we need to go beyond what has been achieved in other fields because it's not good enough. We need more social scientists to pay attention to medical care: It's been a problem that biomedical science has dominated so much in terms of funding for health care research. That situation is starting to change, but it hasn't changed enough. We still need more of a social science orientation in the research we're doing if we're going to understand these application problems.

Diffusion, Dissemination, and Implementation: Who Should Do What?

JONATHAN LOMAS

Centre for Health Economics and Policy Analysis
Health Sciences Centre
McMaster University
1200 Main Street West
Hamilton, Ontario, Canada L8N 3Z5

I wish to discuss and interrelate three processes in this paper: the way in which information flows from a source, the way in which information is received by individuals and organizations and becomes knowledge, and the way in which individuals and organizations turn knowledge into changes in their behavior. Finally, I will discuss the implications of this analysis for assignments of roles to the various parties in the delivery of medical care.

THE FLOW OF INFORMATION FROM A SOURCE

Diffusion, dissemination, and implementation are all terms used, sometimes interchangeably, to denote the idea that information must be part of a communication process before it is available as an input to decision-making. Their connotations are, however, quite different.

Diffusion is a passive concept. Light diffuses from a source; it is not targeted; it is haphazard; it is largely unplanned and uncontrolled. Those who receive diffused messages were likely already open to and seeking out the message. They were active seekers in the face of a passive flow of information. This describes the medical journal and the (increasingly rare) medical journal reader seeking the primary source. In a recent survey fewer than 25% of physician leaders regularly did personal on-line searching of the literature and only 5% of community physicians did so.[1] The probability that the contents of a single article in a medical journal will be recalled is obviously very small. Diffusion is a form of communication that works well only when the potential recipients are highly motivated, when the rewards of finding the information are high (such as clear and unambiguous implications for behavior), and when there is a relatively small pool of information, which minimizes the search costs. These conditions do not hold for today's busy physician faced with conflicting, confusing, and voluminous findings from research.

Dissemination is a more active concept. It not only implies a more aggressive flow of information from the source, almost a launching, but it also implies targeting and tailoring the information for the intended audience. Secondary sources such as meta-analyses, overviews, practice guidelines, consensus statements, and seminal or compelling primary studies are most likely to receive such treatment. Although medical journal publication may be part of a dissemination process, such messages will also be relayed by press coverage, targeted mailings, orchestrated campaigns of oral presentation, and even formal advertising. If the message is relevant for the physician's practice, there is a good probability that she will be exposed to the message whether she wants such exposure or not. If awareness of a message is the goal, the audience is identifiable and the message tailored to its needs, dissemination is an effective form of communication. For instance, awareness of one consensus statement after a comprehensive dissemination process to all members of that particular specialty was nearly 90%.[2]

Implementation implies that the goal of the communication is, however, to do more than increase awareness. Not only is the message tailored to the needs of a general audience, but also the implications of the message for the specific practices of a specific audience must be highlighted. Implementation involves identifying and assisting in overcoming the barriers to the use of the knowledge obtained from a tailored message. It is a more active process still, which uses not only the message itself, but also organizational and behavioral tools that are sensitive to the constraints and opportunities of identified physicians in identified settings. It is a *local* process of communication in which appreciation of the research findings is a necessary but not sufficient condition to bring about changes in decision-making that reflect the message from research. It is a persistent process that seeks to communicate the findings from research through numerous routes and in numerous ways that make it difficult for the physician to ignore as she goes about her day-to-day activities.

The public policy decisions of governments are diffused through technical, legislative and regulatory statutes available to the knowledgeable and motivated interests. Dissemination of public policy relies, however, on the media and targeted information campaigns originating with government to communicate the intent and practical implications of a legislative statute. Implementation of these same decisions is dependent on a complex framework of sanctions and incentives, reinforced by monitoring and adjustment, and often adapted to fit differing environments at more local levels.

Similarly in medicine, the "statutes" of valid and reliable research findings require more than diffusion—publication of the technical details in a journal rarely leads to changes in decision-making. Diffusion, dissemination, and implementation are not interchangeable terms; they are phases in a process of increasingly active and more focused intents, with each subsequent phase dependent on the success of its predecessor phase.

THE RECEIPT OF INFORMATION BY A TARGET AUDIENCE

In the previous section I have argued that diffused information is unlikely to reach most physicians until it has been adopted by the small number of active information-seeking practitioners and organizations, tailored to their needs, and disseminated in a modified and more relevant form. But what is the impact of this disseminated information when it does reach the physician? Do they become widely aware of the information? Do their attitudes to the relevant area of practice change? Is there an increase in their knowledge? Does their behavior change?

These questions have been addressed in a few recent studies, but I will use our own work on cesarean section rates in Canada to illustrate the impact of disseminated information on cognitive and behavioral outcomes.[2,3] First, however, I will relate these potential cognitive and behavioral changes to a model of physician behavior change initially developed from psychology to inform work in the area of health promotion and patient behavior change. Green and colleagues highlight the importance of classifying messages (and activities) as predisposing, enabling, and/or reinforcing changes in behavior.[4] Relatively "weak" messages from outside the physician's immediate environment may generate cognitive changes in awareness, attitude, and knowledge that predispose them to consider altering behavior, but these factors may not be enough to generate the actual alterations. Behavioral change relies on more potent enabling factors, such as those encountered in a local environment on a day-to-day basis that capitalize on previously generated predispositions. Finally, enabled changes are sustained by reinforcing factors from both the local and the more distant environments.

Dissemination activities for practice guidelines, consensus statements, and other forms of tailored information appear to fall into the category of predisposing activities. They are received by the relevant audience as importance contributors to changed awareness, attitudes, and even knowledge, but are not sufficient to enable changes in behavior. In our study of cesarean section practices, the targeted dissemination of a practice guideline resulted in high levels of awareness, a significant change in attitudes, somewhat less impact on knowledge, but a widespread self-declared intent to change practice. Unfortunately these good intentions did not translate into any observable changes in the use of cesarean section.

As a follow-up to this we focused implementation (rather than just dissemination) efforts, in a randomized controlled trial, on local enabling factors to bring about the implied changes in behavior. Where the enabling technique relied on more than traditional information and education approaches (i.e., the empowerment of a local opinion leader), we were successful in bringing about at least some of the desired behavioral change.[5]

Thus emerges some identities between the process of information flow *to* physicians and the process of information receipt *by* physicians. Diffusion of "raw" information through medical journals leads to uptake by highly motivated physicians, researchers, and their organizations. These parties, in turn, produce synthesized and tailored information which is disseminated and received by physicians in a way that predisposes them to consider, but not actually engage in, changes in behavior. Finally, implementation efforts at the local level, with the disseminated information tailored further and embedded in a larger communication process, capitalize on the predisposition and are received by physicians as enabling and eventually reinforcing the implied changes in their practices.

INSIDE THE BLACK BOX OF BEHAVIOR CHANGE

So far I have presented the "magic" of implementation as something of a black box, referring in passing to the importance of the local environment and of enabling and reinforcing factors. In this section I will review four areas of study that have contributed significantly to our understanding of this process whereby disseminated research information is translated into local knowledge and thus implemented as changed practices.

Lessons about how to flow research findings into practice can be extracted from the "social influences" literature, studies of the diffusion of innovations, adult learning theory, and marketing theory.

The social-influences model finds roots in psychology and sociology and the concept of local norms. "The behavioral models of decision-making underlying the social-influence perspective holds that peers' judgement and beliefs play a major role in an individual's evaluation of new information and that peers' beliefs and attention patterns help determine the salience of information and provide interpretations and judgements regarding its implications for behavior" (p. 414).[6] In contrast to isolated diffusion or dissemination processes, social-influence approaches point to habit, socially accepted norms of appropriateness, and peer acceptance as the motivators for behavioral change, rather than such rationality as cost-benefit analyses and imputed impacts on patient outcomes. Modelling behavior as a member of a social grouping takes precedence over acquiring and applying information as an isolated individual.

The second area, studies on the diffusion of innovations, has largely been the domain of sociologists such as Coleman and colleagues,[7] Rogers,[8] Stocking,[9] and Greer.[10] In this field the term "diffusion" is used in a less restricted way than in my definition. It refers to the general process of adopting and incorporating innovations into routine practice.

By observing how medical innovations actually find their way into local practice, investigators in this field have highlighted three important considerations. First, the closed nature of most medical communities and the importance of local product champions and opinion leaders: "the central theme of medical diffusion studies is that physicians act as communities rather than aggregates of unrelated individuals and that medical behavior is literally contagious" (p. 208).[11] Second, the dynamic nature of diffusion, wherein modification and adaptation to the local circumstances occurs as part of a staged process of adoption: "if the innovation is defined too explicitly with too many restrictions on its modification, then its diffusion may be hindered" (p. 75).[9] Third, and in contrast to the social-influences model, diffusion theory isolates important characteristics of an innovation (rather than the practitioner's environment) that influence the diffusion process: its "relative advantage" (for the adoptee and for patient care), its "compatibility" (with personal and local norms), its "complexity," its "trialability" (or extent to which it can be tried temporarily and discarded if found wanting), and its "observability" (or how easily one can see whether the expected results are being achieved) have been identified.[8]

Adult learning theory also focuses on the characteristics of the expected behavior change (or innovation) as well as of the practitioner's environment. Based on interviews with 356 physicians, the book *Changing and Learning in the Lives of Physicians* by Fox, Mazmanian, and Putnam[12] isolates three areas of consideration in understanding the behavior change process for already-practicing physicians:

(1) the force for change—personal and internal catalysts appear to be better motivators than professional, which in turn are preferable to external and social motivators;

(2) the mode of learning—once a decision to change has been made, the mode of learning is influenced by the catalyst: experiential or informal learning is more likely in addressing personal motivators; formal and deliberative learning is associated more with professional catalysts; and compliance (not necessarily accompanied by learning) is often associated with social or external pressures for change; and

(3) the size of expected change in behavior—this will influence the probability of embarking upon the change process: four categories range from small "accommodations," through larger "adjustments" or "redirections," to complex and major "transformations."

Adult education approaches highlight the importance of personal motivation rather than coercion in achieving sustained behavior change, and the fact that "learning sometimes . . . was used to help prepare to change, and to verify that the change was positive and valuable" (p. 174).[12] Education and the consequent learning are not, therefore, useless, but they contribute to predisposing practitioners to consider change and reinforce that change once it has occurred; however, they rarely enable the actual change.

Finally, change in physicians' behavior is now being addressed by marketing approaches, following the development of social marketing techniques to sell health promotion to the general public.[13] Many of the principles for this approach are derived from advertising and the literature on persuasive communication: "it distinguishes five attributes of communication that are consistently important: the "source" or originator of the communication; . . . the "channel" or medium of presentation; the "message" content itself; the characteristics of the "audience" receiving the communication; and finally, the "setting" in which the communication is received" (pp. 314–315).[14] This literature also makes a distinction between communications that merely increase awareness and those that may actually bring about changes in behavior. The latter consists of a more restricted set of influences that focus on influential persons as the source, personalized interactions as the channel, local anecdote or experience as the message, opinion leaders as the audience, and informal environments as the setting. It is noteworthy that few, if any, of these considerations are to be found in the traditional educational communication of research findings, although most *are* found in the promotional and marketing efforts of pharmaceutical companies.[15]

Each of these four approaches makes both unique and common contributions to our understanding of the process of actually implementing research findings into physicians' practices. A focus on social influences underlines the need to view physicians as members of small, locally based, and closed medical communities in which research findings must find resonance with existing norms and values. Studies on the diffusion of innovations also emphasize the importance of the local medical community and its influential members, but in addition draw attention to the need to disseminate modifiable messages from the research that can be adapted to fit the local environment. Adult learning theory highlights the need for the physician to be predisposed to accept change before efforts are made to implement it, that is, behavioral change is a dynamic process, and not an overnight event or coercive act. Finally, the marketing literature once again stresses the value of using local agents-for-change as part of the dissemination process for the research message as well as ensuring that the message itself is tailored to the concerns of the target physician.

The physician is, therefore, not a *tabula rasa* waiting to be informed. She has existing beliefs, practice policies, and habits, and these are reinforced by the numerous routes of influence in her local environment. Common to all four of the approaches reviewed in this section is the message that physicians are subject to powerful and potentially determining influences in their local environments. In broad terms these influences are mapped in the coordinated implementation model (FIG. 1) as educational, administrative, personal, patient-based, community-based, and economic. Even with research information that, after diffusion, has been synthesized and then disseminated by a credible body, its impact is likely to go no further than the awareness, attitude, and knowledge of the physician without active and coordinated implementation efforts. Finding ways to ensure that the research information flows as freely through the administrative, economic, community, and patient routes of influence as it does through the educational route will

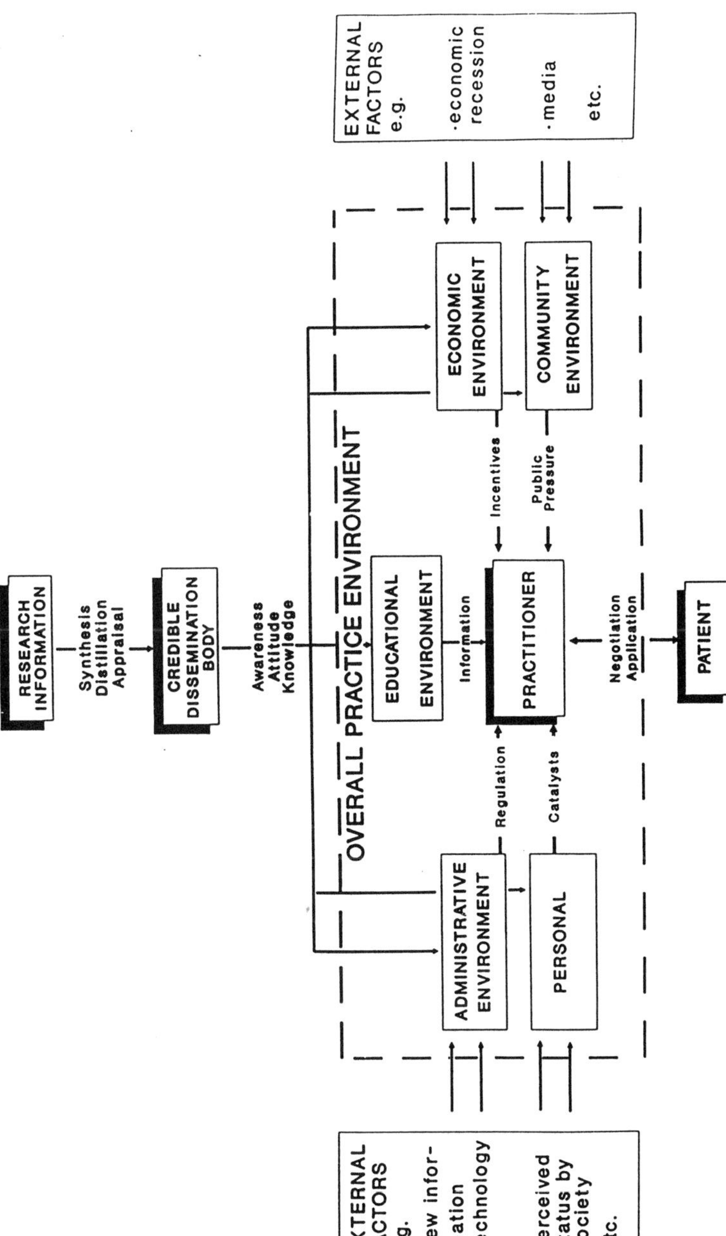

FIGURE 1. The coordinated implementation model.

significantly enhance the probability of successful implementation through changes in the behavior of the physician.

In summary, research findings are most likely to be implemented into practice when most or all of the following conditions hold:

- the diffused research is synthesized by a credible and influential body and disseminated in a "user friendly" format with a message that justifies the need for change by comparison with existing approaches, norms and concerns (i.e., it is a persuasive communication);
- the implied change is implementable within flexible parameters and implementation is within the power of the target physician without the need for extensive collaboration and cooperation with others;
- the existence and importance of the research findings are communicated to the physician from a variety of sources both within and outside the local community;
- there are respected and influential local exemplars considering or actually adopting the findings for their own practices;
- there is an opportunity to explore the implications of the research findings in a personal encounter with either an influential local colleague or respected outside authority; and
- adoption of the findings will not come into conflict with the economic or administrative incentives of the physician's working environment, nor with the expectations of his patients or the communities from which they come.

ASSIGNING ROLES

Although the previous section makes it clear that extensive implementation activities are required in the local environment, it also emphasizes the importance of the prior predisposing activities of diffusion and dissemination. Given the different skills and tools required for each of these three activities—diffusion, dissemination, and implementation—it would be reasonable to assume that different types of individuals and organizations are appropriate for the lead role at each stage.

Diffusion activities require extensive attention to the validity and reliability of the research information because this information is the core building block around which further efforts will be built. It is for this reason that primary research studies should not be excessively marketed and highlighted, but rather left for the "experts" to find based on a study's methodologic quality rather than its promotional prowess. Biomedical journals are potentially well suited to continue their role as the agents of diffusion, although as Haynes points out,[16] there is still room for improvement in how well they both assure validity and reliability of published studies, and differentiate the types of communication (hypothesis-generating versus hypothesis-confirming, for instance). The extent to which pharmaceutical or other narrow interests acquire control over this diffusion role is also of obvious concern.[17]

Insofar as there are still imperfections in the "quality assurance" processes of journals for the studies they publish (diffuse), dissemination agents should have ethical, as well as methodologic and communication expertise. Indeed dissemination can be seen as at least a three-stage process:

(1) a decision on the methodology for synthesizing the information;
(2) the decision of what is ethically defensible as a message, given the state of the evidence; and
(3) the communication of the message, preferably by a credible body.

There are few organizations or individuals in whom all three skill areas reside. Most academic medical centers contain the first two, but not the last. Most medical societies and specialty groups may contain the last but not the first two. The implication is that collaboration is required (and is emerging) between academics on one side and various medical societies, medical specialty groups, and even government agencies on the other side. Practice guideline and consensus statement programs have sprung up under the sponsorship of numerous groups, and perhaps the pressing issue now is how to distinguish between the ethical and the unethical, the valid and the invalid, messages that are being disseminated by this variety of sponsors. It is unfortunate that validity of the disseminated message and credibility of the disseminating agent are not always positively related.

Assignment of responsibility for implementation of these disseminated messages has to incorporate the observation that it is the physician's local environment of daily or weekly contacts that principally determines final adoption decisions. Disseminated research findings have to be adapted to the local norms and values, the systems and incentives in place in the local hospital or health care facility, and the attitudes and expectations of the immediate community and its patients. This cannot easily be done by some outside agent, but rather requires local agents knowledgeable about, and credible within, the specific medical environment. The appointment by medical authorities of local "geographic scholars," who continue to practice but are also paid to be a conduit between the disseminating agents and the community, is one potential model. Such geographic scholars could be responsible for set communities, empowered with resources and encouraged to undertake whatever local educational, administrative, economic, or public information measures they deemed necessary to implement the disseminated research. They would be unlikely to be successful if their sponsors were government or payers, but might well garner the necessary support if they were seen as specialty society- or medical society–sponsored, with a link to a designated academic center.

To an extent continuous quality improvement (CQI) incorporates many of the principles of a successful local implementation initiative.[18] Its focus is on administrative as well as educational incentives and it recognizes the physician as a fallible member of an operating local system. Thus the increasing focus of local institutions in the health care field on CQI may well become a major vehicle for implementation of research findings. Familiarity with CQI principles may become an expectation for health care managers at all levels of the system, and they may thus become active agents of change by capitalizing in their own institutions on the predisposing activities of dissemination agents outside the community.[19]

Yet to be assigned a role in the diffusion, dissemination, and implementation process is government. The principal tools at its disposal are economic and regulatory—both tools with a strong coercive element. Although government can potentially use these tools in an effective way—altering the economic incentives within a fee schedule, for instance—perhaps their preferable role is merely to exist, at least for the time being, as a visible entity holding these *potential* powers. The "threat" value (somewhat coercive in itself) may be the catalyst needed to ensure that physician organizations and local health care facilities take seriously their role in using diffusion, dissemination, *and* implementation to more effectively flow research findings into practice. If these roles are not taken seriously, no one could blame government for exercising fully the tools at its disposal by making the incentives of medical care remuneration and regulation policy more responsive to and reflective of valid research findings.

SUMMARY

The concepts of diffusion, dissemination, and implementation are distinguished as progressively more active steps in the process of flowing valid and reliable research information into clinical practice. Using a staged model of behavior change, diffusion is seen as a precursor for dissemination activities, which in turn "predispose" physicians to consider change in their practices. Local implementation activities capitalize on this by "enabling" and subsequently "reinforcing" the desired behavior change. Different skills are needed for each activity. Biomedical journals, with some improvements, are identified as diffusion agents. Collaboration between academics and medical organizations is best suited to the dissemination stage. Local agents, empowered by resources, are best equipped for implementation activities.

REFERENCES

1. WILLIAMSON, J. W., P. S. GERMAN, R. WEISS, E. A. SKINNER & F. BOWES. 1989. Health science information management in continuing education of physicians: A survey of U.S. primary care practitioners and their opinion leaders. Ann. Intern. Med. **110:** 151–160.
2. LOMAS, J., G. M. ANDERSON, K. D. PIERRE, E. VAYDA, M. W. ENKIN & W. J. HANNAH. 1989. Do practice guidelines guide practice? The effect of a consensus statement on the practice of physicians. N. Engl. J. Med. **321:** 1306–1311.
3. LOMAS, J. 1993. Making clinical policy explicit. Lessons from legislative policy for the development of practice guidelines. Int. J. Technol. Assess. Health Care **9:** 11–25.
4. GREEN, L. W. & ERIKSEN, M. P. 1988. Behavioral determinants of preventive practices by physicians. Am. J. Prevent. Med. **4**(Suppl. 1): 101–107.
5. LOMAS, J., M. W. ENKIN, G. M. ANDERSON, W. J. HANNAH, E. VAYDA & J. SINGER. 1991. Opinion leaders vs. audit and feedback to implement practice guidelines. Delivery after previous cesarean section. JAMA **265:** 2202–2207.
6. MITTMAN, B., X. TONESK & P. JACOBSON. 1992. Implementing clinical practice guidelines: Social influence strategies and practitioner behaviour change. Qual. Rev. Bull. (December): 413–422.
7. COLEMAN, J., E. KATZ & H. MENZEL. 1966. Medical Innovation: A Diffusion Study. Bobbs-Merrill. Indianapolis, IN.
8. ROGERS, E. 1983. Diffusion of Innovations. Free Press. New York.
9. STOCKING, B. 1985. Initiative and Inertia. Case Studies in the NHS. The Nuffield Provincial Hospitals Trust. London.
10. GREER, A. L. 1988. The state of the art vs. the state of the science: The diffusion of new medical technologies into practice. Int. J. Technol. Assess. Health Care **4:** 5–26.
11. DIXON, A. 1990. The evolution of clinical policies. Medical Care **28:** 201–220.
12. FOX, R., P. MAZMANIAN & R. W. PUTNAM. 1989. Changing and Learning in the Lives of Physicians. Praeger. New York.
13. KOTLER, P. & E. ROBERTO. 1989. Social Marketing. Strategies for Changing Public Behavior. Free Press. New York.
14. WINKLER, J., K. LOHR & R. BROOK. 1985. Persuasive communication and medical technology assessment. Arch. Intern. Med. **145:** 314–317.

15. Avorn, J., N. Chen & R. Hartley. 1982. Scientific vs. commercial sources of influence on the prescribing behaviour of physicians. Am. J. Med. **73:** 4–8.
16. Haynes, R. B. 1990. Loose connections between peer-reviewed clinical journals and clinical practice. Ann. Intern. Med. **113:** 724–728.
17. Berd, L. A., A. Galbraith & D. Rennie. 1992. The publication of sponsored symposiums in medical journals. N. Engl. J. Med. **327:** 327–340.
18. Kritchevsky, S. & B. Simmons. 1991. Continuous quality improvement: Concepts and applications for physician care. JAMA **266:** 1817–1823.
19. Laffel, G. & D. M. Berwick. 1992. Quality in health care. JAMA **268:** 407–409.

DISCUSSION

Robert Brook (*UCLA, Los Angeles, California*): Professor Lomas—I'm assuming that you're an economist and not a behavioral scientist—when DRGs (diagnostic related groups) were implemented in the United States, overnight from June 30 to July 1, the length of stay in the hospitals fell for common chronic conditions by 25% in exactly 24 hours without a single additional randomized controlled clinical trial's being performed. When payment for injections was denied in the state of New Mexico, the injection rate from everything from vitamin B_{12} to lincomycin fell by 80% in the course of 3 months. So I would ask you whether you find any hope in changing doctors' behavior quickly in the current technological environment if we don't reward the profession in some way for performing better—either by more money or by a higher market share—and whether that reward does not occur at a public level. In other words, is there any hope that the doctors will quickly follow the results of trials if they can't be guaranteed that they will have either a higher market share or still be in business?

Jonathan Lomas (*McMaster University, Hamilton, Ontario, Canada*): Let me interpret your questions as showing how important the economic incentives are because it seems to me that that's what you're focusing on. Yes, economics are important but not overriding. As an example the provinces of Alberta and Quebec provided a significant economic incentive to physicians for vaginal birth after cesarean section, but it didn't make any difference.

Brook: Did they publish the results of which doctors did which? How do you know whether the incentives worked?

Lomas: You are talking about combining an administrative and an economic incentive, and I'm saying for now that I'm happy that there aren't any *disincentives* in this environment. We shouldn't use the incentives aggressively at the present time because this is largely a professional responsibility, a responsibility that can act best in nontraditional educational ways such as through geographic scholars, educational influence, the administrative environment, and, to an extent, a greater role in educating the public and the community. But for now talking about economic incentives is like waving a red flag at a bull for most physician groups. They don't like the idea, but they do respond, even though they don't like admitting that they respond to an economic incentive. But at the moment I don't think that we're ready for it in Canada, although maybe you are in the United States.

Elaine Power (*Office of Technology Assessment, Washington, D.C.*): In your figure, Professor Lomas, you emphasize the credibility of the dissemination body, but you didn't discuss what lends credibility to that body. If the credibility of the dissemination body is related in some fashion to the particular group of practitioners that one is intending to affect, how do you account for the fact that different credible bodies come out with different guidelines?

LOMAS: First, it's important for us to realize that the credibility of the dissemination body is randomly distributed with regard to a comparison of the credibility and validity of the recommendations. That is a problem, and its solution is the same as the solution to the problem that you have, that different audiences will be appealed to by different kinds of bodies. We need guidelines for guidelines. We need a much better way of assessing the validity of synthesis of information. I started by saying I'm presuming that we've solved those problems, but in reality we are quite a long way from solving that particular problem. But once we've assessed who the credible dissemination body for a particular audience is, then we can ask whether this body has got a guideline and whether it is valid. If they don't, then the question arises as to who is the second most credible body for this audience. But there is that interaction between the quality of the guideline that has to be taken into account and, as I said, I skipped over it, and I think you raised an important point.

THOMAS CHALMERS (*Harvard University, Boston, Mass.*): It seems to me that you've underemphasized a very important part of the loop in changing behavior—and that is the patient. Patients need to be educated to ask about the clinical trial evidence of one proposed treatment over another—is one any better or worse then another? So when the physician proposes a treatment—say transurethral versus suprapubic prostatectomy—the patient should ask what the clinical trial evidence is and where the physician got his information. If we could train patients to ask and physicians not to consider their patients hostile for doing so, we'd make a lot more progress.

LOMAS: You're exactly right—I show a two-way arrow here. One of the concerns, however, is that the nature of randomized control trial information, as we just heard from the thrombolysis example, does not give you the correct thing to do for this patient. It gives you a set of parameters to work with, and I am concerned that the extent to which we wish to empower patients has to be that the nature of randomized control trial research and how it is reported should move away from reporting "this is the correct answer" to "here is the information that the trial produced about the relative risks and trade offs for particular classes of patients." We still have to contend with the legacy of the logical positivist view of the world, which says there is a correct answer when very often there isn't.

I'm glad you asked the question because I would like to quote from John Ralston Saul in a recent book, *Voltaire's Bastards—The Dictatorship of Reason in the West*, which for me sums up one of my concerns about the mismatch between the reality of a practitioner's environment on the one hand and the search for the correct answer from the research community on the other. He says "we must alter our civilization from one that seeks definitive answers to one that feels satisfaction rather than anxiety when doubt is established." He says that "we should be comfortable with panic when it is appropriate. If ours is the advanced civilization we pretend it is, there should be no need to act as if all decisions were designed to establish certainties."

RICHARD PETO (*University of Oxford, Oxford, England*): That reflects Keats's concept of "negative capability." One thing that seemed to be missing in talking about communication is the question of whether the therapeutic information that is to be communicated actually answers medical questions reliably. For example, even in Iain Chalmers' excellent book on pregnancy and childbirth, most of the therapeutic questions that are addressed by trials he reviews aren't answered reliably by those trials. So what is this therapeutic information that one is communicating? It's actually quite rare that one has got anything really very definite to say that doctors don't already know. So perhaps the time to worry is when you've got something very definite and important about the effects of therapies that isn't getting across.

I'd be happier if all the way through your presentation there had been one or two particular, striking examples illustrating the problems of getting clinicians to respond to definite evidence. There are a few cases where there's very definite knowledge that's ignored by many doctors, but half the time so much of what is supposed to be communicated isn't well-established or interesting. Even if you take all of the best clinical trial knowledge available it still answers only a limited number of questions reliably.

LOMAS: Could you give me some examples?

PETO: One example is the use of hormonal treatment for early breast cancer. The tendency in many parts of the United States is still to give cytotoxic chemotherapy even to a 60-year-old woman with early breast cancer rather than a hormonal treatment that would be at least as effective and much less toxic.

LOMAS: If I take that example, then I would say that to publish that in a journal or have a very credible body do an excellent job of meta-analysis and synthesis and practice guideline development on it, and then have the findings mailed out to every practitioner is a very ineffective, inadequate, inappropriate, and naive way to go about transferring that research into clinical practice. We should be thinking about how to put that message in the practitioner's administrative *environment*, into the public through the media, into the community, to particular patient advocacy organizations, through the professional bodies that are respected and thought to be influential on that particular group of practitioners, through the CME route, and through the local physician, who is an influential person. It's not enough merely to publish the information and hope it gets disseminated. For a handful of findings that are so compelling, passive diffusion works and you don't need the rest of the dissemination and the implementation. But there aren't that many penicillins left in the world. . . .

General Discussion: II

Argye Hillis (*Texas A&M Health Science Center, Temple, Texas*): As we move towards managed care, we have a window of opportunity to deal with the question of assuring that whatever system we're moving toward provides for scientific testing of new interventions—so that medicine does not become stuck in the status quo—and some way of sorting out which interventions are good, which are useless, and which actually do harm. We have three choices: One is to give up on randomization, as has been discussed, but since I'm from the field of clinical trials, I don't like that route any more than Richard Peto does. The second is to resist change, which we hear a lot of from my camp. And the third choice is to develop a new paradigm.

Some suggestions have been made—Dr. Silverman has already mentioned simple design, minimal data, and a low budget in carrying out trials so that there is minimal or no disruption of clinical care; we need to focus on that. Other important suggestions include discussion of paying for experimental treatment only in the context of a planned randomized comparison; in that regard we need to consider whether such trials should be large or small or whether they should be evaluated in the context of registries. Firms were mentioned earlier but not discussed, and early randomization is something that needs to be brought in unless we're going to choose one of the other alternatives.

Action is needed now by this group to speak with a clear voice on this point. I would like to see something like a consensus conference model so we could make one statement on something that we can agree upon. We're never going to agree on all of these issues—there's room for 20 more years of work, for lifetimes of work, if we addressed all the issues. But as we move towards some kind of paradigm of managed care, the question of how we are going to allow for development of new interventions becomes an extremely important one.

Kenneth Warren (*Picower Institute for Medical Research, Manhasset, N.Y.*): I agree with you and I'd like Tom Chalmers to say a few words since he is proposing early randomization for all new interventions.

Thomas Chalmers (*Harvard University Medical School, Boston, Mass.*): My idea that randomization should begin with the first patient came from the fact that early in the uncontrolled development of a new technology the people testing it become convinced that it's either good or bad and then either abandon it or adopt it and are unable to do the randomized trial that is necessary; in other words there are three possible outcomes of the uncontrolled pilot trial, which is why I'm against all pilot trials. Either the treatment is so effective that the person doing the pilot trial cannot do a randomized trial; or the treatment is so ineffective that the person cannot undertake randomization because it would be unethical to do so; or the treatment is just "so so" and it would be a waste of time to do a decent trial and so it's abandoned. So we end up with a system whereby uncontrolled data get into the literature and new technology is adopted by the medical community before it has ever been adequately tested. That is why one ought to be forced to do randomized control trials early, and one of the ways to do that—and I have to agree with Robert Brook on this—is to use a financial incentive. The best way to control the situation is to decree, probably by law, that if you want to try a new technology, especially an expensive one that hasn't been established as effective by adequate randomized trials, you randomize the patient or you don't get paid for using the new technology. That was tried once by the Eye Institute when they advised the Health Care Finance Administration not to pay for radial keratotomy because it was still under exploration. The doctors went to court and got a restraint-of-trade decision making the agency pay, which takes education all the way down the line.

The main reason why I've had trouble "selling" the idea of early randomization is not medical or scientific, but political. I'm told that you have to develop the treatment before you can start testing it, which begs the question of how it can be developed without testing it first. And the surgeons say there's no point in randomizing patients to evaluate the new operation against the old until they've developed the new operation so that it has a good chance of being comparable to the old. I then ask the doctors how they get informed consent from the patient not to randomize. In other words, do they say to the patient "I'm not giving you a random chance to get standard therapy because I think my new therapy is going to kill you until I've done a better job of working out the technique. Once I've worked out the technique then I'll do a randomized trial. I'd like your permission to volunteer for me so I can work out the technique, and then I'll try it again on some other people in a randomized trial."? *That* is truly informed consent, and obviously nobody does it. So that is why you should randomize the first patient, and by that I mean the first patient in which the outcome is a variable that you are going to measure. I'm not speaking of pharmacologic studies, although random order of drug dosages would certainly be important. I mean that once you decide to do a pilot trial to see whether a particular drug has any hope of being effective or not or might require a much bigger trial, then that patient should be in a randomized trial.

WARREN: This seems reasonably clear, but I would like to do something a little unusual in a meeting like this and ask all those who agree with Dr. Chalmers' proposal to raise their hands. As new diagnostic tests appear, as new pharmaceutical agents appear, as new vaccines appear, as new operations appear, within the realm of feasibility, should all patients examined from the beginning be randomized? [*Hands are raised.*] I think we have a really powerful consensus here. I would say that at a glance it seems that 90% of you raised your hands showing that you agree with the proposition.

I once ran a meeting entitled "Good Health at Low Cost," a title that evoked the cavil that it was oxymoronic. So I asked whether we should have called it "Relatively Good Health at Relatively Low Cost," and I made my point. The book that came out of that meeting had some influence, but it wouldn't have had the *relatively*s been in the title.

GEORGE SILVERMAN (*General Accounting Office, Washington, D.C.*): Since I'm a government official I want to disavow any claim that I ever said anything ought to be done simply! I'd like to utter a word of caution here, or rather make a suggestion for where to go from here. In December I attended a meeting that the Agency for Health Care Policy and Research held on methods for forming practice guidelines. In February the OTA held a meeting on technology assessment in medicine, and at this meeting again the subject is evaluating medical interventions. Yet, ironically, the organization in this country with the longest history of practical evaluation of medical interventions—the Food and Drug Administration—was absent from the agenda of all three meetings. This is not to criticize those who put these conferences together, for they were all very enlightening, but we do have to look to the experience of the Food and Drug Administration, which has a 30-year history of dealing with very practical issues about how to make decisions about medical interventions.

However, I think that there are two reasons why we have not tapped the FDA's wisdom. One is that the legal notion about the proprietary nature of the information the FDA deals with makes them largely invisible to people outside the government who don't have access to that information; but that situation may be changing. The other reason is of greater concern: it may be that the FDA economic lesson is a scary one in that it's a situation in which tens of millions of dollars are spent to answer essentially very small questions. This gives some sense of how costly it is to embark on a large-scale effort to evaluate all interventions in order to significantly increase the level of certainty in medicine, and that great cost is sort of frightening. So we also need meetings about methods for dealing with uncertainty because we're greatly concerned about how to determine what evidence is good, what evidence is less good, what methods produce good evidence, and what a clinician should do in situations where there is no evidence or only bad evidence. Those concerns may in fact describe the majority of clinical situations.

WARREN: And that's why we have to get answers. Let me note that I tried and failed to get David Kessler from the FDA to come to this meeting, but a previous commissioner, Jere Goyan, will be here tomorrow. And we tried but failed to get several people from the pharmaceutical industry, to whom this conference should have a great interest. I would also note that the Environmental Protection Agency is having similar problems in trying to decide about issues like lead and asbestos, and the mistakes that they have made provide a lesson for all of us.

UNIDENTIFIED SPEAKER: The question was posed about how we can continue to evaluate maneuvers within managed competition. I'd like to remind us all that managed competition itself has never been evaluated, has never been put into a single state, and has never been studied in any systematic way. And it seems as if we're about to embark on a 100-million-dollar experiment in this country without any evidence that it will be of any benefit. So my question is: how can we intervene in this process at this point to try and build some evaluation into this locomotive that's now going full speed ahead towards managed competition? Maybe the United States is the first patient—but I don't know who the second patient will be.

RICHARD PETO (*Radcliffe Infirmary, University of Oxford, England*): We're suffering from that process in Britain as well.

WARREN: Let me just make one point about that: the British have made vast changes in their educational and health structures on a nationwide level time and time again, which have often not worked out. The United States, on the other hand, has the advantage of being able to experiment with different methods and approaches on a state-by-state basis. One of the more important experiments just approved is the Oregon experiment.

PETO: To argue for almost mandatory randomization in various circumstances is to invite unnecessary confrontation with the medical profession, whereas to say that one aims to randomize whenever there is substantial uncertainty is perhaps to encourage collaboration with the medical profession. If you have many different trials running, trials on many different questions, the eligibility criterion for each trial is simply *uncertainty*. If you want to do a trial on whether or not to start antiretroviral therapy, then if you're *reasonably certain* you want to start such treatment, then go ahead and start it and the patient stays out of the trial. If you're *reasonably certain* you don't want to, then again the patient stays out of the trial. But if you and the patient are both *substantially uncertain* whether to start now or much later, then that trial is for you.

I think that *uncertainty* is actually the appropriate fundamental criterion for randomization rather than whether things are new or whether they're regarded by some official or unofficial body as being evaluated. If you say that the doctors and patients are *substantially uncertain,* then randomization is both ethical and helpful to them. The point to emphasize if you want randomization is that, where there is substantial uncertainty, the scale of randomized evidence should be increased by an order of magnitude. That is a more practical thing to try to impose or introduce because you're running with the profession rather than trying to confront them. That should be the principle that we use to expand the process of randomization; this uncertainty principle has been used in many trials and has proved to be practical.

WARREN: Dr. Chalmers, are you going to take up the cudgels on that one?

IAIN CHALMERS (*The UK Cochrane Centre, Oxford, England*): I'm really touched by Richard's concern for the sensitivities of my profession. As far as I'm concerned I am not in the least bit uncertain that if I have a coronary episode this evening I do not wish to receive TPA from a doctor in this city who is uncertain whether or not to give me streptokinase or TPA. I think the uncertainty principle is an extremely good one, but to consider only the uncertainty in the heads of medical people is completely wrong.

PETO: Yes, but uncertainty comes between the doctor and the patient. Doctors talk to patients and if at the end of that process there is substantial uncertainty, then randomization is practical.

CHALMERS: If, when you mention the uncertainty principle, you always talk about uncertainty that involves both the patient's and the doctor's being informed by whatever evidence is available, that would be a very good practice. Unfortunately, this touching sensitivity that you have to the feelings of the medical profession seems to dominate. Now whether that's because you're a statistician rather than a doctor I have no idea but it's not good enough.

Introduction to the Panel on Education

HENRY WALTON

President, World Federation for Medical Education
The University of Edinburgh
Centre for Medical Education
11 Hill Square
Edinburgh EH89DR, Scotland

This panel on education is of importance to my Federation because it deals with concerns which will be central to the World Conference on Medical Education, entitled *"The Changing Medical Profession,"* to be held in Edinburgh on August 8–12, 1993. In accepting with the greatest pleasure my task as chairman, I want to use this opportunity to acknowledge Dr. Ken Warren's profound contribution to the previous World Conference of the WFME, also at Edinburgh in 1988.

The conclusions of the 1988 World Conference, which were expressed in the Edinburgh *Declaration*, are the mandate for reforming the training of medical doctors worldwide. The Edinburgh *Declaration*, endorsed on May 19, 1989 by the World Health Assembly in its Resolution WHA 42.38, is recognized to have the place in medical education which the Alma Ata Declaration has in the field of health care.

The twelve principles of the *Declaration* are the mandate for reforming how doctors are educated and trained. Five years later, all of these principles carry the authority and urgency which derived from their grass-roots origin. First, deans of medical schools responded to 32 urgent issues. Then national conferences were held, leading to six Regional Conferences: in Africa, the Americas, Europe, the Middle East, South-East Asia, and the Western Pacific.

THE DECLARATION

All medical schools are revising their medical curricula, inevitably so: the Edinburgh *Declaration* is their framework for change.

The twelve principles of the *Declaration* are great pointers to reconstruction.

1. Widening educational settings in which medical education now has to take place: the ivory tower "teaching hospital" in lofty isolation has had its day, and future doctors must be taught in all health care settings in which patients are seen.
2. National health priorities as the context for education: each country's national health plan must be reflected in the educational program of the medical school.
3. Active learning throughout life (with appropriate reforms of the examination system): the medical schools start the learning style of a doctor's lifetime; only activated students can become life-long self-directed learners.
4. Professional competence as the purpose of all learning: not memorization of facts soon to be forgotten and superseded as science advances, but clinical ability of relevance to the social responsibility of doctors.

5. Training of medical teachers as educators: their educational duties are as important as their scientific or clinical work.
6. Health promotion and prevention of illness: an essential component of the new medicine, which is not only curative or rehabilitative.
7. Integration of science and clinical practice: the sciences are no longer to be taught only at the start, as theory, and then displaced by clinical work with patients.
8. Selection of entrants, for noncognitive as well as intellectual attributes: those personality qualities which are innate, and cannot be conferred by medical education itself (such as ability to communicate, interest in people, motivation) must be screened-for at admission.
9. Coordination of education with health delivery services: a serious obstacle is that the university system is unrelated to the health care systems of countries, the one a Ministry of Education concern, the other looked after by the Health Ministry, and the two are rarely coordinated.
10. Balanced production of the national need for doctors: the great numbers of unemployed doctors demonstrate by their very existence the irrationality of medical education as a system.
11. Cooperation of the health professions (the issue of multiprofessional training): teamwork is now inescapable where care of patients is concerned.
12. Continuing medical education as a main sphere of medical education: all doctors have to maintain their competence at their work place, and the resources have to be provided which enable them to do so.

In the five years during which the *Declaration* has been implemented, an enormous explosion of reform is in progress, more vigorous than at any time since the start of the century, where the milestone had been Abraham Flexner's *Report* of 1910.

THE 1993 WORLD SUMMIT

The curriculum is not enough. Attention must now be given to the interface between the medical education system on one hand, and the health care delivery services on the other.

Three great themes will be dealt with at Edinburgh later this year:

1. *The wider context*: patients' rights; empowerment—enabling patients to take more responsibility for their own health; the economic crisis; the role of governments; poverty; social breakdown; war, famine, and mass migration.
2. *The changing nature of medical practice*: including payment issues, privatization and health care reform; quality care; new diseases and morbidity patterns; and the ethical and moral basis of medicine.
3. *Coping with the growth of knowledge and technological advance*: the sciences of clinical practice; communication skills of doctors; and the swing to health promotion and prevention of illness.

The Summit will end with a *Communiqué* on August 12. Almost certainly, a global strategy will be instituted, for generating worldwide the changes in the training of the doctors needed for the future. The six Regional Conferences in

1994 will implement the Summit's resolutions. The administrative framework is in place. Main partners with WFME are the WHO, UNICEF, UNESCO, the United Nations Development Programme, and the World Bank. The auspicious tide in medical education will be surveyed at the Summit and encouragement given to its surge around the world.

Using Evidence to Teach Effective Use of Health Interventions

HAROLD C. SOX, Jr.

Department of Medicine
Dartmouth-Hitchcock Medical Center
Lebanon, New Hampshire 03756

The translation of research results into clinical practice is a complex, imperfect process. The purpose of this article is to describe methods for teaching effective use of health interventions, to describe the outcome of teaching, and to speculate about the future.

SCOPE AND DEFINITIONS

The scope of this article is undergraduate and graduate medical education up to the completion of residency training. The output of technology assessment could be either the results of an individual clinical trial, a summative evaluation of several studies, in the form of a meta-analysis or decision analysis, or guidelines for medical practice.

In this article, the goal of the education process is to alter knowledge of the output of technology assessment so that patient care changes. The main outcome measure is change in medical practice. This definition is somewhat restrictive, but changed behavior is the important outcome that is most pertinent to today's health care system.

WHAT ARE THE IMPORTANT DETERMINANTS OF ADOPTION OF TECHNOLOGY?

To change behavior, one must first know what motivates physicians to abandon old practice habits and adopt new ones. Fineberg lists several elements that contribute to the decision to adopt a technology.[1]

- Concordance with prevailing medical theory. Conversely, discordance with prevailing theory or having to learn a new theory may reduce the propensity to change.
- Ease of making the change. A new practice is easier to adopt if it is easy to remember.
- Exposure to added risk because of failing to change. A medical problem that exposes one's patients to death or disability gets a physician's attention. Conversely, a practice style change that exposes one to risk is hard to adopt.
- The physician's ability to change. A prior education that prepares one to grasp new ideas and see their implications will facilitate change.
- A practice setting that encourages change. Availability of the technology, peer pressure to conform to prevailing practice, and financial incentives or disincentives all encourage change.

- Well-designed, credible studies of the technology.
- Effective channels of communication of research results. Ideally, the findings are available at the moment of decision. Our health care system falls far short of this ideal.

This listing provides some insight into the conditions for teaching medical students and housestaff to transform the results of research into the best use of tests and treatments. The students must have a context that supports their learning: a theory (decision theory), a supportive environment (a society that values cost control), and access to pertinent knowledge at the moment of decision.

STUDIES OF LEARNING AND CHANGE IN THE PRE-COMPUTER ERA

Traditional methods for teaching appropriate use of tests and treatments have failed at least as often as they have succeeded. Eisenberg reviewed the literature on this topic in his book *Doctors' Decisions and the Cost of Medical Care*.[2] A selective review of some of the highlights will underscore the methods and the problems.

Marton studied inpatient test-ordering by internal medicine residents by comparing a control group, a fiscal-incentive group, and a chart-review group.[3] Every week each resident in the chart-review group and a preceptor discussed each test ordered for one inpatient. The endpoint of the study was the number of tests ordered. The chart-review group reduced their test-ordering by 30%, significantly more than either of the other two groups. The authors speculated that the weekly chart-review sessions altered behavior by repeated exposure to a value system about the use of tests, rather than by imparting specific information.

A second controlled study of inpatient test-ordering by medical and surgical housestaff came to diametrically opposite conclusions.[4] Among the surgical housestaff, there was an intervention group and a control; the same was true for the medical housestaff. The intervention was a mixture of weekly lectures and chart audit with feedback, similar to Martin's study. The lectures covered ethical, economic, decision-making aspects of test-ordering, and clinical indications for testing. There were no differences in test-ordering between the intervention group and their corresponding control groups.

Marton studied test-ordering in the outpatient clinic at a university hospital and its affiliated VA Hospital.[5] There was a control group, a group that received periodic feedback about their test-ordering relative to other participants, a group that received an 80-page book that taught principles of test-ordering and gave advice about specific tests, and a group that received both interventions. Outcome measures included test-ordering, attitudes toward testing, and knowledge of test-ordering principles. During the intervention period, control group residents ordered $31 worth of tests each visit, the feedback group $21, the manual group $23, and the combined intervention group $21. The authors speculated that their success was due in part to studying the outpatient setting, where the individual resident controls testing decisions.

Williams studied simulated test-ordering by inpatient medical students following an intensive intervention that included a seminar, simulated patient-care exercises, a newsletter, and review of patients' hospital bills.[6] The outcome measure was a test that measured knowledge of test-ordering principles and test-ordering on a series of 10 patient-management questions. The pre-intervention test scores of the intervention group and the control group did not differ from the post-intervention test or from each other. Apparently, no one learned anything.

These studies had very mixed results. An intensive inpatient program was effective in Boston and a failure in San Francisco. A relatively weak intervention was successful in the outpatient setting. All of the investigators were highly competent faculty who were part of the power structure of the study subjects' world. In many cases, the interventions were both extensive and intensive. No one understands why these interventions failed.

STUDIES OF LEARNING AND CHANGE IN THE COMPUTER ERA

The Regenstrief Institute at the University of Indiana has been the site of a sustained two-decade effort to make the computer into an integral part of the patient-care process. The success of recent efforts suggests that the investigators have discovered an important principle of clinical education.

In 1976, McDonald reported the effects of a reminder system for conditions caused by or managed by drugs.[7] Certain findings in the computer-based medical record triggered a "rule" which in turn generated a suggestion for managing the finding. For example, when the computer record contained the information that the patient was on digitalis and that the patient had >2 premature ventricular contractions per minute, the physician received the "suggestion" that the patient might have digitalis toxicity. The nine study physicians responded more appropriately when reminded of the event than when the investigator withheld the reminder.

In 1984, McDonald reported the results of using an expanded version of the reminder system.[8] The reminders included disease prevention and health promotion tests needed to complete the initial database or tests needed to evaluate abnormal findings. The study intervention was providing the reminders. The investigators randomly assigned twenty-seven patient-care teams of faculty and house-staff to intervention or control groups. The outcome measure was the rate of response to the condition that triggered the rule. In the two years of the study, the computer found indications for action in 90% of patient encounters. The response rate for the houseofficers was 49% in the intervention group and 29% in the control group ($p < .00001$).

In 1987, Tierney reported the effect of displaying the results of prior tests.[9] The key feature of the computer in this and subsequent studies was that all test-ordering required using the computer. Therefore, the computer could remind the resident of pertinent information at the very moment that the resident was about to order a test. In this study, depending on the randomized assignment of the patient, physicians either received the results of previous tests at the time of ordering a test or did not receive this information. Test costs were lower by 13% in the intervention group.

In 1988, Tierney reported the effect of displaying a prediction of the results of a test prior to allowing the resident to order the test.[10] The investigators developed logistic regression equations that predicted the results of eight commonly ordered diagnostic tests. The night before a scheduled visit, the computer searched the patient's chart for the data that the predictive equations needed to predict test results. When the resident ordered the test, the computer displayed the probability that the test would be positive. Depending on the randomized assignment of the patient, physicians either received the prediction or did not receive this information. Residents' test charges were 10% less when they received the prediction of test results ($p < .05$).

In 1990, Tierney reported the effect of informing outpatient physicians of the charges for the tests they were about to order.[11] The investigators randomly assigned 121 physicians to intervention or control status. Depending on their randomized assignment, physicians either saw a display of the cost of the test they were about to order or did not receive this information. During the 26-week intervention period, intervention physicians ordered 14% fewer tests than the control group physicians ($p < .005$) and the charges for the tests were 13% lower. The two groups did not differ in test-ordering during the post-intervention period.

In 1993, the Regenstrief group moved to the inpatient setting. Tierney reported the effect of using a microcomputer workstation on test-ordering by resident physicians. When physicians used the workstation to order tests, they received information about test costs, appropriate testing intervals, and cost-effective alternative tests. The investigators assigned residents and faculty attendings to one of six inpatient services in a way that insured that a given physician would be on an intervention service or a control service but would not cross over from one to the other. Total charges per hospitalization were $887 less (12.7%) for intervention teams. Total hospital costs were $594 less in the intervention group. In a 10-hour observation period, the intervention interns spent 33 more minutes writing orders, according to a formal time-motion study, than did control interns (59 vs. 26 minutes).

CONCLUSIONS

This survey suggests that integrating the computer into the process of test-ordering is a more effective way to alter behavior than traditional education methods. Although there is a great deal of work involved in creating a system such as the Regenstrief medical record, replication of the system at other institutions should be relatively inexpensive, at least as compared with the cost of intensive teaching programs.

There are reasons to be cautious in interpreting these studies. The study design of the Regenstrief experiments leaves no doubt about the key role of the computer in achieving the results in that environment. However, the Regenstrief may be a special place in which to learn, so that factors other than the computer are necessary for replication of the findings of their studies. The Regenstrief studies occurred somewhat later into the era of serious national efforts at cost control than the pre-computer era studies, so that the context for learning may have been more favorable to changing behavior at the time of the computer studies.

The list of factors required for adoption of new practice habits includes both credible information and effective channels to communicate that information. Both are increasingly available in this era of technology assessment and computer medical records. This essay has called attention to the importance of having the information available to the physician at the time of the decision to order a test.

REFERENCES

1. FINEBERG, H. V. 1985. Effects of clinical evaluation on the diffusion of medical technology. *In* Assessing Medical Technology. F. Mosteller, Ed.: 176–210.
2. EISENBERG, J. M., 1986. Doctor's Decisions and the Cost of Medical Care. Health Administration Press Perspective. Ann Arbor, MI.
3. MARTON, A. R., M. A. WOLF, L. A. THIBODEAU, V. DZAU & E. BRAUNWALD. 1980.

A trial of two strategies to modify the test-ordering behavior of medical residents. N. Engl. J. Med. **303:** 1330–1336.

4. SCHROEDER, S. A., L. P. MYERS, S. J. MCPHEE, J. A. SHOWSTACK, D. W. SIMBORG, S. A. CHAPMAN & J. K. LEONG. 1984. The failure of physician education of a cost containment strategy: Report of a prospective controlled trial at a university hospital. JAMA **252:** 225–230.

5. MARTON, K. I., V. TUL & H. C. SOX. 1985. Modifying test-ordering behavior in the outpatient medical clinic: A controlled trial of two educational interventions. Arch. Int. Med. **145:** 816–821.

6. WILLIAMS, S. V., J. M. EISENBERG, D. S. KITZ, J. G. CARROLL, L. H. BECK, S. I. RUBIN & G. E. RUFF. 1984. Teaching cost-effective diagnostic test use to medical students. Med. Care **22:** 535–542.

7. MCDONALD, C. J. 1976. Protocol-based computer reminders, the quality of care, and the non-perfectability of man. J. Engl. J. Med. **295:** 1351–1355.

8. MCDONALD, C. J., S. L. HUI, D. M. SMITH, W. M. TIERNEY, S. J. COHEN, M. WEINBERGER & G. P. MCCABE. 1984. Reminders to physicians from an introspective computer medical record. Ann. Intern. Med. **100:** 130–138.

9. TIERNEY, W. M., C. J. MCDONALD, D. K. MARTIN, S. L. HUI & M. P. ROGERS. 1987. Computerized display of past test results: Effect on outpatient testing. Ann. Intern. Med. **107:** 569–574.

10. TIERNEY, W. M., C. J. MCDONALD, S. L. HUI & D. K. MARTIN. 1988. Computer predictions of abnormal test results: effects on outpatient testing. JAMA **259:** 1194–1198.

11. TIERNEY, W. M., M. E. MILLER & C. J. MCDONALD. 1990. The effect on test ordering of informing physicians of the charges for outpatient diagnostic tests. N. Engl. J. Med. **322:** 1499–1504.

12. TIERNEY, W. M., M. E. MILLER, J. M. OVERHAGE & C. J. MCDONALD. 1993. Physician inpatient order writing on microcomputer workstations: Effects on resource utilization. JAMA **269:** 379–383.

Public Health Education

JULIO FRENK[a]

National Institute of Public Health, and
Mexican Health Foundation
Tlalpan, Mexico

INTRODUCTION

Health care faces today, like never before, the challenges of complexity and change. In the search for innovative answers to the new epidemiologic transitions[1,2] and to the unsolved problems of effectiveness, efficiency, and equity, public health has always played a leading role. It has done so in two forms. First, since the nineteenth century the public health movement has articulated the voice for the primacy of preventive, community-based actions, which have proved to count among the most cost-effective interventions.[3] Second, public health research has provided a major part of the intellectual impetus for evaluating the performance of health care practices.

Yet there has been a tendency to fragment the health field and to relegate public health to a secondary role *vis-à-vis* individual medical care. In this paper I will argue that such fragmentation has impoverished both clinical medicine and public health. Much is to be gained from an integrative view that takes advantage of the essential unity of health processes. This is even more important now, because the past few years have witnessed a renaissance of public health, as the limitations of the fragmentary model have become evident in the light of the growing complexity of health problems.

A new public health is emerging.[4] Its main challenge is to build the four elements of any vigorous intellectual field: (1) a **conceptual base,** which makes it possible to define the field; (2) a **production base,** that is, the set of institutions where a critical mass and a critical density of researchers come together to generate the body of knowledge that gives substantive content to the intellectual field; (3) a **reproduction base,** to ensure the consolidation and continuity of the field through educational programs, publications, and professional associations; and (4) a **utilization base,** which makes it possible to translate knowledge into technological developments and scientifically informed decision-making.

This paper deals primarily with public health education, which is part of the reproduction base. However, it is impossible to understand the educational dimensions without referring to the conceptual base, which is the foundation for the new public health. Hence, we will briefly examine the problem of defining public health. Next we will sketch an educational strategy that incorporates public health into the efforts at evaluating interventions.

[a] Address for correspondence: Dr. Julio Frenk, Fundación Mexicana para la Salud, Periférico Sur 4809, Tlalpan, 14610 México, D.F.

DEFINING PUBLIC HEALTH

The term "public health" is charged with ambiguity. Throughout its history, five connotations of the term have been particularly prominent. The first equates the adjective "public" to governmental action, that is, the public sector. The second meaning is somewhat broader, since it includes not only government programs, but also participation of the organized community, that is to say, the "public." The third use identifies public health with "nonpersonal health services," that is, services that cannot be appropriated by a specific individual, since they are targeted at the environment (e.g., sanitation) or the community (e.g., massive health education). The next usage is slightly broader, since it adds a series of personal preventive services for vulnerable groups (for example, maternal and child care programs). Finally, the expression "public health problem" is often used, especially in nontechnical language, to refer to diseases that are particularly frequent or dangerous.

Recently a more comprehensive conception of public health has emerged. According to this view, the adjective "public" does not designate a particular set of services, a form of property, or a type of problem, but rather a specific level of analysis: the population level. In contrast to clinical medicine, which operates at an individual level, and biomedical research, which analyzes the subindividual level, the essence of public health is that it adopts a perspective based on groups of people or populations. This population perspective inspires the two facets of public health: as an arena for action and as a field of inquiry.

As a field of professional practice, the modern conception of public health addresses the systematic efforts to identify health needs and to organize comprehensive services with a well-defined population base. It thus encompasses the information required for characterizing the conditions of the population and the mobilization of resources necessary for responding to such conditions through the health system.

As a multidisciplinary field of research, the new public health can be defined as the application of the biological, social, and behavioral sciences to the study of health phenomena in human populations. In order to visualize the role of public health within the more general field of health research, in a prior article[5] we have related the levels with the objects of analysis, proposing the typology shown in TABLE 1. As regards the first dimension of the typology—the objects of analysis—we define conditions as the biological, psychological, and social processes that constitute the levels of health in a given individual or population. By response we are not referring to the internal physiopathological reaction to a given disease process, but to the external response that society organizes for improving health conditions. As regards the second dimension of the typology, for simplicity's sake we recognize two levels of analysis: one has to do with individuals or parts of individuals (i.e., organs, cells, or subcellular elements), while the other is the aggregate level of groups or populations.

Crossing these two dimensions yields the three principal types of research that characterize the field of health: biomedical, clinical, and public health research. Thus, most biomedical research has to do with the conditions, processes, and mechanisms of health and illness, especially at the subindividual level. Clinical research focuses primarily on studying the efficacy of the preventive, diagnostic, and therapeutic responses applied to the individual. The objects indicated above can also be analyzed at the population level. This is precisely what constitutes public health research, which is subdivided into two principal types, as shown in

TABLE 1. Typology of Health Research, with Examples of Phenomena to be Studied

Level of Analysis	Object of Analysis	
	Conditions	Responses
Individual and subindividual	*Biomedical Research* (Basic biological processes; structure and function of the human body; pathological mechanisms)	*Clinical Research* (Efficacy of preventive, diagnostic, and therapeutic procedures, natural history of diseases)
Population	*Epidemiologic Research* (Frequency, distribution, and determinants of health needs)	*Health Systems Research* (Effectiveness, quality, and costs of services; development and distribution of resources for care)

TABLE 1: epidemiologic research and health systems research (HSR). The first studies the frequency, distribution, and determinants of health needs, defined as those conditions that require care.[6] Health systems research can be defined as the scientific study of the organized social response to health and disease conditions in populations.

Naturally, the typology proposed here represents a mere abstraction for synthesizing distinctions that in real life are never so clear-cut. In particular, the four boxes in TABLE 1 should not be seen as mutually exclusive compartments. To the contrary, there are numerous connections among the major types of health research. Thus, for example, various emerging fields (such as bioepidemiology, clinical epidemiology, decision analysis, and technology assessment) deal with interfaces among the four types. Indeed, the principal message of TABLE 1 is integration: the essential difference between public health research, on the one hand, and biomedical and clinical research, on the other, is not in the objects, but in the levels of analysis. It is possible that a great part of the isolation of traditional public health has been due to a conception that postulated that it should study objects other than those examined by the biomedical and clinical sciences, thus erecting an insurmountable barrier. The future of public health will depend on its ability to build bridges with the other types of health research, making its specific and irreplaceable contribution to this undertaking, namely, analysis at the population level. Thus, the challenge is to integrate levels and objects of analysis in order to achieve a full understanding of the broad health field. Clearly, this also requires integration among scientific disciplines.

THE EDUCATIONAL CHALLENGE

Building those bridges is a key feature of a new educational strategy for public health. For at least 80 years, formal programs in public health education have been at the forefront of training leaders to address the changing realities of health conditions and responses. As the complexity of health care arrangements has increased, schools of public health and related programs have trained most of the researchers and professionals in the fields of epidemiology, biostatistics, and management.

Today, when the assessment of interventions has become a pressing requirement in both developed and developing countries, schools of public health are called upon once again to provide educational leadership. The population perspective defining public health is conducive to the kind of rational probabilistic analysis of health care practices that underlies such emerging fields as clinical epidemiology, decision analysis, technology assessment, and quality assurance. It is therefore natural for schools of public health to lead in the educational effort to reproduce the knowledge generated by these fields.

Two main efforts are required in this respect. The first one is to train future researchers who will be able to sustain and enrich the scientific tradition of health care assessment and evaluation. The second effort is to train future leaders in the practice of health policy and management who will make decisions informed by the results of scientific research. This demands an educational effort that to date has been neglected: the introduction of research topics in the educational programs for those who are not going to be researchers but users of research. Such topics would have two essential purposes: to learn to value the contribution of research to decision-making and to gain a mastery of the minimal criteria for judging the quality of results. A strategy is needed to train "informed consumers" of research products.

As can be seen, education in public health is faced with a challenging agenda. To be successful, programs will need to harmonize two values: academic **excellence** and **relevance** to decision-making. The balance between these two values is the key to a successful utilization of knowledge.[7]

CONCLUSIONS

In the relatively short period of time since World War II the social arrangements for dealing with health have been transformed radically. Nowadays, most people come into contact, whether regular or sporadic, with doctors, nurses, technicians, hospitals, clinics, health centers, pharmacies, clinical laboratories, insurance companies, vaccines, drugs, equipment—all the vast and differentiated set of persons, organizations, and technologies that specialize in health care. A growing proportion of people are born, die, and spend considerable periods of their lives in health-related institutions.

Today, health systems simultaneously represent: a source of institutional differentiation in society, taking over functions previously carried out by the individual and the family; an expanding set of complex organizations with *sui generis* authority structures; a source of income and employment for an array of professionals, managers, and technicians who function within an elaborate division of labor; a channel for mobilizing, exchanging, and redistributing large sums of money, both public and private; a focus for technological innovation and a prime site where the common citizen comes into personal contact with science; a vigorous sector of the economy, with important effects on macroeconomic variables such as productivity, inflation, aggregate demand, employment, and competitiveness; an arena for political struggle among parties, interest groups, and social movements; a set of cultural meanings for interpreting fundamental aspects of human experience, such as birth and death, pain and suffering, normalcy and deviance; a space where many of the key ethical questions of our times are framed and sometimes answered.

There is no *a priori* reason why we should assume that this vast apparatus produces tangible benefits for health. An explicit effort must be made to assess to what extent and at what cost health is advanced by interventions. Armed with an integrative strategy for building bridges towards biomedical research, clinical practice, the social sciences, policy analysis, and managerial leadership, the new public health will no doubt be a key piece in our search for better interventions.

ACKNOWLEDGMENTS

Most of the ideas presented here have evolved over several years of organizational development of the National Institute of Public Health of Mexico, and have been greatly enriched by discussions and joint projects with many mentors and colleagues, especially Guillermo Soberón, Avedis Donabedian, Harvey Fineberg, José Laguna, Jaime Martuscelli, José-Luis Bobadilla, Jaime Sepúlveda, Enrique Ruelas, Lilia Durán, Carlos Santos-Burgoa, and Miguel A. González-Block. The Pan American Health Organization supported parts of this work through its project entitled "Development of the Theory and Practice of Public Health in the Americas." Portions of the present paper derive from my article "The new public health," initially prepared for that project and subsequently published in *Annual Review of Public Health* (1993; **14**: 469–489). This paper was prepared during a sabbatical stay at the Harvard Center for Population and Development Studies; I acknowledge the support of the Center, the Harvard School of Public Health, the National Institute of Public Health of Mexico, the National Council for Science and Technology, and the Rockefeller Foundation. Notwithstanding my gratitude to the aforementioned persons and organizations, the contents of the paper are solely my responsibility.

REFERENCES

1. OMRAN, A. R. 1971. The epidemiologic transition: A theory of the epidemiology of population change. Milbank Mem. Fund Q. **49**: 509–538.
2. FRENK, J., J. L. BOBADILLA, J. SEPÚLVEDA & M. LÓPEZ-CERVANTES. 1989. Health transition in middle-income countries: new challenges for health care. Health Pol. Plann. **4**: 29–39.
3. JAMISON, D. T. & W. H. MOSLEY. 1991. Disease control priorities in developing countries: health policy responses to epidemiological change. Am. J. Publ. Health **81**: 15–22.
4. FRENK, J. 1993. The new public health. Annu. Rev. Publ. Health **14**: 469–489.
5. FRENK, J., J. L. BOBADILLA, J. SEPÚLVEDA, J. ROSENTHAL & E. RUELAS. 1988. A conceptual model for public health research. Bull. Pan. Am. Health Organ. **22**: 60–71.
6. DONABEDIAN, A. 1976. Aspects of Medical Care Administration: Specifying Requirements for Health Care. Harvard University Press. Cambridge, MA.
7. FRENK, J. 1992. Balancing relevance and excellence: Organizational responses to link research with decision making. Soc. Sci. Med. **35**: 1397–1404.

Using Evidence To Teach
Clinical Epidemiology

ARTURO MORILLO

International Clinical Epidemiology Network
3600 Market Street
Philadelphia, Pennsylvania 19104-2644

This conference has systematically reviewed the sources of scientific evidence from observation through various experimental designs, culminating with the overviews, reviews, and meta-analyses. Appropriately, it has extended into discussions of the dissemination and implementation of evidence. Medical associations, insurance companies, HMOs, pharmaceutical houses, and educators have all used this evidence. It may be significant that no time was given for a discussion of how health policymakers can apply the same evidence. I was invited, however, not to discuss the content of the program, but to talk about how the International Clinical Epidemiology Network, known as INCLEN, which is engaged in an international program of clinical epidemiology, uses such evidence to teach the students in our program.

INCLEN is dedicated to teaching the methods of epidemiologic research, biostatistics, health economics, and social sciences to clinical specialists teaching at medical colleges in developing countries. In each medical school, we train a core group of approximately ten faculty members that staff a clinical epidemiology unit or CEU. During the initial phase of CEU development, we train students at medical schools in the United States, Canada, and Australia. Some clinical epidemiology units have now developed to a point where they have assumed responsibilities as training centers in their own right. Three training centers now operate in Southeast Asia. Latin American training centers will soon begin admitting their first students.

INCLEN training emphasizes expertise in the critical appraisal of medical evidence, in generating high-quality research, and in interacting with health policymakers. We train clinicians to gather evidence with the purpose of applying it to solve problems in the communities their medical colleges serve.

Strong critical thinking skills give clinicians a powerful tool to make intelligent decisions based on evidence from medical literature. Instead of passively accepting what they read in medical journals, students are able to critically appraise the literature, leading to an intelligent selection of information and decision-making.

Our program uses evidence to influence policy. We encourage CEUs to address research questions relevant to their communities. The research results generate evidence with sufficient weight to affect policies. Through research, we are trying to establish partnerships among medical schools, health authorities, and communities. Identification of risk factors and determinants of behavior, attitudes, and beliefs has proved valuable in enabling clinicians to better understand and modify the underlying determinants of diseases.

Faculty members in developing countries are closer to decision makers than they usually are in industrialized countries. They are more likely to be consulted by health authorities and hospital directors on matters of policy. With the formation of CEUs staffed by clinicians of high reputation, we are influencing the medical curriculum, medical practices, and health policies of these countries. This influence comes from our use of evidence in training clinicians in epidemiologic research methods. The classroom lecture is giving way to small group seminars with active interaction between students and teachers. The quality of the evidence generated has improved significantly, and journal clubs provide exciting opportunities for students to actively analyze the medical literature in a way without precedent in our academic environments.

In one of our training centers "a new approach to teaching the practice of medicine" has been developed, with a "commitment to produce practitioners of evidence-based medicine."[1] The emphasis in the internal medicine residency is on critically evaluating the evidence from clinical research.

Introducing clinical epidemiologic research has inspired an interest in the economic burden of diseases and the economic implications of clinical interventions. Cost-effectiveness and efficacy are becoming subjects of discussion at the bedside. The new perspective is based on the use of evidence produced by health economists to make clinicians aware of cost-effective analyses. In countries where available resources are so scarce, this new attitude is crucial for a more rational use of meager budgets to cope with the needs of the population. The introduction of evidence from health economics has for the first time influenced clinicians to prioritize problems before making decisions to allocate resources and analyze cost benefits before deciding on alternative interventions.

All these strategies for using evidence as a tool to broaden the perspective of medical educators has created an interest in producing local evidence. The international literature does not always address questions of immediate relevance to developing countries. When it does so, the results may not be applicable because of economic constraints. After an initial period when research was repetitious of what was done in industrialized countries, clinicians are now shifting toward using appropriate methodologies to investigate the most pressing health problems at the local level.

In summary, INCLEN is using evidence in education as a tool to increase critical thinking and critical appraisal of the literature and to generate research addressing the needs of the communities. As a result, we perceive a change in the strategies of health education, in medical practice, and in health policymaking.

REFERENCE

1. EVIDENCE-BASED MEDICINE WORKING GROUP. 1992. Evidence-based medicine. A new approach to teaching the practice of medicine. JAMA **268**(17): 2420–2425.

Continuing Education for
Medical Practice

DENNIS K. WENTZ

American Medical Association
515 North State Street
Chicago, Illinois 60610

Continuing education for medical practice is a major concern of organized medicine and should similarly be of great concern to society at large. That concern has only been intermittently articulated, and the public certainly has a misconception of what occurs in the continuing education of practicing physicians. What is not yet a true continuum of education begins with undergraduate medical education, the 4 years leading to the M.D. degree, continues into graduate education, occupying from 3 to 7 years of additional training and education, and then culminates in the 30 to 40 years spent in delivering medical care, the years of medical practice. In order to do more good than harm, physicians must continually refresh their knowledge base in the context of actual patient care, and integrate new knowledge while discarding the old as necessary. The physician must be aware of the evidence for and against a decision for therapy and treatment: this has been the supposed world of continuing medical education (CME).

CME: THE WAY IT IS

Continuing medical education (CME) in 1993 is very much like it always has been: George Miller described it well in 1987: "In most of the world, CME is content-oriented: everywhere, it is teacher-dominated. On the other hand, it is not continuing, but usually episodic: it is rarely education so much as instruction."[1]

Very little has changed in the actual delivery of CME since the AMA's Council on Medical Education commissioned the first national study on CME in 1955. In a report authored by Douglas Vollan, M.D., the Council found that most physicians viewed CME as formal lectures and predicted as the future: "Medical education is continued in practice mainly through reading, professional contacts, attending medical society and hospital staff meetings, and attending formal postgraduate courses."[2]

Perhaps one thing has changed: in the 1990s, most physicians participate in some CME activity. The 1955 study reported that almost a third of the physicians studied in the survey reported received no formal postgraduate education in the previous 5 years. Today, because of requirements from hospitals for medical staff membership, most physicians must produce documentation of formal CME sessions attended. In addition, 28 states require evidence of CME for re-registration of the license to practice; the preponderant evidence is that only a small percentage of physicians in 1990 ignore CME activities altogether.

However, the enterprise remains content- and teacher-oriented: driven by a funding source that is largely based on registration revenue and industry support, about 2,400 accredited providers of CME operate on the premise that "the course must break even." No other funding sources are usually available, and as a result, innovative CME, and CME directed toward individual physicians working alone, is scarce. There has been no groundswell for change.

Physicians, like others, have great resistance to change. In 1990, the AMA House of Delegates accepted a Council on Medical Education recommendation, after 2 years of study, that the AMA Physician's Recognition Award be changed to require an equal amount of informal, self-directed learning (Category 2). The Council believed that the CME enterprise was heavily focused on formal courses, lectures, and seminars (Category 1).[3] A major furor developed as physicians discovered that they were being challenged to change: after further study, two AMA Physician's Recognition Awards have been created: one which can be met totally by reporting formal learning, and another "With Special Commendation for Self-Directed Learning," which requires physicians to report their individual, informal learning activities.[4] Only time will tell whether or not this will be successful.

CME: THE WAY IT SHOULD BE

In the future, continuing medical education must be reflective of the real work doctors do: CME must be related to medical practice and patient care outcomes. For this reason, a new name is proposed to describe the activities better: Continuing Education for Medical Practice. Such continuing education for medical practice must really reflect, as Manning observed, three overall approaches: (*a*) traditional education, which keeps the physician informed of the current state and cutting edge of medical knowledge; (*b*) education directed toward "specialty-specific" aspects of the physician's own practice, reflecting the most common diagnoses made, the major risk factors of patients, and patient outcomes; and (*c*) instantaneous information, needed "on-the-spot," to answer specific questions that arise while the physician is seeing individual patients.[5]

This is, in reality, a broadened concept of CME. Just as Davis *et al.* had to broaden their horizons to answer the question "Does CME work?," all who consider this area must also broaden their concepts about CME. In their 1992 landmark article, these authors stated: "these randomized controlled trials provide new evidence supporting the effectiveness of broadly defined, complex, practice-linked CME. Based on this evidence, we urge the development of an improved, evidence-based CME delivery system and further research into this last and most complex arena of physician education." They concluded: "Broadly defined CME interventions using practice-enabling or -reinforcing strategies consistently improve physician performance and, in some instances, health care outcomes."[6]

The roots of practice-linked CME go very far back in history, but were recently restated by Manning.[7] The oft-forgotten 1917 recommendations of Dr. E. A. Codman, who was drummed out of the Boston medical establishment, are also more relevant than ever. Said Dr. Codman as he described his End Result System:

> . . . the Trustees of Hospitals should see to it that an effort is made to follow up each patient they treat, long enough to determine whether the treatment given has permanently relieved the condition or symptoms complained of. . . . That they should give the members of the Staff credit for taking the responsibility of successful treatment and promote them accordingly. Likewise, they should see that all cases in which the treatment is found to have been unsuccessful or unsatisfactory are carefully analyzed, in order to fix the responsibility for the failure on:

> (1) The physician or surgeon responsible for the treatment;
> (2) The organization carrying out the detail of the treatment;
> (3) The disease or condition of the patient;
> (4) The personal or social conditions preventing the cooperation of the patient.
>
> This will give a definite basis on which to make effort at improvement. The idea is so simple as to seem childlike. . . .
>
> It is idle to say that we have not already much Truth at our disposal, but it can be said that we should find more Truthful ways in which to use it.[8]

The continuing education of the future thus is related to using evidence related to one's practice, and reflective of personally identified learning needs derived from a study of that practice. It is what Sir William Osler described years ago:

> Begin early to make a threefold category—clear cases, doubtful cases, mistakes. And learn to play the game fair, no self-deception, no shrinking from the truth; mercy and consideration for the other man but none for yourself, upon whom you have to keep an incessant watch.[9]

Physicians must and will be taught the critical evaluation of interventions during the continuum of medical education, but it will be most useful during the practice years.

Rootenberg recently surveyed 126 U.S. medical schools to ascertain how computer-based technologies are being taught and used. Not one school of the 73 responding required students to be instructed in computers as a data management and analysis tool. Fifteen, or 16.3%, offered electives on the topic. A clear obstacle is the fact that only 3.3% of the schools have guidelines that place development of computer-based educational materials on a level with other scholarly and research activities, thereby removing a significant faculty incentive.[10]

Feedback about performance is the most significant motivator of physician learning, and comparison of clinical performance with that of one's peers has been repeatedly shown to increase learning and change behavior. One profile of a practice was created by asking physicians to dictate notes about actual patients as they were being seen; the tapes were returned to the university, assigned ICDA codes, and an examination developed based on the profile. The results were positive and exciting.[11] Manning *et al.* in 1986 provided feedback to individual physicians about prescriptions written and 30% of the group receiving feedback changed their prescribing practices.[12] Berwick and Coltin, also in 1986, reported a reduction in test usage by physicians who received confidential feedback on their individual rates of test use compared with those of peers.[13]

Continuing education for practice relies heavily on reading the medical literature; however, that medical literature is often not completely helpful.[14] Even cumulative meta-analyses are not the final answer in many cases: a modicum of clinical judgement is still required. For example, the clinician is likely to use combinations of therapy and it is just as likely that these combinations of therapy have not been studied in the same manner, and findings are thus unavailable.

I have tried to describe the emergence of what was once called "continuing medical education" from lectures and seminars to an area of serious inquiry and research. This has led several of us to call for the evolution of a new paradigm: practice medical education, or the term I prefer, continuing education for medical practice.[15] This new paradigm not only describes the 30-year block of time covered by education during the practice years, but also establishes a discipline for study and research. This discipline combines the multiple factors involved in medical practice and physician performance: competent patient care, knowledge of medical outcomes, and self-directed education to meet actual and perceived learning needs. This is the world of CME in the future.

REFERENCES

1. MILLER, G. 1987. Continuing Medical Education: What it is and what it is not. JAMA **258:** 1352–1354.
2. VOLLAN, D. D. 1955. Postgraduate Medical Education in the United States: A report of the survey of postgraduate medical education carried out by the Council on Medical Education and Hospitals. American Medical Association. Chicago, Illinois.
3. Council of Medical Education Report D. 1990. American Medical Association 1992 Policy Compendium. :300.977. Chicago, Illinois.
4. Report FF of the Board of Trustees. 1992. American Medical Association. Chicago, Illinois.
5. MANNING, P. R. & D. W. PETIT. 1987. The past, present, and future of continuing medical education. JAMA **258:** 3542–3546.
6. DAVIS, D. A., M. A. THOMSON, A. D. OXMAN & R. B. HAYNES. 1992. Evidence for the effectiveness of CME: A review of 50 randomized controlled trials. JAMA **268:** 1111–1117.
7. MANNING, P. R. & L. DEBAKEY. 1987. Medicine: Preserving the Passion. Springer-Verlag. New York.
8. CODMAN, E. A. 1918. A study in hospital efficiency: as demonstrated by the case reports of the first five years of a private hospital. Privately published. Boston, MA.
9. OSLER, W. 1905. The student life. *In* Aequanimitas and Other Papers That Have Stood the Test of Time.: 185. Norton. New York.
10. ROOTENBERG, J. D. 1992. Information technologies in U.S. medical schools. JAMA **268:** 3106–3107.
11. SIVERTSON, S. E., T. C. MEYER, R. HANSEN & A. SCHOENENBERGER. 1973. Individual physician profile: Continuing education related to medical practice. J. Med. Ed. **48:** 1006–1012.
12. MANNING, P. R., P. V. LEE, W. A. CLINTWORTH, T. A. DENSON, P. R. OPPENHEIMER & N. J. GILMAN. 1986. Changing prescribing practices through individual continuing education. JAMA **256:** 230–232.
13. BERWICK, D. M. & K. L. COLTIN. 1986. Feedback reduces test use in a health maintenance organization. JAMA **255:** 1450–1454.
14. BORZAK, S. & H. ROSMAN. 1993. Letter to the editor. JAMA **269:** 214.
15. WATTS, M. S. M. 1990. CME or PME? J. Continuing Med. Ed. Health Prof. **10:** 129–136.

Panel Discussion 2

HENRY WALTON (*University of Edinburgh, Edinburgh, Scotland*): Dr. Sox has helped us to remember the way in which the computer is transforming education and training. Some say that its impact is akin to that of the microscope in the last century. Julio Frenk reminded us of the great importance of public health, which should inform all branches of medicine, and has updated us in our concept of what public health should be. Dr. Morillo drew our attention to clinical epidemiology and mentioned how complacent and sometimes parochial an audience in the West can be with respect to the developing world. And Dr. Wentz has spoken to us about the imperative of lifelong learning.

Our four speakers have thus emphasized aspects of medical education directly related to the concerns of this conference: information processing, people in populations, the sciences of clinical practice, and the imperative of maintaining doctors' competence throughout their professional lifetime.

The medical educators participating in this conference have the responsibility to ensure that the important methods basic to these deliberations are made central in the educational structure for training in the health professions. The principles emerging from this conference have to be brought actively to the attention of those responsible for the medical schools and other medical education institutions so that valuable impetus will be added to the active educational reforms now in progress.

We now welcome the questions and comments of our audience.

ALAN MORRIS (*LDS Hospital, Salt Lake City, Utah*): I'd like to pick up on Dr. Sox's introduction of digital system use in the delivery of medical care. It is there that one can examine our common concerns for definitive outcomes research and guideline generation and the very sticky problem of how one actually executes and carries out, in the clinical care delivery site, the important implications of these research tools. I think it was Boswell who said that man more often needs to be reminded than instructed. So I'm not so concerned about the comment by Dr. Sox that McDonald's work suggests that the people whose behavior was influenced did not, in fact, learn, because it was probably that they forgot quite quickly. The important element is that the behavior was influenced at the appropriate place and at the appropriate time.

In our institution we have utilized computerized protocols generating instructions at the bedside to actually control therapy in critically ill people 24 hours a day with not reminders but actual instructions carried out in an open-loop system. It clearly works. It may, in fact, have had a favorable impact upon survival—that's being reviewed right now. This is the place where we may get some idea about why there's such a gap between knowledge and performance, and we may in fact find a solution. The delivery of the content of guidelines in a digital system as an instruction that can remind physicians or other caregivers during the performance of work is, in our experience, a profoundly effective way to change behavior.

One implicit question that hasn't been formally articulated is this: If we are to encourage the educational system or introduce into the system the fundamental elements of decision analysis and the tools necessary to deal effectively with complex information and outcomes research, how are we going to get the current emphasis on reductionist science to yield and give time to the constructionist, holistic approaches that have been the focus of the last couple of days of discussion? No one has yet addressed the time constraints in medical education, both formal and postgraduate. I hope that this question can be dealt with without precipitating an open battle between our reductionist colleagues and ourselves.

HAROLD SOX (*Dartmouth Medical School, Lebanon, N.H.*): In the United States about half of the medical schools are currently involved in curriculum reform and I know that our efforts at Dartmouth are very much informed by the world around us and the need to prepare students to make appropriate decisions when they don't have a blank check. I'd be interested in knowing about the experience from the LDS Hospital with maintenance of a program like this. I know that system-building is not an academically very glamorous endeavor and that system maintenance, that is, keeping a system up to date, is a little bit like housekeeping. It is pretty tedious activity and one that is not particularly conducive to promotion or any of the other things that drive people in academic medicine.

WALTON: The problem of a performance gap between what physicians know to do but don't do is a grave problem.

RICHARD PETO (*University of Oxford, Oxford, England*): I felt uncomfortable with some of the presentations at this meeting—even from some very sensible people there has been too much abstraction and philosophy and not enough real results. Now, abstraction and philosophy are fine as long as whatever is presented is less than 50% philosophy and at least 50% real, important examples. For example, Dr. Frenk, you were talking in *general* terms about what public health was and what it wasn't, but you were not providing any specific details. You would have been perfectly capable of doing so, but you didn't do so, and that made what you were saying unnecessarily empty. You could instead have talked about real, particular things that you want to try to introduce in Mexico. The presentation on randomized trials included many real examples of treatments that had previously been thought not to work, but really did work, and for which overwhelmingly clear evidence that they worked had been produced either by large randomized trial or from large overviews of trials. Thus, the talk about the need for more really large randomized trials was illustrated by real examples of clear answers that would not otherwise have been obtained.

In contrast, when we got to the talk about the (rather misnamed) effectiveness research and outcomes research, no such examples were given. Examples were given showing that treatments were not being used that are known to be effective, but when it came to the question of how we are going to find out what is and what is not effective, it was noteworthy that no real examples were given where the analyses of these nonrandomized data sets had actually yielded any important conclusions as to what treatments work and what treatments don't.

Turning to other questions, there is the same need for real examples. Thus, Dr. Sox's presentation was strengthened by containing an important, real example: you can save a lot of money just by integrating computers into the process of test ordering. But many other talks did not give such examples—there's a danger when one discusses medical education and philosophy of public health without offering concrete instances of where things are wrong but rectifiable. If you don't give real examples, you'll move away from public health and from real medicine into some sort of abstract space in sociology and philosophy. Sensible doctors will then quite rightly come to despise the whole enterprise.

WALTON: That's a very trenchant point.

JULIO FRENK (*National Institute of Public Health, Cuernavaca Morelos, Mexico*): Science is the merger of two fundamental traditions. One is a tradition of ideas and—forgive me for being philosophical—the other is a tradition of confronting ideas with empirical reality. We impoverish science whenever we decide to obliterate either of these two. I think our field needs much *more* theory and that just the search for data when not guided by adequately formulated theories simply bastardizes the essence of scientific research. So I don't accept those dichotomies. If there is anything rich about scientific research, it is exactly the blending of the rationalistic constructions of the human mind and the confrontation with something that we believe is an objective world. Even the most apparently concrete exercises, like carrying out a specific randomized clinical trial, ought to be solidly grounded on that ideational rationalistic component of scientific research. We are not truly scientific if we despise the theory building.

I was given only 10 minutes to try to make a point. I did bring to this meeting the report from my institution that gives specific examples of programs and how they have been working. I have my own personal, very practical experience, which is summarized in this 5-year report of the National Institute of Public Health. In the educational training of doctors we do emphasize the need for philosophy of science and theory building as well as for sound empirical methods because you cannot do science with only one of these two. It is as negative to deny the empirical component as it is to obliterate the development of theory and reflection on our common endeavor.

WALTON: Speaking for some of the audience, we would have been profoundly deprived if Julio Frenk didn't, in fact, demonstrate to us this capacity for novel concept building.

MICHELE ORZA (*General Accounting Office, Washington, D.C.*): One perspective that's been given short shrift is that of the consumer. Could we spend some time thinking about the ways in which patients might actually be a positive force for the education of the physician? And to make Richard Peto happy I'll give two quick examples: I find that the ECPC makes a wonderful present for friends who are considering getting pregnant, and what's remarkable is the number of times that they wind up lending their copy to their gynecologists. The second example comes from my grandmother, who lives here in the Bronx and gets her medical coverage from her union. They recently sent her a printout of all the drugs that she was given in the past year and the costs for all of them, as well as what the costs might have been had she been prescribed generic drugs, and she promptly went back to her doctor and requested all the generics. This is remarkable for two reasons: first, she's not a highly educated person—she has only a high school degree—and second, she got no direct financial benefit from her action—the medications are covered no matter which ones she gets. So even though there was no financial self-interest she was persuaded that this was the right thing to do. So maybe we can step away from thinking of patients as passive and begin to think about ways in which they could be a positive force for making physicians do the right thing when they don't want to.

SOX: At Dartmouth Dr. Jack Wennberg and Dr. Alfred Mulley have been engaged in a quasi-experiment of the application of videodisc technology to informed patient decision-making. Recently I've had the opportunity to refer several of my patients to see a videodisc which describes patient-specific risks and benefits regarding the outcomes of various treatments for benign prostatic hypertrophy. In addition, the videodisc gives an opportunity to hear patients who have had various outcomes of prostate surgery and watchful waiting describe what their lives are like in an effort to try to help the patient walk in the mocassins, so to speak, of the persons who have experienced the outcomes, good and bad. This method is currently undergoing a trial in Group Health Cooperative of Puget Sound, with the outcome measure being the number of patients who are getting prostate surgery per year. It's a very exciting technology for engaging patients in decisions which concern them. There are now videodiscs for hypertension, back pain, and breast cancer.

JEROLD LUCEY (*Medical Center Hospital of Vermont, Burlington, Vt.*): I'm a neonatologist. We're all concerned by the muddling around about continuing medical education, which many of us find unsatisfying. The ideal way to continually educate yourself is to participate in trials. I've been particularly upset by the fact that the funding and specialty boards in my own field, neonatology, will give no intellectual credit for participation in a randomized control trial unless you are the leader of the trial! A way of staying alive intellectually in practice is to participate in trials and probably in the ideal Peto–Chalmers' world all clinicians would be participating in trials. This kind of challenge is fun, gives you a chance to learn, lessens your sense of isolation, and allows you to take pride in the results. Let me give you an example.

Surfactant took 30 years to be developed. When the clinical trial phase of it was entered, two companies organized large trials and within 2 years or so 100% of the 3,000 neonatologists practicing in the United States were familiar with the drug and had participated in its randomized trials. So it wasn't necessary to educate these doctors about surfactant—they had developed the market and performed adequate testing at the same time. This is a nice model to show that you can use individuals willing to participate to very good advantage, and you won't have to sell the results to them.

RICHARD DOLL (*University of Oxford, Oxford, England*): I would like to ask the panel to give some examples of the routine use of computer interaction with doctors in the ordering of tests and prescriptions and medicines. Twenty-seven years ago I was appointed as deputy director of a clinical research center, a newly established hospital with a special concern for research in England, and I visited MIT in order to find out how computers could be used in helping doctors decide on prescriptions for patients. They had a splendid program which questioned the doctors, who could only prescribe through the computers, and the program always challenged the doctors as to whether they meant to give that particular dose, and whether they knew that another drug with the same effect cost half the price. I've been out of medical practice for some years, but I've heard many other examples of the way computers can help doctors to decide upon tests and drugs to use, but can anyone tell me where such programs are actually routinely being used in hospitals?

WALTON: We'll take the remaining two questions and then ask the panel to reply.

DIXIE SNIDER (*Centers for Disease Control and Prevention, Atlanta, Ga.*): I would like to make two points: First I'm troubled that at this meeting we're focusing almost exclusively on physicians, for there are many other health care givers besides physicians in this country such as the public health nurse. And from a global perspective one can't identify physicians as even the major health care providers in the world. We need to keep that in mind when we think about trying to transfer new information and new technologies.

My second point concerns public health interventions such as requiring vaccination prior to school entry. That is one instance in which we didn't need any randomized clinical trials to prove effectiveness. As soon as states started passing laws requiring pre-school vaccination, the measles rates, for example, started to decrease and eventually all the states got on board. Examples like that from the public health arena illustrate what can be done without randomized trials when interventions are dramatically effective.

BRIAN HAYNES (*McMaster University, Hamilton, Ontario, Canada*): I want to comment on the issue of changes in medical education. Very few attempts have been made to compare students who have been through differing types of medical education, a situation that is confounded by the fact that nobody has come up with a plan to randomize medical students to different medical programs. Also, graduates from the medical schools that have had problem-based learning are just now getting into the middle of their careers. McMaster has one of the longest traditions in problem-based learning, but our longest graduates are about 18 years after their graduation. Nevertheless there appears to be some evidence that problem-based learning does affect the way that young physicians interact with new information. For example, the graduates of our medical school are more likely than students from traditional schools to maintain some sort of academic affiliation, whether as a faculty member in a medical school, holding a research grant, or having at least a part-time clinical affiliation with a medical school while remaining in private practice. More recently, one of our studies, which has just been published in the *Canadian Medical Association Journal*, compares primary care physicians from the University of Toronto with those from McMaster University. This comparison was based on knowledge of current recommendations for the management of hypertensive patients, and it shows a significant difference for the McMaster graduates not with respect to knowledge retained but with knowledge of current management. The interesting feature of all studies relating time of graduation to knowledge of current management principles is that there's a steep negative slope. The farther you are from graduation generally the less knowledge you have of current information. But the slope for the McMaster graduates is zero—there isn't a slope. The implications of this are interesting, but we still can't say what these physicians do in actual practice with their patients. We need to put more research funds into documenting the differences in the educational approaches that are currently available, but at least there is hope that in undergraduate experience learning by inquiry as opposed to didactic learning may result in practitioners' keeping up to date with new information as it is published.

KENNETH WARREN: (*Picower Institute for Medical Research, Manhasset, N.Y.*): To respond to Richard Peto's plea indirectly, I'd like to ask Arturo Morillo to comment on the International Clinical Epidemiology Network that he runs. This network, which is a major force throughout the world, now includes a large number of clinical epidemiology units in Latin America, Asia, and Africa, as well as the original training units from Australia, Canada, and the United States. Are any of your units involved in randomized controlled trials on interventions of any types and are any of your units involved in meta-analyses?

ARTURO MORILLO (*International Clinical Epidemiology Network, Philadelphia, Pa.*): We have 27 units in 16 countries and at least 20 of these units are engaged in randomized trials, which are one of the most common activities that they develop; however, I am not aware of their participation in meta-analysis, which in any case is made more difficult because of the relative paucity of library resources in those countries. But we are interested in linking with the Cochrane Centre to see how we can cooperate in developing these kind of activities in the future.

With regard to how we influence politics, I will cite a situation in Thailand, where a clinical epidemiology unit conducting studies comparing different kinds of tuberculosis treatment showed that the one suggested by the government was not as effective as another in the trial. This finding influenced the Thai government to change its policy for treatment of tuberculosis.

SOX: In response to Sir Richard's question about computers and routine use, I'm aware that the HELP system, developed by Homer Warner and his colleagues, is in routine use at the LDS Hospital in Salt Lake City. I believe that a number of the features of the Indiana University Regenstrief system are in routine use. The Harvard Community Health Plan has used a reminder system for disease prevention and health promotion.

This symposium seems to be a celebration of achievement in technology assessment. The next step, translating evidence into patient care outcomes, has proved to be very difficult. One of the first steps is to put the same kind of energy and creativity into improving medical education that has been put into improving technology assessment.

FRENK: Dr. Morris mentioned the need for the synthesis of knowledge and the integration of findings, which I believe is both the challenge and the beauty of the field of health. I have tried to present a way of thinking about how those integrations are to occur. This involves the selection of a particular health problem, and then approaching it by integrating the two objects: understanding the condition itself and its frequency and distribution in the population. It is then necessary to understand the response to that particular problem both through clinical research and the study of efficacy of interventions and to see through health systems research how those interventions that have proven efficacious are actually carried out in particular settings and in particular organizational arenas. This kind of analysis involves integration among levels of analysis—we have to take health problems from the subindividual to the population level. And that requires integration among disciplines.

We don't do that now, however: we have been much better at building barriers rather than bridges between the various areas of the health care field. We can only understand it in taking a problem-centered approach, which is not a weakness of the health field, but its most interesting feature. The problem is a crossroads where the biological and the social factors connect these various levels of analysis. At the National Institute of Public Health in Mexico we select a particular problem and try to understand it from the very basic biomedical evidence all the way to its social and economic implications. Human reproduction is another example that can be viewed from a minute understanding of its physiology to its broadest economic and social repercussions.

I agree with the plea for an integrative review, especially when we're dealing with interventions, which are part of the social response. The assessment of interventions is triggered by the randomized clinical trial, which allows us to estimate efficacy. But our job does not stop there—we still have not fully answered the question of where we do more good than harm because the "answer" has to be translated into particular organizational arrangements and research. There's still a patient population that's not simply a passive recipient of our interventions but that reacts. We have to understand those complexities with the same rigor we use to evaluate efficacy. The research agenda is broader and in that sense we cannot reach full understanding.

DENNIS WENTZ (*American Medical Association, Chicago, Illinois*): The fact that so much medical science is reported in the daily newspapers and in the *Wall Street Journal* can irritate physicians, especially when their patients know the information before the doctor him- or herself has read the journal. So obviously the press, and television, and other media drive some continuing education programs because doctors feel that they have to keep up in a very competitive world. I agree with Dr. Lucey that it is an excellent idea to keep physicians participating in research and trials and in teaching—if you want to count credit hours you put that kind of activity in the category 2 section, which is self-directed physician-verifiable learning. We've got to put more emphasis on that kind of learning, for its outcomes can only be positive.

I agree with Dixie Snider that we are focusing too much on physicians. However, we've recently had an opportunity to look at the literature in continuing education across all the professions, and the literature in medicine exceeds by 10-fold everything else so it's not altogether inappropriate at this stage to focus on the doctor. And, finally, I agree with Brian Haynes' comment on the need for more research into the outcomes in the practice years for physicians who are trained in different modes. We've got to build in money up front for this sort of research.

The Clinical Efficacy Assessment Program of the American College of Physicians

JOHN R. FEUSSNER[a] AND LINDA JOHNSON WHITE[b]

[a]Division of General Internal Medicine
Duke University Medical Center
Durham, North Carolina 27710; and
Center for Health Services Research in Primary Care
Department of Veterans Affairs Medical Center
Durham, North Carolina 27705

[b]American College of Physicians
Health and Public Policy
Independence Mall West, 6th Street at Race
Philadelphia, Pennsylvania 19106-1572

BACKGROUND

The American College of Physicians (ACP) initiated its Clinical Efficacy Assessment Program (CEAP) in 1981.[1] The goals of this program were to: (1) assemble and review the clinical literature on a specified topic; (2) identify the best scientific papers; and (3) analyze, reformulate, and present such information so that practitioners can readily determine the usefulness of diagnostic tests, procedures, or treatments.

The Institute of Medicine defines practice guidelines as systematically developed statements that assist practitioner and patient decisions about appropriate health care for specific clinical circumstances.[2] As such, practice guidelines as currently developed represent point estimates reflecting current scientific evidence or expert opinion concerning the use of diagnostic technologies or medical or surgical therapies.

The Clinical Efficacy Assessment Program focuses on several dimensions of diagnostic test use and treatments that include safety, relative and absolute contraindications, efficacy (preferably as demonstrated by experimental studies), limitations, and their costs to patients.

Development of practice guidelines should not rely on the weight of medical information, which can be ponderous, but on the weight of scientific evidence. During the CEAP process, experts in research methods collaborate with content experts to identify salient clinical issues and to generate recommendations or guidelines based on the best research products. Therefore, the CEAP process emphasizes the quality, not the quantity, of the evidence.

PROCESS OF GUIDELINE DEVELOPMENT

TABLE 1 show the process used by the ACP to develop clinical practice guidelines. A CEAP topic guideline survey is conducted among members of the College. High-priority diagnostic technologies or therapies are considered and

TABLE 1. Process for Development of Practice Guidelines

Topic survey of practitioners
Expert consultants identified
Review of project scope
Guideline background paper produced
Internal peer review
External peer review

topics for guideline development are chosen. The ACP identifies expert consultants to develop practice guidelines. The College internally reviews the project's scope and plan. Then the expert team prepares a background paper that reviews the literature comprehensively. The Clinical Efficacy Assessment Subcommittee (CEAS) reviews the background paper through several iterations. After revisions are completed, the manuscript is reviewed externally by other content experts and medical societies. For example, guidelines developed for magnetic resonance imaging of the brain and spine have been reviewed by as many as six external expert reviewers. These reviewers represent specialty societies including the American College of Radiology, the American Academy of Neurology, the American Association of Neurological Surgeons, and others. Authors of the original guideline paper and the American College of Physicians CEAS members review the critiques from the external reviewers. A consensus is reached on all issues raised by internal and external reviewers.

The Clinical Efficacy Assessment Program is an evidence-based process. The CEAP process collates the existing medical literature, usually limited to English-language papers. An expert team provides a methodologic review of pertinent manuscripts. The literature is summarized using techniques of information synthesis, such as meta-analysis, decision analysis, or cost-effectiveness analysis.[3–6] The final product is a concise list of recommendations or guidelines that are useful to practicing physicians. Besides a background paper, a brief summary paper is prepared that enumerates specific guidelines without providing the background justification.

Several strengths of the clinical efficacy assessment program are listed in TABLE 2. The focus of CEAP is on the generalist practitioner. The CEAP process seeks to clarify the complexities of the scientific evidence. All pertinent literature is identified. Scientific evidence is integrated with expert opinion. Because the process is evidence-based, strong guidelines can be developed when scientific evidence is of high quality. When evidence is lacking, guidelines are conservative. Finally, the guideline development process is dynamic, and guidelines are systematically reevaluated, especially when newer information becomes available.

TABLE 2. Strengths of the Clinical Efficacy Assessment Program

Focus on clinical practioner
Comprehensive literature review
Evidence-based guidelines
Integration of expert opinion
Conservative guidelines when evidence is incomplete
Dynamic process with systematic review

The CEAP process, as with other guideline development processes, has limitations (see TABLE 3), including use of only published literature and use of methodologic criteria that, while reasonable for an individual project, are not standardized across projects. The developed guidelines are frequently based on a few quality research products. When evidence is limited or of low quality, a compromise must be made between the paucity of scientific evidence and the surfeit of expert opinion. In addition, conflict management among experts is *ad hoc*; conflict occasionally becomes irreconcilable.

RESULTS

Products of the CEAP process include the development of credible guidelines free from conflict of interest and the possibility that such guidelines will improve physician knowledge or, at least, enhance physician acceptance of guideline statements. Finally the CEAP process clearly exposes information gaps in the scientific literature.

On a health policy level, CEAP has influenced such agencies as the Health Care Financing Administration (HCFA), health maintenance organizations (HMOs), and third-party insurers. For example, the HCFA applied ACP guidelines for phonocardiography use with a large reduction in reimbursement levels. A large

TABLE 3. Limitations of the Clinical Efficacy Assessment Program

Only accesses published literature
Scientific criteria for quality are not standardized
Guidelines are based on a few quality research products
Compromises with expert opinion
Conflict management among experts is *ad hoc*

West Coast HMO applied ACP-generated guidelines on the use of hyperbaric oxygen pressurization treatments resulting in reduced expenditures. Under these circumstances, guideline use has been directed toward elimination of unnecessary procedures or therapies with consequent cost savings.

On the physician level, opinions on guideline impact have been obtained through physician surveys. The ACP completed a nationwide mailed survey of a random sample of 2,600 members and associates. While most internists said they had positive impressions about guidelines, one-third of the respondents reported significant concerns such as a potential loss of autonomy from increased guideline use. The survey results also showed that fewer than 15% of internists reported that guidelines greatly affected their clinical practice. Clearly, concerning guideline dissemination, the survey results are mixed.

The ACP has disseminated its guidelines through continuing medical education programs that include national meetings, audiotapes, and presentations of guidelines by expert physicians on medical television.

DISCUSSION

While the ACP has maintained the Clinical Efficacy Assessment Program for the past decade, the CEAP process continues to evolve. Beyond actively updating previous guidelines, the ACP is also making a concerted effort to prepare succinct, informative summaries for patients, as well as its physician membership. The ACP continues to cooperate with other efforts by other agencies (e.g., the Agency for Health Care Policy and Research) and Medical Societies (e.g., the American Medical Association).

Still, as so aptly put by Paul Simon and Art Garfunkel, "a man hears what he wants to hear and disregards the rest." Changing the fundamental truth of this statement should be a major goal of any group seeking to influence medical practice through the use of practice guidelines.

SUMMARY

The experience of the American College of Physicians (ACP) in evaluating the clinical literature and publishing clinical guidelines spans more than a decade. The ACP uses an evidence-based method for the development of clinical practice guidelines for diagnostic technologies and treatments. The approach of the Clinical Efficacy Assessment Program (CEAP) involves collation, methodologic review, and analysis of the clinical literature. The process focuses on the safety, contraindications, efficacy, limitations, and cost of diagnostic technologies or treatments. To ensure a balanced perspective of the evidence, methodologic and content experts cooperate to prepare a summary paper. Strengths of this evidence-based approach include: (1) focus on the needs of practicing internists; (2) identification of all pertinent clinical literature; (3) integration of expert opinion when literature is inadequate; (4) recommendations based on high-quality scientific evidence; (5) preparation of conservative guidelines when evidence is lacking; and (6) reevaluation of past guidelines as new evidence becomes available. Limitations of the process include: (1) access only to published research; (2) use of criteria for scientific quality that are not standardized across projects; (3) published recommendations based on small numbers of high-quality research products; (4) compromise with expert opinion when evidence is limited; and (5) *ad hoc* management of conflict between experts when scientific evidence is sparse. The process produces credible recommendations that may improve physician knowledge and acceptance of practice guidelines.

REFERENCES

1. SCHWARTZ, J. S. & J. R. BALL. 1982. Safety, efficacy and effectiveness of clinical practices: A new initiative. Ann. Intern. Med. **96:** 246.
2. FIELD, M. J. & K. N. LOHR. 1992. Guidelines for Clinical Practice: From Development to Use. National Academy Press. Washington, DC.
3. GOLDSCHMIDT, P. G. 1986. Information synthesis: A practical guide. Health Serv. Res. **21:** 215–237.
4. L'ABBE, K. A., A. S. DETSKY & K. O'ROURKE. 1987. Meta-analysis in clinical research. Ann. Intern. Med. **107:** 224–233.
5. SOX, H. C., M. A. BLATT, M. C. HIGGINS & K. I. MARTON. 1988. Medical Decision Making. Butterworths. Boston, MA.
6. WARNER, K. E. & B. R. LUCE. 1982. Cost-benefit and Cost-effectiveness Analysis in Health Care: Principles, Practice, and Potential. Health Administration Press. Ann Arbor, MI.

Using Evidence for Utilization Management: An HMO Manager's Perspective

STEPHEN C. SCHOENBAUM

Harvard Community Health Plan
10 Brookline Place West
Brookline, Massachusetts 02146

Health maintenance organizations (HMOs) combine payment of covered medical care expenses for a population with a medical care delivery system for that same population. HMOs do not just obtain volume discounts for care. Staff and group model HMOs especially pride themselves on their ability to manage processes of care, a major component of which can be called "utilization management."

Not all utilization management depends upon evidence. Indeed, the most effective intervention for HMOs has been having a different set of incentives than fee-for-service delivery systems. In staff and group model HMOs the physicians are usually salaried. In group network HMOs, the physicians, whether or not they individually are salaried or compensated on some other basis, belong to groups which are capitated as a whole to provide care to a specified population. In either structural arrangement there is little economic incentive to hospitalize patients. Not surprisingly, hospital utilization rates in such HMOs have been a fraction of those seen in fee-for-service settings. This has generated an economic advantage for HMOs. Only as controls on hospital utilization have been imposed on the fee-for-service sector have HMOs begun seriously to address management of utilization of other types of health care services.

Utilization is managed when a "manager" insists that the services being ordered or provided by clinicians be ones for which there is evidence that the benefits exceed the risks. Another level of utilization management is to require that the benefits be worth the cost. In other terms, in the context of utilization management, practices should be effective and cost-effective; they should be "essential" or "medically necessary."

Despite the economic incentive structure of HMOs, there is substantial variation in utilization within them. There is variation between physicians or between sites such as health centers or medical groups. Absolute levels of utilization may be less than in fee-for-service practice. Nevertheless, the variation which occurs in HMO practice has similar sources to those in fee-for-service practice. They include different responses to incentives (largely non-economic in HMOs), lack of knowledge of existing evidence, differences in practice style which arise in the absence of any evidence, scientific disagreements among knowledgeable practitioners, and different patient preferences. Only the last two might be considered justifiable sources of variation.

Evidence is clearly important to clinical managers in HMOs who are interested in managing utilization and managing variation in practices. It is understandable that patients may differ in their values and respond differently to evidence about their medical choices. This is the basis of the principle of informed consent. Nevertheless, in how many instances in which informed consent is obtained is an unbiased presentation of the available evidence and lack of evidence given to the patient? The probable answer is "very few." This is leading HMOs to be interested in the work of Wennberg and colleagues on shared decision making,[1] a process in which interactive videodisk technology has been employed to present evidence and opinion about important medical decisions to patients. This process should enhance the likelihood that informed consent is obtained. The programs for shared decision making are quite recent, and evidence about the value of the process itself is being awaited eagerly.

Scientific differences do occur, but they are relatively few and far between. Scientific differences delineate clear-cut targets for future research; and ultimately, if the research is done, there will be evidence to resolve the controversy and guide clinical decision-making. Clinical controversies often arise when the benefit-risk or benefit-cost differences of alternative approaches are qualitatively dissimilar. Decision-analytic techniques have been helpful in elucidating some of these controversies. The most important issue for those interested in utilization management is whether the clinical controversy is really just due to a difference in values of different clinicians. An objective of utilization managers should be to help physicians distinguish their own values from those of their patients and help them learn to frame choices for patients in ways in which it becomes the patients' values not the physicians' values which are dominant (*vide supra*).

Differences from lack of knowledge of existing evidence do exist. It is essential to be able to package evidence in ways that are most interpretable and usable by clinicians. Utilization management may require that evidence be presented in particular ways, for example, by giving an indication of the absolute magnitude of a treatment effect not just the relative magnitude of the effect.[2] Very large HMOs may be able to undertake their own educational programs and may be able to review and package existing evidence. Most HMOs, however, do not have the capability of doing the literature syntheses and meta-analyses necessary for appropriate packaging of available evidence. Accordingly, HMOs become important customers, rather than suppliers, of such information.

It is regrettable how little evidence on the effectiveness and cost-effectiveness of medical practices is available. This is the major problem in basing utilization management upon evidence. The work of Adams *et al.*[3] has quantitated the poverty of good information on cost-efficacy that has been derived from clinical trials. An additional problem is that efficacy, as determined in clinical trials, does not always translate into clinical effectiveness[4]; and relatively few studies have been done to document effectiveness of practices that have been shown to be efficacious in small trials.

Perhaps as a backlash to the recent onslaught of the quality management movement, there are many health care organizations in which people now consciously avoid using the term "quality." Utilization management is an even more highly charged concept than quality management. The notion of utilization management always brings up the spectre of rationing; but utilization management is not synonymous with rationing. In fact, utilization management and higher quality of care are quite compatible—particularly when the utilization management is based upon evidence. It is not rationing to withhold treatments that are not known to be effective. Conversely, providing treatments that are supported by evidence of effectiveness and cost-effectiveness should be the desired goal of any health care delivery system. Evidence-based utilization management requires the tools of clinical guidelines, review criteria, performance measures, and standards of quality. No HMO or other managed care organization should be uncomfortable about the fact that other organizations, such as government or specialty societies, are developing evidence-based guidelines. Indeed, one extremely important job of HMOs is to implement such guidelines and to do so more effectively than has been done in the past by unmanaged health care delivery components.

In short, HMOs are consumers of medical effectiveness and cost-effectiveness evidence. HMOs need an academic community which is oriented towards producing such evidence. In return, HMOs can provide populations from which such evidence might be obtained.

REFERENCES

1. WINSLOW, R. 1992. Videos, questionnaires aim to expand role of patients in treatment decisions. The Wall Street Journal. February 25: B1, B3.
2. NAYLOR, C. D., E. CHEN & B. STRAUSS. 1992. Measured enthusiasm: Does the method of reporting trial results alter perceptions of therapeutic effectiveness? Ann. Intern. Med. **117:** 916–921.
3. ADAMS, M. E., N. T. McCALL, D. T. GRAY, M. J. ORZA & T. C. CHALMERS. 1992. Economic analysis in randomized control trials. Medical Care **30**(3): 231–243.
4. GOTTLIEB, L. K. & S. SALEM-SCHATZ. Anticoagulation in atrial fibrillation: Does efficacy in clinical trials translate into effectiveness in practice? Arch. Intern. Med. In press.

The Role of Evidence in the Approval of Pharmaceuticals

JERE E. GOYAN

Alteon Inc.
165 Ludlow Avenue
Northvale, New Jersey 07647

The title of this volume implies that it may be possible for us to do more harm than good when we use drugs. And when we consider doing more good, the basic question that we immediately face is: Are we talking about more good than harm, individual by individual, or on a public health basis? For example, the sweetener, aspartame, cannot be used by persons with the metabolic disease known as phenylketonuria. If one were concerned only about the effect on an individual-by-individual basis, one would not approve the product. On the other hand, assuming that a noncaloric sweetener is useful to the public, the FDA chose to approve aspartame with labeling warning phenylketonurics of the danger. Similarly, the patient who has a massive gastrointestinal bleeding after taking a non-steroidal anti-inflammatory drug would probably argue that the drug should have been banned, although *over all* it is undoubtedly doing more good than harm.

Similar arguments have dominated the rhetoric of the drug-approval process for several years. Those who claim that a delay in the approval of the first beta blocker "killed" many Americans (a public health argument) are rebutted by those who say that many individual patients were spared from blindness by the FDA's refusal to hurry that approval.

While serving as Commissioner of the Food and Drug Administration, I used to argue that I would take a 10% cut in the agency's budget in return for a 10% better understanding of statistical concepts by the American people. As I have reflected on that argument over the years, I have reached the conclusion that it was probably wrong. For example, I buy lottery tickets from time to time realizing full well the odds against winning, taking into account the even smaller odds of any risk. If a new drug has a risk of some side effect of one in one thousand, and only one in one million chance for a potential benefit, would I take the drug? Well, if the alternative is certain death, as it is today with a disease like acquired immune deficiency syndrome (AIDS), I have the feeling that I would. On the other hand, I certainly would not accept the same odds for a purported cure for male pattern baldness.

The problem, of course, with this sort of thinking is that we never really know all of the potential risks and we tend to romanticize the potential benefits. Perhaps the best-known example of an unknown risk, which has come to haunt society, is clear-cell carcinoma of the vagina induced by diethylstilbestrol in the daughters of women who took the drug to prevent spontaneous abortion during their pregnancy. This is a particularly egregious example since the unknown toxic effect was so devastating and the purported benefit turned out to have been totally illusory.

When I left the agency in 1981, I left believing that there was a societal contract relative to the drug-approval process which had been agreed to by most of those interested in the process, whether from academia, the pharmaceutical industry, or the Food and Drug Administration. However, it was only a couple of years later when that societal contract was ripped asunder by the advent of AIDS.

There had previously been questions raised about the process of drug approval, especially in areas where adequate drugs were not available, such as for many forms of cancer. However, the arguments put forward by many of the people at this conference and others had held sway emphasizing the importance of a sound scientific approach to proving drug efficacy, because it is so difficult to know whether a drug works or not, and there are so many potential pitfalls on the road to knowing, as detailed in the book by Bill Silverman on human experimentation.[1]

Everyone in this room probably agrees that sound statistical methods are a must for scientific credibility. Unfortunately I would maintain that such scientific credibility is almost irrelevant from the public viewpoint. Many of you will remember the full-page advertisements taken out by the soft drink industry showing the hundreds of cans of soft drinks a consumer would have to drink per day to reach the level of risk found in the rodent studies of saccharin demonstrating carcinogenicity. These advertisements were successful in trivializing the argument, and allowed the American people to laugh at the "foolishness" of the FDA in trying to ban saccharin. With sand recently identified as a potential carcinogen in labelling required by the State of California one must wonder, where will it all end?

What can be done to minimize risk and maximize potential benefit, at least on a public health basis? As a former regulator, I believe that one must first recognize the fact that decisions will always have to be made on inadequate data and that every statistical analysis is open to second guessing and criticism by other statisticians. I have endured several hours of argument between my friends who are committed "intent to treat" advocates and those who are committed to analyzing only those patients who "have received the drug," and I am convinced that agreement will never be reached between the contending parties, although both groups certainly support the need for statistical analysis of the data. But insofar as we continue to have such battles, we allow those who care not one wit for either approach to occasionally carry the day.

For example, during the past ten years we have observed the spectacle of the drug Bendectin being driven off the market by plaintiff lawyers using so-called "expert witnesses." Their arguments never would have been accepted in a peer-reviewed journal. Indeed, meta-analysis of all of the studies addressing the possibility of Bendectin-induced teratogenicity has shown that Bendectin in all probability is not teratogenic. Nevertheless, the drug is no longer available in this country. The U.S. Supreme Court is presently considering an appeals court decision which rejected a re-analysis of 30 epidemiologic studies finding Bendectin to be a teratogen on the basis that their analysis had not been peer-reviewed.

What then, might be done? Perhaps it is time that those of us interested in the problem accept the burden of attempting to challenge bad science in the court of public opinion. You may recall that for many years, no one challenged the claims of those who were bending spoons by their thought processes and carrying out other equally inplausible stunts. I have always thought that those magicians who took on the burden of unmasking such charlatans and showing that they could do the same thing by legerdemain have done the public a great service. If a similar approach could be used challenging the bad science presently used as a basis for tort claims and wild public charges, it could be a major contribution to "doing more good than harm" both on an individual-by-individual and a public health basis.

However, challenges must be based on solid evidence and I trust this conference will assist each of us in assessing the value of interventions such as drug therapy and prepare us to mount such challenges.

REFERENCE

1. SILVERMAN, W. A. 1985. Human Experimentation—A Guided Step into the Unknown. Oxford University Press. New York.

Panel Discussion 3

ARGYE HILLIS (*Texas A & M Health Science Center, Temple, Texas*): I will preface my remarks by saying that I have not been able to sell some of these ideas in my own HMO, which is run by Scott and White. But, addressing the question of clinical trials in HMOs, I was glad to hear the evidence that patients are better cared for in clinical trials and better informed as well. And the physicians themselves are better cared for and better informed when they participate in clinical trials. From that standpoint I would like to raise this question: Don't the HMOs have a responsibility not only to implement the guidelines but to help produce them as well.

I support the comments about clinical trials needing to address common problems; they need to address problems in the real world, which the HMO context can provide. Those of us in large clinical trials are worried that managed care, HMOs, and that kind of delivery system will cut out clinical trials because of the payment issues. So I would much rather see clinical trials brought into the fold of the HMOs and managed care systems because that's where they can be done best. The HMOs need the clinical trials for their physicians and for their patients, and certainly the clinical trials need the HMO context.

STEPHEN SCHOENBAUM (*Harvard Community Health Plan, Brookline, Massachusetts*): The largest HMOs, such as Kaiser-Permanente and Group Health Cooperative of Puget Sound, and ourselves, have a long history of participation in clinical trials, some of which have been about the health care system itself (such as Group Health Cooperative's participation in the health insurance experiment, which was really a randomized trial of HMO care versus other delivery systems). The payment issue is an important one: HMOs, like most insurers, say in their benefits contracts that they don't pay for experimental treatments.

In fact, however, most HMOs that I know of pay routinely for participation in such trials; they may not pay for the experimental drug, but they pay for trials. Our Institutional Review Board has this year 60 protocols in active use just by our oncologists. Now I know that some insurers don't pay for experimental oncology regimens, but that is not the case in our HMO at least. This is not an issue that has to remain unresolved forever. If the world is headed towards uniform benefit packages, it ought to be fairly easy to include participation in responsible, approved research. It does need some advocates, but I don't think you'll find the HMOs on the *con* side of the issue. By and large the persons I know in the HMO industry favor the generation of new knowledge.

IAIN CHALMERS (*The UK Cochrane Centre, Oxford, England*): I'd like to comment on Dr. Goyan's presentation. I was glad to see him, after seeming to have reservations about the public's involvement, take a more optimistic tack. It reinforces Michele Orza's earlier comments on just how important the public is in supporting research of the kind we're talking about. Adrian Grant has also spoken about how consumer groups in the United Kingdom gave very explicit support on television, on radio, and in the newspapers to the randomized evaluation of chorionic villus sampling versus amniocentesis. Another consumer organization is running its own multicenter trial to address an issue of concern to it. So the public should be regarded as an important ally in this enterprise and it is very important to involve members of the public in the health care research endeavor.

Dr. Schoenbaum referred to the classic conceptual distinction between efficacy and effectiveness trials, which goes back to the work of Schwartz and Lellouch in France, who made a distinction between explanatory and pragmatic trials. This distinction was reinforced in the late '70s and early '80s by the very important documents produced by the WHO and the Office of Technology Assessment. But it has to be recognized that the distinction between efficacy and effectiveness studies is blurred. When, for example, in GISSI-1 90 percent of the coronary care units in the whole of Italy collaborated in the trial of streptokinase it is not an issue whether or not the results are relevant to general clinical practice—they were derived from general clinical practice, so of course they are.

When Richard Peto was concentrating on the issue of reducing statistical imprecision in getting estimates of moderate treatment effects, he may have under-stressed the importance of the generalizability of the results when a trial has had very wide entry criteria from community hospitals, from academic centers, from many countries, and so on. The sort of network that Dr. Jerold Lucey and his colleagues at the University of Vermont have developed for neonatal trials is a good example of one that will generate information that is far nearer to the *effectiveness* end than to the *efficacy* end of the spectrum.

Finally I'd like help with the following question: One hears the statement made with confidence and fairly repeatedly that the results of randomized controlled trials are often not applicable in practice. Does Dr. Schoenbaum or anyone else know of a systematic review of the evidence which supports that often-made statement? I'm not aware of such a review, although I would love one to be done. We need to know the quality of the evidence upon which that statement has been made so confidently. Does anyone know of any reviews?

SCHOENBAUM: I don't know of such a review, but the point I was trying to make is that it is not necessarily the case that the effectiveness one sees in use will be equivalent to the efficacy demonstrated in a clinical trial. The question I'm asking relates to your observation that in one study 90% of the coronary care units participated. The question is, how can we make our effectiveness come closer to efficacy? There are two components to the answer: one is to treat restricted populations as in the applied clinical trial or, conversely, to include broader populations in the trial so that the results are more generalizable; and the second is to adopt treatment methodologies that are closer to those that are adopted in the trials. It is often said almost disparagingly that those trials put so much effort into getting the treatment right. And I'm saying that a good health care delivery system ought to be able to do the same thing. So our target is to close the gap between the results of clinical trials and the results of use of the same treatments in "usual" care.

CHALMERS: I agree absolutely with the second point, but I'm concerned about the unwillingness to extrapolate beyond the population that was in a particular trial. We have heard about the ill-considered exclusion of elderly people from controlled trials and how older people can benefit more from a particular intervention than younger people. I think that restrictive entry criteria, which are often plucked out of the air—such as you shouldn't allow someone over 65 to go into the trial—are unfair unless such exclusion can clearly be shown to be justified. The entry criteria should be wide, which is another message of these large, simple trials.

JOHN FERGUSON (*NIH, Bethesda, Maryland*): I was glad to hear Dr. Goyan talk a little bit about the other segment of our society that does technology assessment, namely, the courts. We've studied a number of issues, such as immunoaugmentative therapy and Laetrile, relative to how the courts arrive at their decisions about them; our findings are going to be published next month in the *Journal of the*

American Medical Association. In that article we suggest that the courts use better science and published peer-reviewed science. I note in the case of *Daubert* versus *Merrill Dow Pharmaceuticals* that's coming up before the Supreme Court that friend-of-the-courts briefs have been filed on the part of the National Academy of Sciences, the American Association for the Advancement of Science, the *New England Journal of Medicine*, the *Journal of the American Medical Association*, and the AMA. If the defendants win, then, as I understand it, information, to be allowed as evidence in court, will have to have been published in a peer-review journal. This then makes the editors of medical science journals the arbiters of what is allowed into court as evidence. I wonder how these editors view that change in their job description!

JEROLD LUCEY (*University of Vermont, Burlington, Vt.*): It's a shocking thought. Actually I've always had the feeling that everything eventually gets published if somebody is driven enough to persist. There are 40 journals in the pediatric world, and it's no secret among editors that there's a pecking order, and that one of them will eventually publish whatever it is the person wants to have published. The journals give some protection from the pseudoscientists who show up on television talk shows. Then they appear in court as "experts." Some of these people are much better presenters than true scientists and prevail over the honest folks. Some protection will be afforded, but not an awful lot.

JERE GOYAN (*Alteon, Inc., Northvale, N.J.*): I suspect that some of you noticed the article in *Newsweek* this week relative to this very issue of junk science. I found myself a little surprised to be in complete disagreement with Stephen J. Gould and some others who argue that almost every generally accepted view was once deemed eccentric or heretical and consequently that we should not rule these odd notions out of the courtroom because they may be right. But I have trouble with that opinion. If the science is right, it will eventually be acknowledged as right. Indeed the examples that Gould and others cited were things like the Krebs cycle, Barbara McClintock's work with jumping genes, and other ideas that had trouble at first getting acceptance by the scientific community. But I think that we ought to let science make those decisions, rather than allow the courts to make decisions based on inadequate evidence.

HAROLD SOX (*Dartmouth Medical Center, Lebanon, N.H.*): I wanted to make a brief comment on Dr. Feussner's presentation about the American College of Physicians Clinical Efficacy Assessment Program or CEAP. I also spent some time on that and I want to be sure that the audience does not get the impression that the people who develop these background papers were content experts. Quite the contrary: as a matter of policy, the ACP program has sought out general internists with the skills of the clinical epidemiologist to write these papers, sometimes in collaboration with a sympathetic open-minded content expert, but often alone. This strategy has allowed the ACP program to approach the technology of the problem from an entirely fresh point of view and thus may be one of the reasons why those recommendations frequently are countercultural.

JOHN FEUSSNER (*Duke University Medical Center, Durham, N.C.*): I agree with that, Dr. Sox. One of the difficulties with trying to marry the content expert with the methodological expert is that while the methodologist may not have an axe to grind, the content expert frequently does. Those differences have marked some of the conflicts that we've experienced in the process.

I'd like to take that observation further. Dr. Goyan talked about establishing efficacy for drugs and part of the CEAP process looks at establishing efficacy for diagnostic tests and new technologies. There appears to be, at least in the past, a substantial double standard for accepting or for creating evidence to demonstrate the efficacy of pharmaceuticals versus evidence demonstrating the efficacy of surgical therapies, rehabilitation therapies, alternative therapies, and new technologies especially in this country. There may well be more MRI scanners in the state of North Carolina than in the country of Canada, and I suspect that something is remiss there. When we've recently been engaged in the CEAP process looking at MRIs, a potential replacement for CT scanning, we saw that there are fewer than three studies published in the English language that experimentally address the efficacy of those two competing technologies. There's also a dramatic paucity of evidence that increased diagnostic precision is often, occasionally, or rarely translated to better patient outcomes.

LAWRENCE ALTMAN (The New York Times, *New York, N.Y.*): Given Dr. Ferguson's comments about a change in the job description for editors, it is prudent to remember their vested interests. Some journal editors have written that no medical or scientific information should be presented to the public until it is published in a peer-review journal. They have developed strict embargo policies based on a belief, not on data showing that such a practice is dangerous. It is simply scoop journalism. Several points about journal peer review: First, a standard definition of a peer-review journal is lacking. No dictionary that I have consulted defines a peer-review journal. Since science prides itself on precision, we will need to define a peer-review journal—and a peer as well. The National Library of Medicine has no criteria for defining a peer-review journal. And the National Library of Medicine, as publisher of *Index Medicus,* is the arbiter of what a peer-review journal is. When I last checked, the Library had no standard definition, no official criteria, and no checklist of what constitutes a peer-review journal. The Library has its own process for listing a journal in *Index Medicus.* Second, much that appears in a peer-review journal is not peer-reviewed, and that adds a misleading aspect to the issue. Third, if peer reviewing becomes the criterion, why not consider publishing the criticisms, caveats, and other pertinent remarks made by peer-reviewers so the reader could benefit from such comments. Fourth, we will need to have a better understanding of the number of reviewers used in a journal's peer-review process because the number varies widely among journals, from one or two to into the teens. Fifth, journals will need to periodically publish information about their peer-review process, something very few journals now do. I could go on with this list. Instead, I will refer those interested to my paper entitled "The Myth of Passing Peer Review" that was published by the Council of Biology Editors. Finally, in the interests of accountability, I wonder whether the journals will need one of Dr. Codman's end-result cards to assess their performance!

MARY ANN CHIASSON (*New York City Health Department, New York, N.Y.*): There's an additional, serious problem: occasionally papers in peer-review journals are retracted, and while the initial paper becomes part of the standard knowledge base, the retraction is never made well known.

ALTMAN: There's an even more serious problem: some journals will not publish retractions. In the case of Philip Felig and Vijay Soman at Yale with the *New England Journal* a couple of years ago one of the authors wanted to issue a retraction in the *Journal of Clinical Investigation*, but there is no correspondence column there.

KENNETH WARREN (*Picower Institute for Medical Research, Manhasset, N.Y.*): As a professor of information science as well as medicine I've spent 25 years working on issues like the one under discussion. Larry Altman is right. I was on the Medline and MEDLARS committee many years ago and at that time there were no criteria for deciding what journals went into MEDLARS. The

Institute for Scientific Information produces the Science Citation Index and *Current Contents*. They publish good criteria as to what they consider to be a journal that should be admitted into a system.

I've been concerned for a long time as to what makes scientists send articles to certain journals and it's not because they're peer-reviewed or not. What makes the *New England Journal of Medicine* or the *Lancet* two of the premier journals in medicine is that any scientist worth his salt, any biomedical or clinical investigator, who is prepared to publish a paper would die to get in the *Lancet* and the *New England Journal*. So it's not the issue of peer review that determines whether an article will be submitted to the *New England Journal*—it's that the best people, who usually produce the best papers, will send their papers to the best journals that they could possibly get an article into. And if it's an immunologist, he'll send his article to the *Journal of Immunology* and the *Journal of Experimental Medicine* and so on. One time I was trying to devise a strategy for improving a medical journal by just getting a group of people to make a decision that they'd send their articles there if they didn't get into the *Lancet* or the *New England Journal*. I'm sure that is what would happen.

So when you talk about looking at articles in so-called peer-review journals, you need to remember that the best articles get submitted to a very small proportion of journals. I'll make one other point. In my own specialty of tropical diseases, the dean of my medical school asked me why I was publishing all my articles in the *American Journal of Hygiene and Tropical Medicine*, the *Journal of Parasitology*, and the *Transactions of the Royal Society of Tropical Medicine and Hygiene*. So I took his advice and began to publish in the *New England Journal*, the *Lancet*, and the *Journal of Immunology*. And what happened to me was that my papers and my experimental design got better because I couldn't have gotten my earlier articles into the quality journals that the dean suggested. Finally, one of the top investigators in the immunology of parasitic diseases, a man named Andre Capron, initially couldn't speak English and published all his articles in journals like the *Comptes Rendu* and they were mediocre. He forced himself to learn English and then began to publish in journals like the *Journal of Immunology*, and the articles were orders-of-magnitude better. So there are reasons why you would want to accept evidence from certain journals rather than others simply because they're in Medline.

ALAN MORRIS (*LDS Hospital, Salt Lake City, Utah*): I'd like to pick up on the exchange between Dr. Chalmers and Dr. Schoenbaum, and refer to some comments by Dr. Feussner about guidelines. I found the difference between efficacy and effectiveness problematic in a number of circumstances. One wonders why the delivery of good care in situation A doesn't get translated into delivery of good care in situation B, but there are clearly some compelling factors at work to explain it. Two different approaches to this problem have been mentioned. Dr. Chalmers pointed out that if you increase the number of hospitals, you move towards making the sample more and more like the population. Then once the sample becomes the population there's no difference between the two. There are many virtues to that approach and it sounds very exciting.

Dr. Schoenbaum asked why we can't get people in a different setting to deliver the "good care" defined as efficacious by an RCT. I'm going to suggest that one of the reasons is lack of specificity. Most guidelines are quite general in nature. Medical care guidelines are replete with commands like "maximize oxygen therapy" "optimize antibiotic therapy." While these are helpful in thinking conceptually, they are rather useless for executing anything in particular. You couldn't cook a meal with a recipe that only told you to "maximize the taste of the roast."

Guidelines need to be made more specific. Practice under those conditions that generate efficacy results (that is, an RCT) and clinical care practice that generates effectiveness results will thus converge. The ultimate expression of that may be found in computerized guidelines. During computerization of an algorithm people are forced to pay attention at a level of detail that's otherwise humanly impossible. Duplication of practice with computerized protocol-controlled decisions is extremely reliable in different circumstances.

FEUSSNER: To address Dr. Chalmers' question, I can only mention what Schwartz and Lellouch would have called explanatory trials in the development of new drugs. An example might be the case of the drug ticrynafen, which, when disseminated widely to the population, had some disastrous side effects and was subsequently withdrawn from the market. That may be a case of where a more pragmatic trial would have revealed adverse effects. Perhaps post-marketing surveillance could be thought of as an example where problems are sometimes identified that are missed in efficacy or explanatory trials.

GOYAN: I was Commissioner of the Food and Drug Administration when ticrynafen was removed from the market so I have a pretty good sense of what happened. The hepatic problem had not been picked up because of the fact that it was very rare, occurring in something like 1 in 10,000 cases, and no trial is likely to get large enough to pick that up. Consequently it wasn't until it had been approved and on the market for a period of time that there were some deaths attributed to hepatic failure. So we did what the FDA does: we brought in the people from SmithKline and asked them to recall it and they kept refusing to do so until finally, when the stock exchange closed in New York they said they agreed with us, removed it from sale, and made their press announcement at that time.

FEUSSNER: To address Dr. Morris's point that many times guidelines are too general, I think there's a direct relationship between the quality of the evidence and the specificity with which the guideline can be crafted. When the evidence is weak, the guideline tends to be vague. I'm glad Dr. Morris used the analogy of the roast because sometimes clinicians talk about the guidelines very pejoratively as "cookbook medicine"—the fear is that the closer it gets to a recipe, the more resistance there will be to implementing it.

I agree with Dr. Morris and with something that Hal Sox said earlier because I think that the computer can be effective in limiting this problem by providing ready access to knowledge at the decisive moment. If the guidelines were available and user-friendly the next step in the process would be to develop specific decision-support technologies that are computer-based and that have algorithms that physicians can follow. Previous evidence generated many years ago by Hal Sox showed that even written algorithms used by non-physicians diminish the variation in practice and perhaps even improve the quality of care.

MORRIS: I agree with your comments, Dr. Feussner, but would like to enlarge upon what I infer you meant when you said that the quality of the evidence is related to the specificity of the guideline. Certainly that's true when the evidence is clear-cut—in fact it's frequently not necessary to give a guideline, and most physicians don't need a guideline or a cookbook, though that's what they're using when they give a penicillin derivative to a child with streptococcal pharyngitis. That is cookbook medicine, and it's good medicine. Immunization for measles is also cookbook medicine and good medicine; it is medicine based upon actuarial data that convinces most practitioners on a scientifically valid basis that the outcome of the patients will be favorably influenced by the intervention.

On the other hand we have a paradigm that suggests that since individuals are unique psychobiologic units, somehow all interventions in medicine need to be individualized. That paradigm in other human-behavioral activities is anathema. Edwards Deming would object if you suggested to him that you should individualize every automobile door on a production line. He would tell you that the Japanese have pointed out that if you reduce unnecessary variation, the product improves. So I would suggest that even under those circumstances in which we don't know what to do, it's just as important to think of standardizing for the elimination of unnecessary variation. Standardized medical practice will then provide the platform for improvement in the future. We have so much noise of both the random and systematic variety in the delivery of much medical care that the signal-to-noise ratio for outcome data is small. Therapy-induced changes in outcome data are not perceptible and we don't progress. One of the effective ways to reduce noise is to reduce the unnecessary variation in the response of the health care deliverer to the clinical problem. Even when there isn't definitive evidence about what to do there can be a formulation of a reasonable approach, and that reasonable approach, if standardized, will then provide the platform for future progress.

So I can't accept at face value what I infer from your statement that when scientific evidence is absent, we let the system just float freely and leave physicians with independence to do whatever they please.

FEUSSNER: I largely agree with you and certainly didn't mean to imply what you inferred. I have suggested when the evidence is sparse that the guidelines be conservative. Under those circumstances less is more. So when we wrote a guideline some years ago about curing patients with asymptomatic neck bruits by operating on them, we said that those patients should not be studied because there was no evidence that the treatment worked. We were afraid that if they were studied then doctors would make the casual association be a *causal* one and do something that was harmful.

DENNIS WENTZ (*American Medical Association, Chicago, Illinois*): Dr. Feussner, how does the ACP actively disseminate your clinical practice guideline development to members of other primary care specialties such as family medicine? If you've developed the guidelines, but they're not members of ACP they may not see them.

FEUSSNER: As I was listening to the discussion of the peer-review process I was trying to figure out how the ACP got me to invest time in this guideline development process at a reimbursement rate of approximately $0.25 an hour. I realized that it was because they promised me that if I produced an acceptable product they would consider it for publication in a prestigious peer-review journal, the *Annals of Internal Medicine*. I think that there's a fair amount of sharing now going on between the American Academy of Family Practice and the American College of Physicians. My impression is that the processes that the two societies use are slightly different, but there's communication back and forth and they frequently receive a late version of a practice guideline for their review and for their input and vice versa. The ACP gets guidelines that they develop for our review and comments. So there is reciprocal communication between the two groups.

HILLIS: I want to put a quick caveat against the overenthusiastic development of computer-driven protocols. We use them all the time in clinical trials, but having from my perspective of trying to implement them in the practice of medicine for many years, I've come to believe that overselling them will result in a backlash because computers do not make exceptions; they do not have common sense, and any rigidly computer-driven protocol is going to hit exceptions. Anyone who develops these computer protocols needs to allow for a trial period and for loopholes for people to get out or else there is going to be a tremendous backlash against this very useful tool.

FEUSSNER: I'll tell you that I eagerly await the day when they'll be a backlash from the overuse of computers in medicine. In 1969 as a medical student I rotated on a gynecologic service that was fully computerized. I used no paper, I put all my work-ups into the computer, and the computer made me read about the efficacy and side effects of drugs before I ordered them. I was naive enough in 1969 to think that that was how medicine was practiced. That was with the original Weed POMR (or problem-oriented medical record) system at the University of Vermont. I empathize with your viewpoint, Dr. Hillis, but having waited for more than 20 years for computers to really invade my practice, I almost relish the opportunity for the backlash. What computers do much better than doctors can do is to *remember* and to have options that are more than just dichotomous or trichotomous. I don't think doctors do that well and so I view the computer as a potent assist device. I'd like to think that someday the computer will be as commonplace as the stethoscope.

SOX: I'd like to make a brief correction: Computer-driven protocols imply that the computer senses a signal and action occurs. That occurs in some clinical laboratories where the result of a test will drive a sequence of tests, but that is not what I was referring to in the articles that I described. I meant that the computer simply provided reminders and advice—something to aid in a global decision-making process.

CHALMERS: I agree that monitoring for adverse effects of drugs in phase-4 evaluations is a very important example of a general process which is necessary even if a trial has shown efficacy in terms of proximal outcomes. But I was thinking more in terms of extrapolation of evidence of efficacy into general clinical practice. If we take the diethylstilbestrol example, no one could have predicted that there was going to be vaginal adenocarcinoma 20 years down the line, but if they'd looked at the *controlled* clinical trials, the doctors wouldn't have been giving the drug in the first place. In fact, one of the saddest things is to see debates among daughters of women and women themselves who took diethylstilbestrol which make no reference to the very extensive use of beta-mimetic drugs such as terbula-line in pregnancy given chronically over months. This is another classic example of where there is no evidence that the drug is useful. Goodness knows what we're setting ourselves up for in terms of another possible diethylstilbestrol-like tragedy. Yet this connection is not being made at all.

I was thinking of the limitations that people place on the results of controlled trials in terms of effectiveness or evidence of lack of effectiveness. The EC-IC trial is a fairly classic example of a situation where the researchers were blamed for not having studied types of patients that neurosurgeons had not included in the trial. That strikes me as the most extraordinary reversal of responsibility. What was known was that for people entered into the trial there was no evidence that surgical intervention was preferable to conservative medical intervention. If there is a class of patients for whom it is believed that a different result might have been achieved, then the onus is on those people who hold that belief to do a randomized controlled trial to find out whether they're right or wrong. But there's this curious reversal of responsibility back onto the researchers to do a different trial. It is not right and it cannot be tolerated any longer.

That is why I was asking for systematically collected evidence that strong evidence of efficacy from trials (or strong evidence of lack of efficacy) in terms of proximal outcomes is not generalizable. It doesn't matter whether people can't think of an example today—I invite them to write to me, for I'd be very grateful to see whether there's any substance to this oft-made claim that randomized controlled trials, in general, are not applicable in practice—there may be such evidence, but I don't know of it.

GOYAN: I would just make one final comment. A number of suggestions have been made to include additional people such as the elderly, children, and women of childbearing potential in trials. As a person in the pharmaceutical industry today, I can tell you that there are reasons why they're not included in trials which are fairly self-evident in most cases. But the sponsors are anxious to prove that efficacy is there, and so the sponsors are going to do everyting they can to choose a population in which the drug is most likely to be successful. You're not going to change that fact of life no matter how much we ask for additional changes.

Health Care Reform in the United States

The Contribution of Health Services Research to the Debate

KAREN DAVIS

The Commonwealth Fund
1 East 75th Street
New York, New York 10021

Health care reform has again become a leading issue on the national policy agenda. Yet unlike the Carter administration in the late 1970s, the Clinton administration has available to it sophisticated computer modeling capacity and an extensive body of research that clarifies the consequences of most major policy decisions. Development of the Carter National Health Plan was a 2-year effort from 1977 to 1979; the Clinton administration is attempting to develop a plan within 100 days. While such a schedule is ambitious, it would not be feasible without the substantial advances in analytical capacity that have been made in the last 20 years.

This paper summarizes the contribution of health services research to the current debate on health care reform. It reviews the databases, research, and modeling capability that give us a much clearer understanding of the nature and consequences of gaps in health insurance coverage and rising health care costs, as well as the major issues and decisions required to shape health care reform legislation.

HEALTH INSURANCE COVERAGE, ACCESS TO CARE, AND HEALTH CARE COSTS

Health care reform is concerned with two major problems: the lack of adequate health insurance coverage for millions of Americans and the rapid growth in health care costs. Advances in data collection and research in the last 20 years provide us with a much clearer and more current picture of the nature and dimensions of these problems.

The Current Population Survey of the Bureau of the Census now provides annual counts of the uninsured and information on their characteristics. Data are available with approximately a 1-year lag. By contrast, in the late 1970s the primary database on health insurance coverage was the Health Interview Survey of the National Center for Health Statistics. Insurance coverage was not asked every year, and substantial lags in the data often led to use of data that were 3 to 4 years' old. The Survey of Income and Program Participation follows a nationally representative population sample for a period of 28 months, providing current information on turnover in health insurance coverage.

As a result of these data advances, we have learned that 85 percent of the uninsured are in families where someone works full- or part-time.[1] Half of the working uninsured are in firms with fewer than 25 employees or are self-employed.

Loss of health insurance coverage is a major problem. One-fourth of the population is without health insurance coverage for at least 1 month during a 2-year period.[2] Turnover is particularly high among low-income people. One-third of Medicaid beneficiaries lose coverage in 8 months. Half of those leaving Medicaid become uninsured.[3]

The consequences of gaps in health insurance coverage for access to health care are also much better documented today than they were 20 years ago.[4] In the mid-1970s, access to care was measured by comparing rates of physician visits per capita between the insured and the uninsured.[5] One major development has been the conduct of telephone interview surveys that provide much more current information, as well as qualitative information on barriers to care. For example, the Kaiser/Commonwealth Fund Health Insurance Survey of 1992 found that approximately 23 million Americans said that they needed medical care but did not get it in the last 12 months, and 54 million people said they postponed care they thought they needed for financial reasons.[6]

Much more detailed and current information is now available on public programs such as Medicare and Medicaid. Medicare monitors access to care for beneficiaries through the Current Beneficiary Survey. The Kaiser Commission on the Future of Medicaid has compiled extensive current information on the experience of this program.[7]

Similar improvements in information on health care costs have occurred in the last 20 years. Data on national health expenditures have been collected for more than 30 years. However, computer models now generate future projections that dramatically illustrate the consequences of continuing on the current course.[8] Past trends are disaggregated to show the contribution of economic inflation, medical price inflation, population and aging, and increased intensity or utilization of health care services. The relative experience of public and private programs in controlling hospital and physician costs, for example, are now well documented. Despite these advances in research, data, and modeling capacity, much remains unknown about the reasons for the persistence of rise in health care costs or the most effective approaches to slowing growth in outlays.

One major improvement in data in the last 20 years has been the compilation of international statistics on health care expenditures and utilization of health care services. The Organization of Economic Cooperation and Development (OECD) now publishes annual statistics on health care expenditures in all major industrialized nations.[9] Research on health systems in Germany, Canada, Australia, and Japan, among others, provides U.S. policymakers with a wealth of information on the effectiveness of different approaches to assuring universal health insurance coverage within the context of cost containment or global budgets.

PUBLIC OPINION ON HEALTH CARE REFORM

Policy officials also now have the benefit of extensive polls of public opinion on options for health care reform. The Kaiser/Commonwealth Fund survey of health insurance, for example, found that people are divided roughly evenly among their preference for an employer-based system, a single government system, and the giving of tax credits to purchase individual private health insurance.[10] Americans strongly support price controls on hospitals, physicians, and prescription drugs, but are extremely concerned about any approach that would ration health care services or limit choice of physician. International surveys provide comparable information on the attitudes, concerns, and experiences of patients and physicians in major industrialized countries such as the U.S., Canada, and Germany.[11]

HEALTH CARE REFORM ISSUES

Difficult choices will need to be made by policy officials in shaping health care reform legislation. More than three dozen legislative proposals were introduced by members of Congress in the last two years. The first key difference among these proposals is the extent of public vs. private health insurance coverage. Some plans are modeled on the Canadian health care system, with a single government-financed plan covering the entire population. Others are employment-based plans, which require employers to finance health care services for workers and dependents. Others would give individuals tax credits toward the purchase of private health insurance. Computer simulation models developed by government agencies and private organizations are now available to estimate how such plans would affect the allocation of health care dollars among the public and private sector. Extensive research is also available on the relative performance of public and private insurance with regard to administrative costs and control of the cost of health care services.

Perhaps the most significant advances have come in the development of methods of paying health care providers.[12] The research at Yale University on the diagnosis-related groups case-mix methodology for hospital inpatients formed the basis of reform of Medicare's payment of hospitals. Research at Harvard University on a resource-based relative value system similarly formed the basis of reform of Medicare's payment of physicians. These developments in Medicare are the methods most often proposed for payment of hospitals and physicians under a universal health insurance system.

Computer models have also been developed that provide information on the distributional impact of alternative sources of financing health care reform. For example, one recent study found that families with incomes under $75,000 would pay 75 percent of a tax cap on employer health benefits.[13] Similar information is available on the distributional impact of income taxes, payroll taxes, value added taxes, and alcohol and tobacco taxes—all potential sources of financing expanded health insurance coverage.

Modeling the cost of health care reform has been significantly advanced by the Rand health insurance experiment, which was the largest social experiment ever conducted in health care.[14] Information on demand elasticities and the behavioral response of patients to cost-sharing permits much more sophisticated modeling of the likely impact of any given reform proposal. Much remains unknown, however, about the likely supply response of health care providers to assured financing. For example, it is unclear to what extent price controls on physician services will induce physicians to provide more services, offsetting at least in part the effectiveness of cost controls.

Another significant advance in the last 20 years is the development of extensive research on the appropriateness of health care services and on measuring health outcomes. With support from The Commonwealth Fund, Robert Brook at the Rand Corporation has conducted extensive research resulting in the discovery that as much as a fourth of all health care services are of questionable or no benefit to patients. Practice guidelines based on this research could help assure that resources are targeted to effective services.

Decisions on health care reform will not come easily—and the debate within the Congress is likely to be extended. Yet, the ability for decisions to be informed by accurate information is greatly enhanced by developments in health services research over the last two decades.

REFERENCES

1. U.S. HOUSE OF REPRESENTATIVES, COMMITTEE ON WAYS AND MEANS. 1993. Health Care Resource Book. Government Printing Office. Washington, DC.
2. BUREAU OF THE CENSUS. 1992. Current Population Survey. Government Printing Office, Washington, DC.
3. SHORT, P. F., J. CANTOR & A. MONHEIT. 1988. The dynamics of Medicaid enrollment. Inquiry **25** (Winter): 504–516.
4. DAVIS, K. 1991. Inequality and access to health care. Milbank Memorial Fund Quart. **69**(2): 252–273.
5. DAVIS, K. & D. ROWLAND. 1983. Uninsured and underserved: Inequities of health care in the U.S. Milbank Memorial Fund Quart. **61**(2): 149–176.
6. THE HENRY J. KAISER FAMILY FOUNDATION AND THE COMMONWEALTH FUND. 1992. Americans' Health Care Concerns: A National Survey. The Commonwealth Fund. New York, NY.
7. THE KAISER COMMISSION ON THE FUTURE OF MEDICAID. 1993. The Medicaid Cost Explosion: Causes and Consequences. Henry J. Kaiser Family Foundation. Menlo Park, CA; and Medicaid at the Crossroads. Henry J. Kaiser Family Foundation. Menlo Park, CA.
8. BURNER, S. T., D. R. WALDO & D. R. McKUSICK. 1992. National health expenditures: Projections through 2030. Health Care Financing Rev. **14**(1): 1–29.
9. SCHIEBER, G. J., J. P. POULLIER & L. M. GREENWALD. 1991. Health care systems in twenty-four countries. Health Affairs **10**(3): 22–38.
10. KAISER/COMMONWEALTH FUND. 1992. *Op. cit.*
11. BLENDON, R. J. 1990. R. LEITMAN, I. MORRISON & K. DONELAN. 1993. Satisfaction with health systems in ten nations. Health Affairs **9**(2): 185–192; BLENDON, R. J. *et al.* 1993. Three nation physician survey. N. Engl. J. Med. **328**(14): in press.
12. GINZBERG, E. 1991. Health Services Research: Key to Health Policy. Harvard University Press. Cambridge, MA.
13. SERVICE EMPLOYEES INTERNATIONAL UNION. 1993. Taxation of Health Benefits. Service Employees International Union, AFL-CIO, CLC. Washington, DC.
14. NEWHOUSE, J. P. 1991. Controlled experimentation as research policy. *In* E. Ginzberg, *op. cit.*

Using Evidence: The Role of Foundations

BARBARA STOCKING[a]

King's Fund Centre for Health Services Development
126 Albert Street
London NW1 7NF, England

To many people foundations are seen simply as a source of funding and, of course, it is the case that foundations can fund innovative projects or select a particular area of work requiring development and push it forward. Foundations can take greater risks than government funding bodies, for example. They are a source of venture capital and many would see themselves as failing in their responsibilities if they did not support work that everyone else was ignoring or pushing to the margins.

However, because of their independence, foundations play a wider role: They often bring together investigators in a particular area for mutual support. They can also disseminate the findings of research by publications and through meetings. Because foundations are seen as being at the forefront, policymakers do take note, if only to be alerted to activities and trends that may otherwise come upon them unexpectedly. The relationship to government, at least for the King's Fund in the U.K., is a fascinating one. It is usually cooperative, the Fund's being seen as able to do things the government would like to do but cannot be seen to do, or where its motives would be suspect. Occasionally it is seen as an irritant, when the Fund raises questions or exposes gaps the government would rather not acknowledge.

The King's Fund undertakes all these activities in the U.K. Its mission to improve the health care of Londoners (traditionally through the London hospitals) is interpreted broadly. Its unusual feature in the world of foundations, however, is that it has three operating arms:

- the King's Fund College is a management-development college for managers in health, and to some extent social services;
- the King's Fund Centre is a service-development agency in health and social care;
- the King's Fund Institute is concerned with policy analysis in health and health care.

The combination of grant-making with the ability to support and drive forward particular issues through these operating arms, particularly the King's Fund Centre, can be enormously strong.

With that as an introduction to the King's Fund, it is time to look at what the Fund has been able to do to promote the use of evidence, beyond the publication of findings from the grants it has made. This paper comprises four examples of these means.

[a] Present address: Chief Executive, Oxford Regional Health Authority, Old Road, Headington, Oxford OX3 7LF, England.

EXPERIMENTS IN CHANGING CLINICAL PRACTICE

One of the earlier forays into use of evidence was, in fact, in the straightforward grant-making mode. The Royal College of Radiologists in the U.K. has made sterling efforts to define standards for the use of X-rays. One of its best known reports is on the use of the chest X-ray before surgery, indicating the extensive amount of inappropriate test ordering; inappropriate because the results made no difference to whether the operation went ahead or not (and often the results were not provided until after surgery had taken place).

In the early 1980s the Fund supported an experimental trial undertaken by Dr. Gerry Fowkes to examine alternative strategies to bringing about change in the routine ordering of chest X-rays.[1] This was one of the early studies showing that more than just agreement on standards was needed for them to be implemented, feedback and monitoring by peers being more successful. The Fund has since gone on to support the Royal College in other approaches to changing behavior.

The work was a decade ahead of its time, at least in the U.K., in that only now is it being recognized that we need to understand a great deal more about changing clinical behavior, and that this will involve experimentation. The Fund has been one of the active bodies in getting that issue on the agenda.

CONSENSUS DEVELOPMENT CONFERENCES

The first example illustrated the grant-making role, but the other three are all associated with the King's Fund Centre in its more operational mode. Both the experimentation with consensus development conferences and the use of interactive videos are work where we did not support the innovation ourselves, but we have been in a position to spot developments elsewhere (in these cases the U.S.) and experiment with them in the U.K.

Neither the government, research establishment, nor the medical Royal Colleges were prepared to experiment with consensus conferences, although there was little overt antagonism, and the Fund decided to try them in a U.K. setting. In fact, that was a great benefit since, whatever else might be argued, the Fund was seen as "independent [and] with no particular axe to grind." We emphasized heavily the need for the panel to consider the scientific evidence and not to reach a false consensus where this did not exist. In this, though, I do think we were hampered by the title "consensus," which seems to imply the lowest common denominator. Unusually, compared to U.S. panels, our panels only had one or two experts in the particular topic, the rest being experts in various aspects of health care and health policy. I believe that again was a strength, although there is no doubt it was threatening to some experts. We also emphasized the lay input in the audience, in the speakers, and in the panel. I believe this has gone some way towards dispelling the notion that even intelligent lay people cannot understand medical care. They can if the evidence is presented in a jargon-free clear way.

Ultimately I do not think we were as successful with consensus conferences as our Swedish colleagues in particular. SPRI (the Swedish Planning and Rationalization Institute for Health and Social Services), the organization that runs their conferences, is funded by county councils who can request specific topics as the subject of conferences. As a result these Swedish health authorities are even more likely to implement the results in practice. Our conferences did have two major achievements, however. First, they demonstrated that lay involvement in technical issues is both feasible and enormously enhancing. Secondly, they stimulated a number of other bodies, including the Royal College of Physicians and a regional health authority,[2] to hold their own consensus conferences or to develop standards of practice based on evidence. Interestingly, although the government was luke-warm about the conferences while we were running them, mainly on the grounds that we might come up with something that contradicted government policy, they too have now recognized the importance of setting out the evidence and stimulating public debate. Early this month [March 1993] we organized a consensus conference on maternity services on behalf of the Department of Health.

PATIENT INVOLVEMENT IN TREATMENT CHOICES

We are now involved jointly with the Foundation for Informal Decision Making in getting the use of interactive videos established in the U.K. The timing is right in that the government's own Patient's Charter sets out the right for patients to be informed about their treatment and care, including the alternatives. While some clinicians are working towards this goal, there is a very long way to go in the U.K. and the interactive videos are just one of a series of approaches that will be needed. Again, though, the use of these videos has demonstrated that patients can understand treatment alternatives and, as clearly found in the U.S., do make different decisions from those of their doctors, particularly about risks, when they are fully informed. We are evaluating in full randomized trial mode the videos on prostatectomy, mild hypertension, and breast cancer treatment. We hope also to collaborate in the development of new videos, perhaps on hysterectomy and hormone replacement therapy, so that both British and American versions can be produced. In the autumn we would like to move from experiment to a wider promotion of the videos in the U.K.

IMPLEMENTATION OF THE FINDINGS OF EFFECTIVE CARE IN PREGNANCY AND CHILDBIRTH

In 1987, when I was at first director of the Centre, Iain Chalmers's team and I spent about a year debating the researchers' role in implementing findings. We both learned a lot from those discussions, coming to the conclusion that while researchers must make their findings available and disseminate them as far as they are able, implementation requires some different skills. The interest in the Effective Care in Pregnancy and Childbirth (ECPC) program, though, rumbled on until it was stimulated again by another Foundation, the Milbank Memorial Fund, who commissioned me to write a strategy for implementing the ECPC.[3] The strategy summarizes the need to influence the whole range of actors in our health care process: the Health Authority purchasers, who specify what services they will buy; the health care providers, especially the clinicians; women them-selves and their organizations; the media; and above all government, which needs to take the lead in providing a coordinated approach. I do not want to dwell on the strategy, but rather the ability I have had to use resources of the Fund to get this topic moving. Because of the wide networks of the Fund it was easy to bring representatives of all the relevant groups together to discuss what the strategy might be, both in small meetings and then in a wider workshop. It was also pleasing that this work coincided with Professor Peckham's interest in developing a knowledge-based National Health Service, in which evidence is used in policy and practice. He agreed to chair the larger workshop and has since taken the ECPC forward as a test case of the implementation of research findings, which has now been agreed by the Management Executive and with the Regional Directors of Research and Development. This is an example where the "arms-length" relationship of foundations to government can be turned to strong advantage to promote an issue by using the strengths of the different styles of operation.

These, then, are some examples of the way the Fund has operated to increase the use of evidence in health care. With the NHS Research and Development strategy in place,[4] led by Professor Peckham, the Fund will have to decide whether it should continue direct work or whether it is now right that the government take the lead in this area, with the Fund resorting to its "thorn in the side" role.

REFERENCES

1. FOWKES, F. G. R. 1985. Strategies for changing the use of diagnostic radiology. Project Paper Number 57. King's Fund. London.
2. STOCKING, B., B. JENNETT & J. SPIBY. 1991. Criteria for Change: The History and Impact of Consensus Development Conferences in the UK. King's Fund. London.
3. STOCKING, B. 1993. Implementing the Findings of Effective Care in Pregnancy and Childbirth. Milbank Memorial Fund. New York. In press.
4. 1991. Research for Health: A Research and Development Strategy for the NHS. Research and Development Division, Department of Health. Her Majesty's Stationery Office. London.

Financing Medical Effectiveness Research: Role of the Agency for Health Care Policy and Research

J. JARRETT CLINTON

Public Health Service
Department of Health and Human Services
Agency for Health Care Policy and Research
2101 E. Jefferson Street
Rockville, Maryland 20852

This year marks the 25th anniversary of federal support for health services research. In 1968, the National Center for Health Services Research (NCHSR) was established within the U.S. Public Health Service to examine systematically the organization, provision, and financing of health care services. Since then, the field of health services research has grown and matured, both in its methodology and its contribution to improving the nation's health care system.

In December 1989, the Agency for Health Care Policy and Research (AHCPR) was established as the federal government's focal point for health services research, continuing and expanding the work begun by NCHSR. AHCPR focuses its efforts on issues related to cost, quality, and access to health care.

A key component of health services research is the study of "patient outcomes," or "medical effectiveness." Medical effectiveness research is intended to improve the effectiveness and appropriateness of health care by enhancing our understanding of how patient outcomes are related to specific medical interventions. The importance of such work has been highlighted by documentation of wide variations in treatments and services prescribed for similar medical conditions. Given these discrepancies, health services researchers ask the question: "What works best?" Moreover, there are clinical uncertainties about the scientific basis on which many treatments are predicated—and these uncertainties can only be assuaged by further research.

A medical effectiveness research program was formally established within NCHSR in fiscal year (FY) 1988 with the transfer of $1.9 million from the Medicare Trust Fund to NCHSR, earmarked for "patient outcome assessment research." Although some outcomes research was already under way, such studies did not achieve priority status until FY 1988.

The budget for outcomes research received a significant boost in FY 89, to $5.9 million. By the time AHCPR came into being in December 1989, the research portfolio included 13 patient outcomes research projects. These ranged in size from a $1.3 million Dartmouth College study to evaluate outcomes of hospital care using claims data; to a $21,000 Johns Hopkins University study of variations in patterns of primary care among the elderly.

AHCPR's first budget (FY 1990) represented a quantum increase in funds—to $37.5 million—for federally sponsored medical effectiveness research. This level of funding, reflecting Congress's heightened interest in enhancing cost-effective quality care, supported new activities such as facilitating development and dissemination of clinical practice guidelines.

Within AHCPR, research in medical effectiveness and development of clinical guidelines are carried out as part of the Medical Effectiveness Treatment Program (MEDTEP). Other components of MEDTEP include development of health databases and widespread and timely dissemination of research findings and practice guidelines.

Since FY 90, the MEDTEP budget has experienced steady growth, though modest in relation to the program's intent. In FY 91, the MEDTEP budget was $62.7 million; in FY 92, it increased to $67.0 million; and rose to $73.0 million in FY 93.

As indicated, the original budget for medical effectiveness research came from the Medicare Trust Fund. The legal basis for this is the Social Security Act, as amended by the Omnibus Budget Reconciliation Act of 1986 (P.L. 99-509). The rationale for the transfer was the presumption that benefits of medical effectiveness research will accrue to the population served by Medicare. When AHCPR was created, this basic feature of the law was preserved; a relatively small proportion of the MEDTEP budget continues to come from the Medicare Trust Fund.

AHCPR outcomes research focuses on conditions that affect large numbers of individuals; there is uncertainty and controversy regarding effectiveness of treatment; associated risks and/or costs of treatment are high; and, needs of the Medicare program are addressed.

In FY 89, AHCPR began funding Patient Outcomes Research Teams (PORTs), a major component of medical effectiveness research. Each PORT is a multi-year effort that includes data acquisition and syntheses (meta-analysis), development of clinical recommendations, dissemination of research findings, and evaluation of the effects of these findings in terms of change in clinical practice. To date, AHCPR has funded 15 PORTs, including investigations of prostate disease, low back pain, ischemic heart disease, type II diabetes, and prevention of stroke. In addition to PORTs, other research projects address specific health conditions or interventions, and are designed to complement or extend the work of PORTs.

AHCPR-supported clinical practice guidelines are developed by multi-disciplinary panels comprised of private sector experts and by contracts with nonprofit organizations. They are designed to identify the best ways to prevent, diagnose and treat selected clinical conditions. Topics for guideline development are selected on the basis of prevalence of the disease or condition; assessment of the financial burden posed by the illness; and the potential effect that the guideline could have on health outcomes. All AHCPR-supported guidelines are based on the best available scientific evidence, and are revised periodically to reflect advances in their field or topic area.

Through AHCPR's intramural databases, such as the National Medical Expenditure Survey (NMES), information is collected on how Americans use, pay for, and finance health care services. This information is widely used by health planners to determine the cost of various health insurance benefit packages and to estimate the costs of providing coverage for the poor and uninsured. Two NMES surveys have been conducted, and a third is planned for 1996. A second data set, the Provider Studies Program, develops basic information on the use and cost of services related to hospitals and other providers.

New research efforts budgeted under MEDTEP, include: (1) a $19 million 5-year commitment to establish Research Centers on Minority Populations; and (2) studies of the effects of pharmaceuticals on patient outcomes. AHCPR also is working with other public and private entities to develop a research agenda on quality assurance issues.

In conclusion, the decade of the 1980s has left a general legacy of unfinished business and neglect in the field of public health. In its three years of existence, AHCPR has drawn favorable reviews from the health care community and from the general public. But its current budget of approximately $120 million represents a mere 0.02 percent of the more than $650 billion spent for health care in the United States.

The AHCPR budget must be substantially increased if Congressionally mandated goals are to be realized, and if we are serious about identifying the most efficient and effective treatment modalities. Indeed, a compelling case can be made for the concept of "medical effectiveness" as an essential element in health care reform.

Panel Discussion 4

Robert Lawrence (*Rockefeller Foundation, New York, N.Y.*): This panel discussed how to pay for all of the important research undertakings that have been reviewed at this meeting. Involved as I am predominantly with the issues of cost-effective interventions in the context of Latin America, sub-Saharan Africa, and Asia, I want to note that this conference is importantly timed in connection with the release in the next few months of the World Bank report. This year the report is going to focus on the health sector, emphasizing the economic issues of allocative and technical efficiency. Much of what has been discussed at this conference relates to how we improve both allocative and technical efficiency within the context of *northern* health systems.

I want to remind you, however, that of the global economy of 25 trillion dollars, an estimated 2 trillion is now being spent in the health sector, but 1.6 trillion of that 2 trillion, or a full 80 percent of the total, is being spent on the 15 percent of the world's population that lives in the established market economies; this leaves the other 85 percent, the poorest nations of the world, to try to improve health outcomes by utilizing the 15 percent of the global health resources remaining to them. So if we think it's important in our own North American and European context to measure outcomes and be sure that we are getting the optimal benefit for our health dollar investment, you can imagine how much more important this is in face of the daunting problems facing the less-developed countries.

Our first discussant, Karen Davis, is the senior executive vice-president of the Commonwealth Fund here in New York City, but no sooner had she settled into that job than she was recalled to help the new, Clinton administration in Washington.

And Barbara Stocking's presentation restored symmetry to the representation between foundations and governments, because although she's currently with the King's Fund Centre, she is about to become the regional chief executive for the Oxford Regional Health Authority within the National Health Service. Lastly, we heard from Jarrett Clinton, Director of the Agency for Health Care Policy and Research in the U.S. Public Health Service, who told us that five new guidelines per year are prepared in the clinical domain. I remember that the U.S. Preventive Services task force, which met from 1984 to 1989 and then reconvened under Hal Sox's chairmanship two years ago, took five years to produce guidelines on 60 conditions, or about 12 a year, but they were in the domain of *prevention,* where some of the data were a little more clear-cut than they are in the arena of clinical treatment and services.

Frederick Mosteller (*Harvard University School of Medicine, Boston, Mass.*): I got so interested in the descriptions of the AHCPR that I decided to ask a question that has puzzled me for a long time. The AHCPR program has guidelines for benign prostatic hypertrophy and I heard a preliminary presentation about 2 years ago saying the guidelines were to appear very soon, but I haven't seen them yet. Have they actually come out? I have a deeper reason for this question, for we also have a PORT that deals with the same topic, and I keep wondering what will happen to the guidelines in the long pull as the PORTs proceed with their work. I've wondered about this because it didn't seem to me that the PORTs had a mandate to produce guidelines.

JARRETT CLINTON (*AHCPR, Rockville, Md.*): That is a good question and one that puzzles all of us. The PORTs were created before our requirement to move ahead with clinical practice guidelines, and while PORTs willl generate clinical findings, they will not create a guideline. There is a great deal of interaction between a PORT and a clinical practice guideline when the two exist, as, for example, with low back pain, cataracts, and with benign prostatic hypertrophy. In every instance, the PORT contributed to the analysis and interpretation of data and the highlighting of new findings that ought to be included in the guideline. The PORT produces a research report which is distinguished from a guideline, which is the synthesis of everything we know produced in a format useful to a practitioner.

The delay in producing the BPH guideline is a point of considerable annoyance in that the expert panel developing the guideline has taken too long to complete its work. This group is not under my direct command, and although I have persuaded, cajoled, and threatened, the BPH guideline is going much slower than it should have. It seems to be part of human nature for people to wait for the *perfect,* rather than being satisfied with the *good*—I think it's a regrettable tendency. Other guideline panels have moved along quickly with their process and have delivered their product in a reasonable period of time. We are absolutely committed to revision, and I'm arguing that rather than wait for the next clinical trial, which will be ready in 7 months, we should publish what we know, acknowledge that there's more coming, and then revise a guideline when that data become available.

The experience with the BPH panel has taught us how we might leverage the process to some extent—it's one of the reasons we decided to go the contract route, but that won't solve the human problem of procrastination. There is good interaction when research exists, contributing to the synthesis of research, which is a practice guideline.

HENRY GREENBERG (*St. Luke's-Roosevelt Hospital, New York, N.Y.*): I have a question for Dr. Davis, although I think it applies pretty broadly. You have shown that health care expenditures for the United States include many non-medical expenses, and by that I mean expenses that are immune to universal coverage, to managed-care algorithms, and even to bureaucratic reform. Your Medicare totals, for example, include multiple readmissions for many of my elderly, widowed patients in New York with congestive heart failure who come in three extra times a year because we don't have adequate housing facilities for them. Or consider the epidemic of teenage pregnancy, with or without crack babies—this represents an enormous expense that Jackson Hole solutions will not touch; patient education in this context and as you are talking about it isn't going to make a dent. There are major social and cultural issues, major urban issues, and "lifestyle" issues such as alcoholism and smoking that add enormous expense that health care reform *per se* cannot touch. My concern is that the reforms that we are going to have are those that are *do-able,* that is, health care will be rationed for the middle class, but little else will get touched because we will not acknowledge the major social problems we must deal with in other arenas that have a direct impact on health costs. I would like to see a slide at some meeting with a little bar indicating that a certain chunk of the Medicare cost is not a health care issue. I've yet to see that.

KAREN DAVIS (*The Commonwealth Fund, New York, N.Y.*): You raise a point that many of us are sympathetic with, and I did once hear the President ask how much our health care expenditures were related to drug use and antisocial behavior. No one present could answer because although they know the percentage of hospital costs and physician costs, they cannot say how much of it can be ascribed to various social ills. This is something we don't know and haven't examined. There are some things that health care reform can do to address some of the concerns you've raised, Dr. Greenberg, but obviously a lot of it is outside of that debate. Health care reform can address the issue of long-term care so that chronically ill patients are not inappropriately cared for in institutional settings, but have genuine choices for care at home or in community-based settings. And certainly the question of whether or not preventive services are covered has something to do with whether we get at some of the basic causes of health care expenses. Whether funds are set aside to do outreach community-based prevention of some of the problems of substance abuse is an important question. From what I've seen there seems to be a more comprehensive look at that array of issues than is traditionally the case, but this should not raise expectations that health care reform in and of itself will deal comprehensively with the social issues you raise, Dr. Greenberg.

RICHARD PETO (*Radcliffe Infirmary, Oxford, England*): I'd like to raise one fairly fundamental point about the way in which AHCPR works and has worked. The tradition was established before Dr. Clinton became director that the PORTs would try to assess what produces favorable or unfavorable outcomes from nonrandomized evidence, or even from claims-based evidence. In doing this, the PORTs are going to generate grossly misleading information. I'm not saying that randomization can answer everything, but attempts by the AHCPR to determine what works and what doesn't work for serious outcomes, such as death, from nonrandomized evidence does a great disservice to the general public and to the reputation of your agency. You can't change this kind of thing quickly—it's now an established tradition in your agency, but I think that it's a very bad tradition. As director, Dr. Clinton, you should really consider how you can change that tradition.

CLINTON: That's been done.

PETO: Can you give details of that?

CLINTON: You are assuming that something is established in an agency that is only 3 years old. Nothing has been established so far that is cast in concrete. The AHCPR PORT program under the leadership of Dick Green joined with a large number of people about a month ago to discuss limitations of the PORT approach. I didn't design the PORT—some of the best thinkers in America were brought together to design it about 5 years ago, and clearly it has been more of a hypothesis-generating than hypothesis-testing activity. We were constrained when we started this program—we had only 6 million dollars to start. So we recognize the considerable limitations of the PORT even though we have some examples of where it has made considerable contributions. We hope that we can move towards case-control and cohort-control studies, as well as the clinical trials that you've been urging America and the world to consider. We are limited by lack of funds and have an ethos that will not allow us to receive money from pharmaceutical companies to underwrite some of this work. That is a fundamental part of a value system that I live with.

At times we have to perform a balancing act between carrying out congressional mandates in a way that is consistent with the Administration's programmatic and fiscal policies. For example, Jack Wennberg's work makes it clear that we need clinical trials with regard to the various options in the management of a benign prostatic hypertrophy. And, with considerable work on the part of Wennberg and others, the American Urological Association produced a proposal that would have met most of your criteria. But it costs on the order of 20 million dollars and

AHCPR doesn't even have $20 million for new research in any given year. Our study sections gave it a score that is the equivalent to a D−. Because we could not finance that, the investigators came back with a more modest approach, within the funding range of what we might do. But the numbers were so small as to make generalization impossible.

So we are in a great dilemma: We are required to do clinical trials but we do not have the resources. My job then is either to convince my colleagues at the NIH to do the trial or to address the Congress to say that we need a different approach.

PETO: But you don't need to spend 20 million dollars to do a trial comparing one form of treatment of prostatic hypertrophy with another. If you make your trials too expensive then they won't be done. We need large randomized trials and we cannot get them with the American tradition of complexity and high cost per patient. It's quite easy to do trials that are an order of magnitude less expensive per patient than those in the American tradition.

CLINTON: I would welcome your helping American investigators to design that trial and submit it to us.

ALAN MORRIS (*LDS Hospital, Salt Lake City, Utah*): I have a suggestion for Dr. Clinton: Perhaps it would be worth considering appending a caveat to the brief statement of the guidelines, which, I fear will be much of what drives decision-making by policymakers as they rush from meeting to meeting. That caveat would identify the level of evidence and its level of confidence.

CLINTON: This is sometimes done. I would say that the guidelines vary in the degree to which they do that. I think you'll see that strongly done on the depression guideline, which will be out next month. On cataracts it's moderately well done. And it was done with exceptional detail on the guideline on pain. I agree that the scientific evidence citations should be listed—when I don't see a reference, we have a long talk about it.

MORRIS: Will your agency consider establishing a mechanism so that they can capture the data associated with physicians' refusal to follow the guidelines? If you can't learn why physicians don't follow the guidelines and fold that information back in an iterative process, there is no way to actually construct a guideline into a market-ready product that will be useful.

CLINTON: Encourage Senator Hatch from Utah to give us the authority to require that kind of mechanism—we'd be delighted to comply.

MORRIS: The next time he invites me for guidance I'll be sure to bring it up!

CLINTON: I think that he'll be receptive to the idea, but we are a science-based organization and I have authority over nothing. I do have the bully pulpit to influence the Health Care Financing Administration and the insurance companies of America, and I think that some of your suggestions will be enacted but not in the short run.

MORRIS: I'd like to ask Dr. Davis whether she can help us to estimate the potential financial return from eliminating that large fraction of therapy that will undoubtedly, if studied, be demonstrated to be not only ineffective, but also likely harmful. It appears to me that not much attention is being paid to the elimination of unnecesary care as an approach to cost reduction that seems to be more likely to increase quality.

DAVIS: Robert Brook's work on this question is as good as any, and I believe that the numbers given now are something on the order of anywhere from 3 to 15% for harmful or ineffective care. It would seem important to develop a policy instrument that can identify useless or harmful care without eliminating care that is beneficial. As we go forward with health care reform, a better place to start is by a utilization review that is science-based and that would try to deny payment for care that is in violation of guidelines or that is not appropriate given patient conditions; this is more sensible than some of the rationing systems that are not concerned with just eliminating unnecessary or ineffective care, but in even eliminating care that has benefit to patients but is viewed by a lay commission as not worth it in terms of the cost.

I'd like to see all of the multiple utilization review methods that are currently used by insurance companies and other third parties replaced by a single system that is science-based and based upon evidence of appropriateness.

IAIN CHALMERS (*The UK Cochrane Centre, Oxford, England*): I am pleased to hear Dr. Clinton's remarks. The activities of his agency are impressive. I'm particularly heartened by the emphasis on outcomes that patients themselves value as important, and it is disgraceful that you have to pay the NIH to ensure that they, in their trials, measure outcomes that are important to patients. The NIH should take on that responsibility itself and should take a lesson from the National Cancer Institute of Canada, which now requires proponents of cancer trials to give reasons why they are not looking at patient-oriented outcomes in the trials they're considering.

My question, though, is how we can avoid unnecessary duplication of effort internationally in this sort of work. Dr. Clinton produced an impressive list of topics his agency is covering, and I know for certain that some people in other countries are tackling the same issues. The Swedish Council for Technology Assessment in Health Care has had a major initiative in back pain, something that is of great interest in the Netherlands as well. The AHCPR has groups working on cesarean section and low birth weight, topics I've been involved in and I believe, Dr. Clinton, that you've got quite an important initiative starting on depression. Some work has been going on elsewhere on depression and it would be a shame if it wasn't possible to build on the work that's going on under your aegis. As long as there is a willingness to recognize that data derived from human beings involved in research all over the world probably have relevance in most countries, it should be possible to share some of the work load and some of the costs required for these studies.

So, Dr. Clinton, I'd be pleased to hear how you decided to duplicate work that is being done elsewhere and how you see all of us who are interested in producing this information can reduce the amount of unnecessary duplication. And obviously a case can be made for planned replication, where two different groups analyze the same subject but with a view to comparing findings.

CLINTON: We call that prudent redundancy, and I think that a case can be made for it. In the workshop I just referred to in answering Richard Peto's question we had representatives from the U.K., France, Italy, Denmark, and Spain, and we would welcome hearing from any country that would like to participate in our ongoing research workshops and conferences. We like to hear about what you're doing, and to provide a forum like this as a prelude to collaboration. Jack Wennberg probably has the greatest experience in collaborating with his European counterparts with regard to benign prostatic hypertrophy. He has found that in some European nations they're doing much more open prostatectomy, which has posed an intriguing and puzzling dilemma for us in the United States. We welcome that kind of collaboration although we cannot finance research outside the United States unless we can prove that it contributes to the American issue. But there's nothing that prohibits collaboration between those outside the United States and those within, which is why I suggested to Richard Peto that he help U.S. investigators to put together an international trial.

We're a small group with a small mailing list, and I invite anyone interested to get in touch with us for information because this kind of interaction is necessary. Let's think about some way in which we might have an international meeting and decide whether a new entity is necessary or whether it's sufficient just to have people meet. I have some reservations about just transferring this to another institution that has another agenda, but I believe the issue deserves discussion.

Alternative Medicine

JOSEPH J. JACOBS

Office of Alternative Medicine
National Institutes of Health
Bethesda, Maryland 20892

The public response in America to the creation of the Office of Alternative Medicine at the National Institutes of Health has been nothing less than phenomenal, although I suspect that the cognoscenti of the complementary medicine community may not find it surprising. But the fact remains that we are in the midst of a tremendous change in the relationship between complementary and orthodox medicine. This change can only be received in a positive way if we evaluate complementary medicine in a methodical, dispassionate manner, devoid of politics and bias.

The Office of Alternative Medicine is the brainchild of Senator Tom Harkin, who chairs the National Institutes of Health Appropriations Subcommittee in the U.S. Senate. As chair of that committee, he is in a powerful position to influence research directions of the NIH through the appropriations process. As deliberations occurred for the 1992 fiscal year NIH appropriations, language was inserted into the funding legislation directing the NIH to establish an office that would evaluate unconventional medical practices. (The belief in complementary medicine is evidenced by the homeopathic level of funding of $2,000,000.)

The U.S. Congress does not usually establish new programs through the appropriations process, but exceptions are made. New programs are usually left to the purview of the "authorizing committee" chaired by Senator Ted Kennedy. Authorities for programs created in the appropriations process usually last for only one fiscal year and require renewal in subsequent fiscal years. The Office was reauthorized in fiscal year 1993. I am pleased to inform you that the Office has been included in the NIH reauthorization legislation by both Senator Kennedy's Committee in the Senate and Congressman Henry Waxman's Committee in the House of Representatives. When people ask me what I expect the lifespan of the Office to be, I quote the passage that frequently appears in Indian treaties created by the U.S. Congress; "As long as the grass grows and the river flows." What Indian people never anticipated was that rivers might be dammed or that grass may be covered over with concrete!

When the NIH became faced with this Congressional imperative of the creation of this Office, several challenges appeared before it. A large organization like the NIH, with its $10 billion budget, requires a significant amount of bureaucratic effort to initiate a new program direction. This task is not unlike the preparations made by the British government in preparing for the Falklands war or the Allied efforts in the Persian Gulf. Important issues such as determining the magnitude of the assignment and determining the magnitude of the solutions need to be addressed prior to initiating a major campaign. Although defining a research agenda for the NIH may not be on the same scale as the examples cited, it is still a significant undertaking.

The first challenge facing the NIH was in defining alternative medicine. This question was addressed by polling individuals in the various Institutes and Centers

TABLE 1. Classification of Unconventional Medical Practices[a]

Diet/Nutrition/Lifestyle Changes

- Macrobiotics
- Megavitamins
- Diets
- Changes in lifestyle

Mind/Body Control

- Art therapy/relaxation
- Biofeedback
- Counseling and prayer therapies
- Guided imagery
- Hypnotherapy
- Sound/music therapy

Traditional and Ethnomedicine

- Acupuncture
- *Ayur veda*
- Herbal medicine
- Homeopathic medicine
- Native American
- Natural products
- Traditional Oriental medicine

Structural and Energetic Therapies

- Acupressure
- Chiropractic medicine
- Massage therapy
- Reflexology
- Rolfing
- Therapeutic touch

Pharmacological and Biological Treatments

- Anti-oxidizing agents
- Cell treatment
- Chelation therapy
- Metabolic therapy
- Oxidizing agents (ozone, hydrogen peroxide)

Bio-Electromagnetic Applications

[a] Classification has been made to facilitate the structuring of the review process and provides only examples of different interventions. Many other interventions are expected to be candidates for investigation.

of the NIH to determine the scope of activity that might constitute alternative medicine (TABLE 1).

The second challenge was to determine the principal players in alternative medicine. After identifying a number of key individuals, an *ad hoc* advisory panel was established and convened in June 1992 to hear testimony from the alternative medicine community. In September 1992, a larger meeting was held in Chantilly, Virginia, where invited members of the alternative medicine community were asked to participate in drafting a "strategic plan" that would outline a research agenda for the Office. We expect this report to be completed soon.

Under the category of **Diet/nutrition/lifestyle changes** we see *macrobiotic diets* (use of "organic fruits and vegetables" and *megavitamins*. The science of nutrition is rapidly advancing, providing us with greater insight into the value of various nutritional products. A significant example may be seen in the report released by the Division of Cancer Prevention of the National Cancer Institute on the role that various vitamins and minerals have in preventing cancer of the esophagus and stomach among people in a certain part of China. Although this may represent a case of vitamin deficiency, it is an important observation nonetheless in the link between vitamins and cancer. We also see *various designer diets* with a specific therapeutic effect that is hoped for. Finally, with respect to *changes in lifestyle,* we have recently seen in the press the recognition for possible insurance reimbursement of the Dr. Dean Ornish cardiac rehabilitation program by the Mutual of Omaha insurance company. This program uses various modalities such as a low-fat diet, support groups, moderate exercise, and meditation. Each of these components seems to make common sense, but it took support from the NHLBI and years of meticulous data collection by Dr. Ornish to bring it to this point of recognition.

The next major category includes **Mind/body control**. These therapies include: *art therapy/relaxation* and *biofeedback,* which some persons regard as part of mainstream medicine since it is widely recognized as an effective form of therapy; *counseling and prayer therapies,* where we might note that all too often, physicians and other health care providers ignore the beliefs of the patient; *guided imagery,* one form which may be seen in Lamaze training for childbirth. We accept the therapeutic benefits of Lamaze without questioning the physiological mechanisms that work to reduce the reliance on pharmaceuticals to deal with pain; and *hypnotherapy* and *sound/music therapy.*

One characteristic that these therapies may have in common is that they may all be forms of self-hypnosis. We must be open-minded to the possibility of significant clinical benefit despite unknown mechanisms of action.

Another very important category of alternative medicine is **Traditional and ethnomedicine**. This includes *acupuncture,* a significant part of traditional Chinese medicine that is shown to have a strong scientific basis; *Ayur veda,* the traditional healing system of India which we recognize as a significant component of transcendental meditation. Studies are ongoing with support from the National Heart, Lung and Blood Institute on the therapeutic benefits of TM on blood pressure; *herbal medicine; homeopathic medicine,* a system of care widely used in Europe on the theory that microdilutions of substances that cause the symptoms can cure the disease; *native American healing practices,* which focus on prayer and spirituality; *natural products,* which include substances such as bee pollen and shark cartilage; and *traditional Oriental medicine.*

Many of these categories share two very important characteristics: (1) they represent several thousand years of "trial and error" and (2) they are being used by a majority of the world's population.

Another important category is **Structural and energetic therapies**. These therapies represent the laying on of hands to effect the healing process. They include *acupressure,* the use of pressure rather than needles on acupuncture points; *chiropractic medicine,* a therapy used by many people who seek relief from low back pain; *massage therapy* for relief of stress; *reflexology,* or manipulation of the feet to achieve some form of healing; *rolfing,* deep painful massage which is thought to be therapeutic; *therapeutic touch,* a form of energy healing and transfer studied and promoted by some members of the nursing profession.

Another group is **Pharmacological and biological treatments,** which include *anti-oxidizing agents* (some vitamins fall into this category); *cell treatment,* which may include the transfer of normal muscle cells to patients with some forms of muscle disease; *chelation therapy,* which uses a substance called EDTA, normally used to remove lead and other harmful substances from the blood. Some people feel it may be beneficial for heart patients; *metabolic therapy*; and *oxidizing agents* such as ozone and hydrogen peroxide.

Finally, we have **Bioelectromagnetic applications**, which include developments that purport to promote bone healing. Consideration may also be given to the cancer-causing effects of low levels of radiation.

Several functions related to the Office have evolved since I have assumed the role of director on October 26, 1992. These functions have included the following:

1. The Office is serving as a broker between the alternative medical community and the orthodox medical community. We endeavor to foster collaborative relationships between individuals with mutual interest in a particular area. For example, acupuncture as a treatment modality for subacute pain could be included as part of a larger clinical trial by one of the Institutes at the NIH interested in the management of pain in a particular group of patients. The Institutes have larger budgets and staff to execute these types of trials.

2. The Office provides the essential technical assistance to the alternative medicine community aiding them in tasks ranging from filling out an application for funding from the NIH to developing sound research methods for good clinical trials.

3. The Office is a clearinghouse for information related to alternative medicine as well as dissemination of information about its own activities. Queries from numerous sources have come to the Office, especially after media reports on alternative medicine activities.

4. The Office is carrying out field investigations to try to determine the relative clinical benefit of a purported treatment and to determine the level of sophistication of the provider. A methodology developed by the National Cancer Institute called the "best case series" is the model we use in trying to guide our assessment of which investigations to pursue. Several field investigations are about to begin.

5. The primary method of supporting research by the NIH is through the grant-making process. A grant program for evaluations of alternative medical practices has been initiated through the publication of a Request for Applications (RFA) on March 26, 1993. This RFA is intended to solicit applications for grant funds up to $30,000 that can be used for planning for studies of alternative medical practices. These grants will provide for the initiation of "pilot projects" to identify promising areas of research. This program also encourages the collaboration between alternative medical practitioners and health care institutions. To date, we have received more than 800 "letters of intent" to apply for grant funds and more than 400 such applications.

6. The Congressional mandate also includes the establishment of a Program Advisory Council to the Office. This committee is composed of members of the alternative medicine community and will provide advice on program direction as well as perform a "peer review" advisory function.

We hope to provide more attention to issues related to herbal and ethnomedicine. Also, we cannot ignore the tremendous wealth of information beyond the borders and shores of the United States. Part of the task is to go beyond the "ethnocentric" view of American medicine.

The activities of the Office are being done in a changing health care environment in America. The emergence of alternative medicine as a major factor is one of multiple "revolutions" facing U.S. medicine. These other revolutions include:

(*1*) recognition of the importance of primary care;
(*2*) recognition of "small area variations" and emergence of outcomes research;
(*3*) the imperative to manage resource consumption by physicians and other providers; and
(*4*) the emergence of "mid-level" practitioners.

My fears for the Office are the tremendous expectations placed upon it. The American health care system is pluralistic in modes of delivery through different systems of care, levels of technological sophistication, mechanisms of payment, and types of regulation. It is a unique challenge to this Office to maintain a steady course in looking solely at the mandate to evaluate alternative clinical practices for clinical benefit. Holding on to the middle ground will surely advance the cause for advocates of complementary medicine.

DISCUSSION

KENNETH WARREN (*Picower Institute for Medical Research, Manhasset, N.Y.*): I thank Dr. Jacobs for coming to this symposium on such quick notice. His appearance came about because of Natalie Angier's superb article on Dr. Jacobs in the Science section of the *New York Times* last week. A lot of us who have been interested in the Congress's mandating an office to examine alternative medicine feared that if it were done badly it might be a tragedy. But I was convinced by Dr. Angier's article that this might be done very well indeed. And because it's almost impossible to get ahold of Dr. Jacobs we're pleased that he could come and report on the sorts of therapies his office will be investigating.

IAIN CHALMERS (*The UK Cochrane Centre, Oxford, England*). It's going to be very helpful that John Ferguson is trying to get a registry of control trials being funded by NIH because that should help you identify what the other institutes are doing in this field.

In view of your small budget, my question relates to the need to take advantage of work that has been done elsewhere. I'm thinking particularly of the Netherlands, where a group based in Maastricht has done a very thorough search for articles published not just in English, but also in German and French and other European languages. Another group in Germany is also trying to draw together the control trials in alternative medicine. Can you tell me how you intend to "stand on their shoulders" and to build these groups into your process? Obviously a considerable amount of effort has been invested in their work and it would seem a shame not to take advantage of it.

JOSEPH JACOBS (*Office of Alternative Medicine, NIH, Bethesda, Md.*): You're absolutely correct. We have had numerous discussions with people in the Netherlands as well as in England concerning the wealth of literature that's there. We've also been having some intense discussions with representatives of the People's Republic of China with regard to traditional Chinese medicine, and there is a fair amount of data there as well. As you say, with the homeopathic level of money we have we need to take advantage of some of the work that has been done elsewhere.

The fact that we don't readily accept the data that come from other countries is a reflection of our own arrogance and ethnocentricity, but it's something that we want to break through. We've had discussions with the National Library of Medicine concerning a recommendation on changing key words, to reflect findings in alternative medicine. We said to replace the term *alternative medicine* and use the word *complementary* to be consistent with the literature databases in Europe. We're trying to get into lock step with communities outside the United States.

JANE BARRY: Are you thinking of incorporating research with alternative methods into conventional research? Is there enough factorial design, for example, not to have an alternative therapy versus a conventional method, but studied in conjunction with one of the research arms, perhaps using relaxation or meditation along with medication.

JACOBS: That's what we are hoping to do in our negotiations with other institutes. Essentially I would like to be able to get various alternative therapies as part of the research agenda within a particular institute. The most effective way of doing that, of course, is if you have more money and are willing to pay for it because the priorities are established on the basis of resources. Evaluating bee pollen for allergies is one of those things we've been looking at. NIAID may be interested intellectually, but it's not a very high priority so we would have to come in with additional funds and offer to fund an additional arm of a clinical trial to add bee pollen as one of the treatments studied. We're just looking at it in terms of being one part of several things being tested. But are you also asking whether alternative therapies can be complementary or whether they could work synergistically?

BARRY: Yes; and if it wouldn't be interesting to look at them as one arm, then perhaps they could be studied as working in conjunction with the conventional drug.

JACOBS: Part of the conventional wisdom at the NIH is that when you look at the ACTGs, for example, you realize that perhaps the results of a particular clinical trial may be questionable because of the heavy use on the part of AIDS patients, say, of alternative therapies—this may complicate the clinical trial that you're looking at. This is a very important issue. Many of the people who are working with our office feel that these therapies should be looked at as an *adjunctive* modality rather than in the classical way. For example, we don't want to study coffee enemas as a *cure* for cancer, but rather as a significant palliative modality.

In fact, we're trying to ask how we *heal* the patient rather than *cure* the patient. We're trying to instill a rhetoric of *healing* within the other institutes.

Summation of the Conference

SIR RICHARD DOLL

Imperial Cancer Research Fund
Cancer Studies Unit
Harkness Building, Radcliffe Infirmary
Oxford OX2 6IIE, England

Among the many advances in medicine in the last decade, there has been the realization that the expert reviews of a subject that have been regularly published in medical journals constitute an unreliable means of arriving at the truth about a controversial issue. Dr. Tom Chalmers some years ago provided a splendid example when he examined 56 reviews of the value of radiotherapy after mastectomy for stage II breast cancer and found that they were evenly split for and against. More remarkably, he found that the conclusions reached depended on the specialty of the reviewer, with radiotherapists concluding overwhelmingly that the treatment was beneficial and other specialists concluding the reverse. Dr. Oxman analyzed the reasons for this variability and provided conclusive evidence in favor of reviews that provided the detailed evidence and utilized the new method of meta-analysis. When applied by the early breast cancer collaborative trialists' group to the results of radiotherapy, this showed practically no difference in overall survival between all the patients given and not given radiotherapy (because the small decrease in breast cancer deaths was counterbalanced by a small increase in other deaths).

The realization of the partiality of experts constitutes a problem for editors of journals faced with the need to substitute dry statistical analyses for elegant essays, but a still greater problem for someone in my position required to produce a summation of a three-and-a-half-day conference, packed with hard data and the reports of specialists who have presented, in 25-minute papers, the distilled wisdom gained from many years of practical experience. Time and the lack of preprints excludes the possibility of an evidence-based summation and I can hope to avoid the errors that would be likely to be associated with an authoritative summation only by not attempting to give one. In these closing remarks, I shall therefore limit myself to a few points that have seemed to me of outstanding importance, recognizing that the assessment of their importance is subjective and influenced by my own long-standing prejudice.

With that publicly admitted, I can turn to the principal issue raised in this conference: namely, the relative roles of meta-analyses, or as I prefer to call them, overviews, and large-scale simple randomized clinical trials.

Consider first the scientific overviews that were introduced into medicine by Tom Chalmers and Richard Peto and their colleagues, and which have been turned into a tool for reassessing objectively the whole edifice of medical practice by Iain Chalmers. These were introduced to extract the truth underlying, and often obscured by, the results of several small randomized clinical trials; but they have now been extended to the analysis of the results of observational studies of the etiology of disease. Charles Hennekens drew attention to the fact that we still have to obtain most of our information about the causes of disease from observational studies and that the use of randomized clinical trials to test the validity of conclusions about causes by randomly allocated experiments in the prevention of disease is seldom practicable. This does not always matter, as it is sometimes possible to obtain clear and incontrovertible conclusions about the etiology of disease from such observations, as, for example, has often happened with severe occupational hazards; but when the increased risks are small, the interpretation of observational studies may be exceptionally difficult. Inevitably, therefore, there has been a tendency to extend the use of overviews to the analysis of the combined results of many case–control and cohort studies. Unfortunately the results of such studies are liable to be influenced by biases in their design and conduct and by confounding between the agents under investigation and other agents directly responsible for the production of the disease. The overviewer has, therefore, the problem of selecting out the studies that are thought to avoid these difficulties, or which provide enough evidence to enable confounding to be allowed for, and this essentially depends on the subjective assessment of the scientist responsible for the overview. Tom Chalmers has attempted to deal with this problem by laying down criteria for weighting studies according to their scientific reliability, but there is, in my opinion, still a long way to go before such overviews can provide the conclusive answer to a problem that we can now expect to get from an overview of randomized clinical trials. I have drawn attention to this problem, although it has not been discussed in this conference, because of the danger that the extension of overviews to nonexperimental evidence, when they may easily mislead, may bring overviews of experimental evidence into undeserved disrepute.

The important problem concerning overviews that has been discussed at this conference is the extent to which they make large-scale randomized clinical trials unnecessary and unethical. In my opinion the two approaches should be seen as complementary rather than as alternatives. There are two main advantages of the large-scale simple randomized clinical trial. First, it provides evidence that is much more readily accepted by clinicians who have become accustomed, over the past 30 years, to basing their practice on the results of randomized clinical trials, while many clinicians still regard the evidence from overviews as a statistical trick played by backroom statisticians. Secondly, involving large numbers of clinicians in the trial predisposes them to accept the results, as it is a characteristic of human nature to believe what you have experienced in your own life more readily than what someone else has experienced and told you about. Participation in a large-scale controlled trial constitutes, in practice, one of the best means of continuing medical education.

Against this need for a large-scale randomized clinical trial is the idea that the results of a properly conducted overview provide equally sound scientific evidence and that the conduct of a randomized clinical trial when the overview has shown results that would be obtained by chance (say less than 1 in 10,000 times) is ethically unjustifiable. It is not impossible that this may, in the course of time, come to be generally accepted; but that time has not yet arrived. First, it still has to be shown that overviews consistently provide the correct answer and that they are not sometimes vitiated by the selective publication of positive results. The good overviewer takes immense trouble to ensure that the results of all trials are included irrespective of whether they are published, but until we have a register of trials on which ethical committees and funding bodies require the trial to be recorded before it is approved, there is always the possibility that some trials have been abandoned because the results were seen to be unpromising and not been drawn to the overviewer's attention, and there is the virtual certainty that many small trials that showed positive results were stopped when the results appeared positive rather than continued to their planned conclusion, when the results might have been less extreme. This is not a criticism of the trialists' behavior—they had no option if they were admitting patients themselves—but it leads to distortion of the results (like publication bias) in favor of ones that are positive.

As it happens, the overviews of aspirin and thrombolytic agents led to results very similar to those observed in large trials, but it is too early to be sure that this will always prove to be the case.

Despite this concern, some of the proponents of overviews, most notably Tom Chalmers, have argued that the conduct of a large-scale randomized clinical trial is unethical when the results of an overview are clear. I cannot agree with this, as doctors, in practice, are still often unconvinced by the results of overviews and the conduct of a large-scale randomized clinical trial, contrary to what Tom Chalmers argues, does not sacrifice lives since the lives would have been lost without the trial. The large-scale trial actually saves lives, as it changes practice more quickly than would have occurred without it. There is, however, a real ethical issue in the way the randomized clinical trial is conducted in the face of overview evidence. As Chairman of the Data Monitoring Committee of ISIS-2 I made it clear that if I had a myocardial infarct I wanted to have both treatments and agreed to be on the Committee only on the understanding that the trialists made clear to the clinicians what the results of the overview were before they admitted any patients to the trial and that they should admit patients only if, despite the overview, they were uncertain about the correct treatment to give—as hundreds of clinicians apparently were. There was no difficulty about this, as it had been the initial policy of the Steering Committee before I was involved.

What then were the ethical considerations that the Data Monitoring Committee had to have in mind when reviewing the results? In these circumstances the overriding consideration was whether the results, if known to the investigators and taken in conjunction with other existing evidence, would alter clinical practice. When that situation arose, we thought the Steering Committee would want to know the results and we drew their attention to them. There is, in my opinion, a clear distinction between the ethical responsibility of the treating physician who must do the best he can for each patient and, if he suspects the evidence in favor of one therapy is suggestive enough, he must stop randomizing—something that he might want to do when he knew the p value of the difference between the results in the study in which he was participating was near to 1 in 20. The Data Monitoring Committee, in contrast, does not have responsibility for the next patient so much as for the next generation of patients, and it will want to report significant results only when it believes they are likely to alter medical practice. To report them earlier would be to ignore the reason for which the trial was initiated (the failure of doctors to use the promising treatment) and to do a disservice to the public.

These ethical considerations are, I believe, important, as they are crucial to our ability to get the best treatments widely adopted. At present, there has been far too little public discussion of the role of scientific enquiries in relation to medical practice. Randomly allocated clinical trials are, I suggest, in an entirely different category from physiological experiments carried out for the sake of increasing knowledge without any prospect of doing good to the individual experimented on. In these latter circumstances there can be no diminution of the need for the strictest procedures for obtaining fully informed consent. In the case of the randomized clinical trial, the position is different and the treating physician who admits his patient to the trial because he is uncertain of the best way of treating him or her is in no different position from the honest physician treating a patient for the same condition outside the trial who is uncertain about the best treatment to prescribe. The ethical requirements for informed consent are, in my opinion, similar in both situations and should not be made more onerous for the physician admitting to a controlled trial than for a physician treating a patient independently on his own. (We have discussed this more fully elsewhere,[1] with particular reference to ISIS-2.)

I conclude that we have need for both overviews and for large-scale simple randomized clinical trials because they provide the only techniques for making small advances in the treatment of common conditions and, in the current state of scientific development, it is only small advances that we can generally hope to make. Occasionally, brilliant discoveries like the use of platinum drugs for the treatment of testis cancer will be made, and these may need no randomized clinical trial to demonstrate efficacy, but if we wait for such discoveries we shall miss out on many improvements which could be made in the treatment of common conditions. We could fail to save tens of thousands of lives a year waiting for miracles that may never occur.

Outcome research is no substitute for the proper scientific assessment of therapies. It has its place in discovering the extent to which appropriate therapies are being provided and, in certain circumstances, it may help to discover whether care is being delivered with equal competence in different communities and different social groups. It is perhaps of special value in testing whether the delivery of medical care meets the requirements of equity as well as those of cost efficiency. Biases, however, that are inherent in delivery in different circumstances and variation in the selective factors that bring patients to care make outcome research, divorced from random allocation, as inadequate a means for assessing the value of a specific form of treatment as the outdated technique of comparing the results in a current series of patients with those obtained on other patients in the past. The use of outcome research is to be welcomed for the limited object for which it is appropriate, but it provides no useful means of assessing the value of a therapy. Consequently it has been agreed that this conference should send a letter on the subject to Hillary Rodham Clinton.

A great many valuable suggestions were made in this conference about how new knowledge could be transmitted to medical practitioners, so that it quickly contributed to routine daily practice. These will repay study when the report of the conference is published, but I have preferred not to try to summarize them now so that I will not distract from the few subjects of primary interest with which we have been concerned and which, if taken to heart by the profession and by those responsible for providing medical care, will ensure that the conference marks a turning point in the history of medicine in the developed world.

REFERENCE

1. COLLINS, R., R. DOLL & R. PETO. 1992. Ethics of clinical trials. *In* Introducing New Treatments for Cancer: Practical, Ethical and Legal Problems. C. J. Williams, Ed.: 49–65. Wiley. London.

Large-Scale Randomized Evidence: Large, Simple Trials and Overviews of Trials

RICHARD PETO, RORY COLLINS,
AND RICHARD GRAY

ICRF/MRC/BHF Clinical Trial Service Unit
University of Oxford
Oxford OX2 6HE, United Kingdom

Worldwide, hundreds of thousands of premature deaths a year could be avoided by seeking large-scale randomized evidence about various widely practicable treatments for the common causes of death, and by disseminating such evidence appropriately. Likewise, appropriately large-scale randomized evidence could vastly improve the management of many important, but non-fatal, medical problems.

The chief techniques for obtaining large-scale randomized evidence are large, simple trials (or "mega-trials") such as the ISIS[1-4] and GISSI[5,6] studies, and large systematic overviews of trials (or "meta-analyses") such as those from the worldwide collaborative groups of trialists[7-9] or of meta-analysts.[10] Over the past decade the introduction of these complementary techniques has already yielded a succession of striking and definite findings that have improved the treatment of millions of patients. But, what has been achieved so far is only a fraction of what could quite readily be achieved by the wholehearted pursuit of such research strategies.

Inevitably, any review of the need for really large-scale randomized evidence has to discuss to some extent the general unreliability of non-randomized evidence (whether this be called "historically controlled" evidence, "data-base analyses," or, more misleadingly, "outcomes research" or "effectiveness analysis"), and it has to discuss to some extent the general unreliability of small- or medium-scale randomized evidence (whether from one medium-sized trial or from a medium-sized overview of several smaller trials). But, the chief aim of this review is positive, rather than negative: the main question is not whether large-scale randomized evidence is needed; rather, it is how in practice such evidence might best be generated and interpreted. What are the real, practical obstacles and how might they best be circumvented?

Before the obstacles are discussed, however, a few real examples of large-scale randomized evidence will be introduced in sufficient detail to illustrate some of the important achievements of such research and to illustrate the two really fundamental medical assumptions that generally underlie the need for large-scale randomized evidence. These assumptions (which can also help to guide the collection and the proper interpretation of large-scale randomized evidence) are fairly straightforward:

(1) The real differences between two treatments in some important outcome will *probably not be large,* but even a moderate difference in an important outcome may be worthwhile.

(2) If there really is, for some readily identifiable category of patients, a moderate difference between two treatments in their effects on some specific outcome, then this difference might be larger or smaller in other readily identifiable categories of patient, but it is *unlikely to be reversed.*

The medical importance of treatment effects that are only MODERATE in size implies the need for large-scale randomized evidence

Unrealistic hopes about the chances of discovering large treatment effects can be a serious obstacle to good clinical research. For, such hopes may misleadingly suggest to some clinical research workers that small, or even non-randomized, studies may suffice, and this may prevent people from planning the collection of properly randomized evidence from appropriately large numbers of patients. Realistically moderate expectations of what treatment might achieve (or, if one treatment is to be compared with another, realistically moderate expectations of how large any difference between those treatments is likely to be) should, in contrast, tend to foster the design of studies that aim to discriminate reliably between differences in outcome that are **moderate but worthwhile**, and differences in outcome that are **too small to bother with**. Studies with this particular aim must guarantee strict control of bias (which, in general, requires proper randomization and appropriate statistical analysis, with no unduly data-dependent emphasis on specific parts of the overall evidence), and must guarantee strict control of the play of chance (which, in general, requires large numbers rather than a lot of detail).

The logic is obvious: moderate biases and moderate random errors must both be avoided if moderate benefits are to be assessed or refuted reliably.

This leads to the need for large numbers of properly randomized patients, which in turn leads both to large, simple randomized trials, or "mega-trials" (with entry governed by the "uncertainty principle": see the legend to FIGURE 1) and to large worldwide overviews, or "meta-analyses," of the randomized trials. A strategy that pursues such evidence can, by determining reliably whether certain widely practicable treatments for common conditions do, or do not, produce any worthwhile difference in long-term survival, lead to the avoidance in many separate instances of thousands or tens of thousands of premature deaths a year worldwide, and thereby in total avoid hundreds of thousands of such deaths a year. Examples that illustrate these points will be given both from neoplastic and from vascular disease, and the general principles are also of relevance to some aspects of the control of the main infective and parasitic diseases.

In contrast, non-randomized evidence, excessively data-dependent subgroup analyses, unduly small randomized trials, or unduly small overviews of randomized trials are all much inferior as research strategies. For, they cannot discriminate reliably between moderate differences and negligible differences in outcome, and the mistaken clinical conclusions that they engender could well result in the under-treatment, over-treatment, or other mistreatment of millions of future patients. The value of large-scale randomized evidence will be illustrated by citing real examples, in which proof of benefit that could not have been achieved by small-scale evidence, or by non-randomized evidence, leads to widespread changes in practice that save tens of thousands of lives a year.

PART I: FOUR REAL EXAMPLES

IMPORTANT RESULTS IN THE TREATMENT OF VASCULAR AND OF NEOPLASTIC DISEASE THAT COULD HAVE BEEN RELIABLY ESTABLISHED ONLY BY LARGE-SCALE RANDOMIZED EVIDENCE

First Example: Antiplatelet Therapy (Medium-dose Aspirin or Other Antiplatelet Drugs for Patients at High Risk of Suffering Some Occlusive Vascular Disease over the Next Few Months or Years)

In the ISIS-2 trial, among 17,000 patients with suspected acute myocardial infarction (AMI), one-quarter were allocated aspirin (162 mg/day for one month, which virtually completely inhibits cyclo-oxygenase–dependent platelet inhibition), one-quarter were allocated streptokinase (1.5 mega-units of SK infused once only over 60 minutes, in a fibrinolytic regimen that reopens the majority of recently occluded coronary arteries within a median of about 90 minutes of starting the infusion, but that causes a serious hemorrhagic stroke in a few out of every thousand patients treated), one-quarter were allocated both of these treatments (SK and aspirin), and one-quarter were allocated neither. The 1-month mortality results are illustrated in FIGURE 1: aspirin alone and SK alone were both highly significantly better than nothing, and the combination was highly significantly better than either alone.[2] The SK result will be considered later, along with the results of the other main fibrinolytic trials, after this discussion of the aspirin result.

Before 1988, when these ISIS-2 trial results were published, aspirin was not routinely used in acute MI, and no other major trial had (or has subsequently) assessed aspirin in suspected acute MI. But, the effects of 1 month of aspirin were so definite in ISIS-2 (804/8587 vascular deaths among those allocated aspirin versus 1016/8600 among those not) that even the lower 99% confidence limit would have represented a very worthwhile benefit from so simple and inexpensive a treatment. Worldwide treatment patterns therefore changed sharply when these results emerged, and aspirin is now routinely used in many different countries for the majority of emergency hospital admissions with suspected acute MI. (In the U.K., for example, a British Heart Foundation survey[11] showed that routine aspirin use in acute coronary care increased from under 10% in 1987 to over 90% in 1989.) The annual number of patients with suspected MI who would nowadays be given such treatment may well run into some millions worldwide, suggesting that in this clinical context alone aspirin is already saving several tens of thousands of lives a year. Four-year follow-up of the later deaths in the ISIS-2 trial has shown the persistence of significant benefit among those allocated aspirin (unpublished data presented at the 1993 American Heart Association meeting in Atlanta).

Aspirin for suspected acute myocardial infarction has now become widely accepted, but in the mid-1980s it was difficult to get doctors to take it at all seriously. Indeed, many cardiologists were opposed to it, believing only anticoagulants to be of any potential value in an acute heart attack, and it required incontrovertibly strong evidence to overcome these firm but mistaken judgements. ISIS-3[3] and GISSI-2[6] subsequently studied one particular anticoagulant regimen involving seven days of high-dose subcutaneous heparin and, by randomization of 60,000 patients, showed it to have little effect on one-month mortality among patients who had been given an adequate dose of aspirin (FIG. 2). (In contrast, ISIS-2 had shown aspirin to be of substantial additional value among patients who were to receive either subcutaneous or intravenous heparin.[2]) If the ISIS-2 trial had been

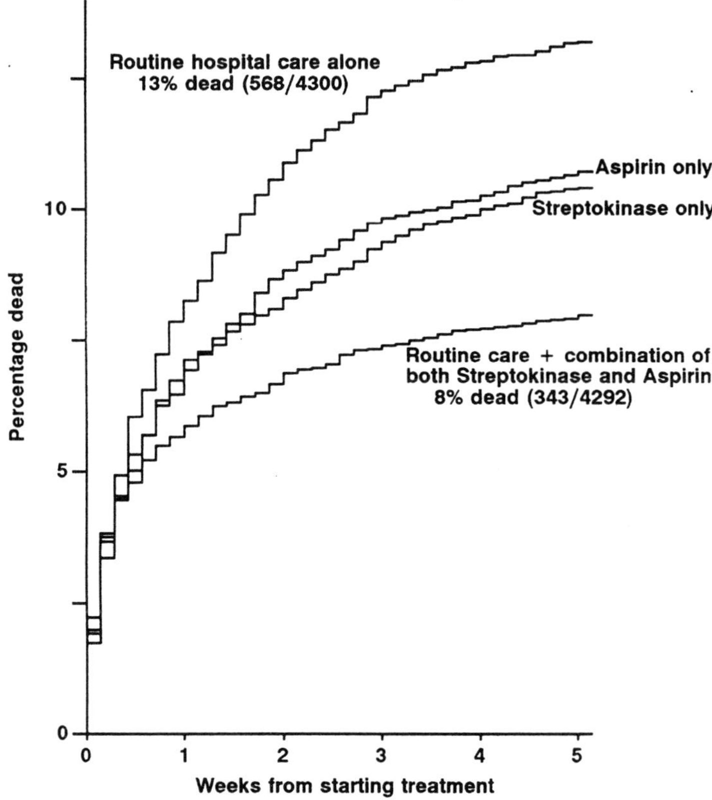

FIGURE 1. Main 1-month mortality results in the Second International Study of Infarct Survival (ISIS-2).[2] Lives saved in ISIS-2 among 17,187 heart attack patients who would not normally have received streptokinase or aspirin, divided at random into four similar groups to get aspirin only, streptokinase only, both, or neither. (Any doctor who believed that a particular patient should be given either treatment gave it, and did not include that patient in ISIS-2.)

ten times smaller (1700 instead of 17,000), then exactly the same overall results as in FIGURE 1 would not have been conventionally significant, and would therefore have had much less effect on medical practice. Likewise, if the ISIS-2 trial had been non-randomized then it might well have got the wrong answer (since in a non-randomized study doctors might tend to give active treatment to patients who were particularly ill, or who were in various other ways somewhat different from those not given active treatment). And, even if a non-randomized study did happen to get an unbiasedly correct answer, it would be impossible to be sure that it had actually done so, and hence again a non-randomized study might have had much less influence on medical practice than ISIS-2 did.

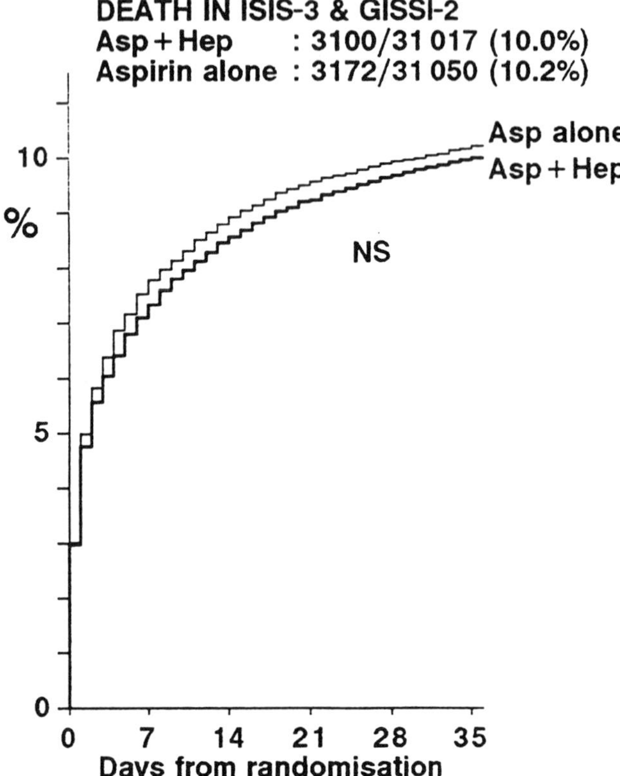

FIGURE 2. Combined 1-month mortality results in the two mega-trials[3,6] of the effects of adding subcutaneous heparin to standard treatments for acute myocardial infarction. (All patients in both trials were to get fibrinolytic and antiplatelet therapy.) This small mortality difference is not conventionally significant.

In the ISIS-2 trial, aspirin significantly reduced the 1-month mortality (FIG. 1), but it also significantly reduced the number of non-fatal strokes and of non-fatal reinfarctions that were recorded in hospital.[2] When all these three outcomes are combined into "vascular events" (stroke, death or reinfarction), 13% of those allocated aspirin and 17% of those not were known to have suffered a vascular event in the month after randomization (TABLE 1: an absolute difference of 40 per 1000—or, perhaps more relevantly, of 40,000 per million).

The randomized trials of aspirin, or of other antiplatelet regimens, in other types of high-risk patients (e.g., a few years of aspirin for those who have survived a myocardial infarction or stroke) have not been as large as ISIS-2, and so, taken separately, most have yielded false negative results. But, when the results from many such trials are combined, statistically definite reductions in "vascular events"—non-fatal MI, non-fatal stroke, or vascular death—are seen (TABLE 1).[7] Since such treatments do not appear to increase non-vascular mortality, all-cause mortality is also significantly reduced. In principle these findings could, if appropriately widely exploited, avoid about 100,000 vascular deaths a year in developed countries alone (FIG. 3), and there are probably at least as many vascular deaths in less developed as in developed countries (TABLE 2).[12]

So, with realistically achievable levels of use of "medium-dose" aspirin (75–325 mg/day) for the secondary prevention of vascular disease, it might well be possible in practice to get enough aspirin used to prevent, or substantially delay, about 100,000 vascular deaths a year worldwide, and such use of aspirin would in addition also prevent an even greater number of non-fatal strokes or heart attacks. (Medium-dose aspirin was the least expensive and most widely tested antiplatelet regimen: it is of proven efficacy, and on review of all the antiplatelet trials no other antiplatelet regimen has been shown to be of greater efficacy in preventing vascular events: see notes to TABLE 1.) This large-scale randomized evidence about medium-dose aspirin is now changing worldwide clinical practice in ways that will, at low cost, prevent much death and disability in

TABLE 1. Summary of Overall Results in Trials of Aspirin (or Other Antiplatelet Drugs)[a] for the Prevention of Vascular Events[7]

Types of Patient Studied	Average Scheduled Treatment Duration (& approx. no. of patients randomized)	Proportions who Suffered a Nonfatal Stroke, Nonfatal Heart Attack, or Vascular Death during the Trial		
		Antiplatelet	Control	Events Avoided in These Trials
High-risk				
Suspected acute heart attack	1 month (20,000)	10%	14%	40 per 1,000 ($2p < 0.00001$)
Previous history of heart attack	2 years (20,000)	13%	17%	40 per 1,000 ($2p < 0.00001$)
Previous history of stroke	3 years (10,000)	18%	22%	40 per 1,000 ($2p < 0.00001$)
Other vascular disease (e.g., angina, peripheral vascular disease, vascular procedures)	1 year (20,000)	7%	9%	20 per 1,000 ($2p < 0.00001$)
Low-risk				
Primary prevention in low-risk individuals	5 years (30,000)	4.8%	4.4%	4 per 1,000 ($2p > 0.05$)

[a] The most widely tested regimen was medium-dose aspirin (involving an average daily dose of 75–325 mg), and no other antiplatelet regimen appeared to be significantly more or less effective than this at preventing such vascular events. By comparison, in the U.K. or U.S. a single children's aspirin tablet includes 75–80 mg of aspirin, while an adult tablet includes 300–325 mg.

Pharmacologic evidence suggests that after the first few days all daily doses of aspirin in the range 75–325 mg are likely to be approximately equivalent in their effects on platelets and on the vascular endothelium. Hence, to limit any gastric discomfort with long-term use, a daily dose at the lower end of this range might be slightly preferable, such as 75, 80 or 100 mg (depending on what is conveniently available). But, in acute emergencies such as suspected myocardial infarction or unstable angina, at least the initial dose should perhaps be at the upper end of the range, such as 250, 300 or 325 mg, so as to achieve a virtually complete antiplatelet effect within less than one hour (which could then be maintained by a lower daily dose).

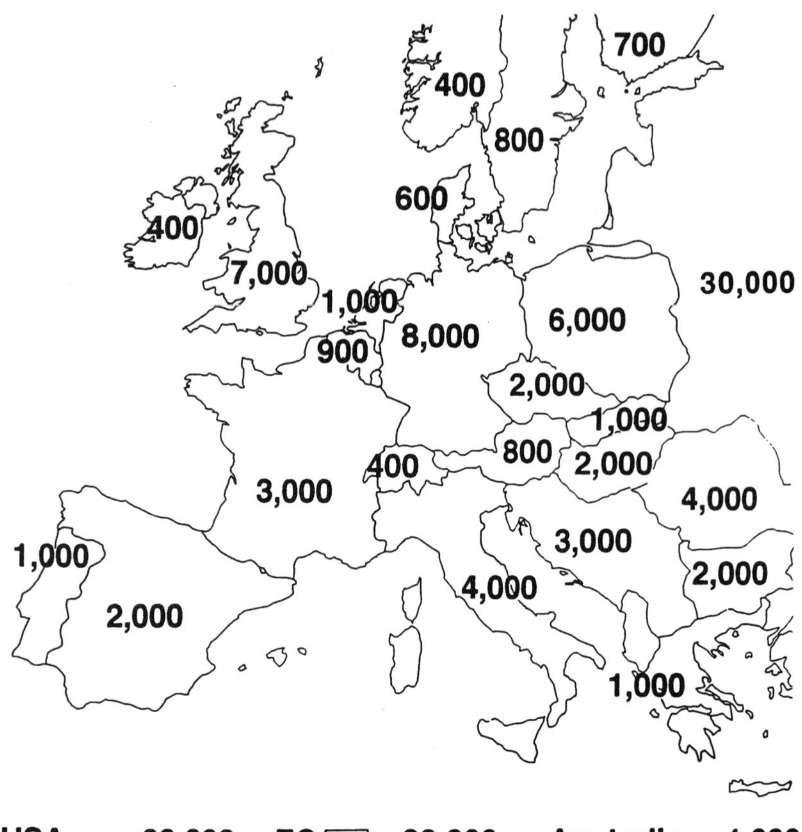

FIGURE 3. Developed countries only: estimated numbers of deaths that could be avoided or substantially delayed by the routine use of antiplatelet therapy[7] in all patients with clinical evidence of occlusive vascular disease. (The estimate was arbitrarily made to equal 10% of vascular deaths at ages 35–69, or 6% of this number in the USSR: see TABLES 1 and 2. Note that there are at present in developed countries three times as many vascular deaths in old age as in middle age.)

high-risk patients. But, small trials, small overviews or non-randomized studies could not possibly have provided appropriately reliable evidence about such **moderate** risk reductions.

An obvious next question concerns the effects of prophylactic antiplatelet therapy among people who have no definite history of vascular disease and are at low risk of suffering a vascular event over the next few years. Some large randomized trials have already addressed this (showing, thus far, a small absolute reduction in myocardial infarction, a possible small increase in hemorrhagic stroke, but little net difference in overall vascular mortality[7]) and others are in progress. The appropriate comparison is between a policy of widespread prophylaxis for such people and a policy of deferring treatment until a definite indications for it arises. Answering this question reliably is difficult even with large-scale randomized trials, and would be virtually impossible without them.

Second Example: Fibrinolytic Therapy (Streptokinase or Other "Clot-busting" Drugs as Emergency Treatment for Patients Who Are Suffering an Acute Heart Attack)

FIGURE 1 illustrated not only the effects of antiplatelet therapy, but also those of streptokinase (SK), a fibrinolytic drug that, within a median of about 90 minutes of starting emergency treatment, dissolves any thrombus that may be blocking a coronary artery and thereby causing an acute heart attack. Such drugs were introduced into clinical research in the late 1950s, but the trials of them in the 1960s and 1970s were too small to be statistically reliable (none involved even 1000 patients), and by the early 1980s the hemorrhagic side-effects were obvious, the benefits had not been convincingly demonstrated, and such drugs were generally considered to be dangerous and ineffective. Overviews, published in the mid-1980s, of those previous small trials (involving a total of only some 6000 patients in two dozen trials[13]) indicated a statistically definite benefit, but were not really believed by cardiologists. So, such treatments were not widely used.

The situation has been saved by two large randomized trials, GISSI-1[5] and ISIS-2[2] (FIG. 1), both of which involved more than 10,000 patients, and by the aggregation of seven medium-sized randomized trials that each involved more than 1000 patients. Taken separately, even ISIS-2, the largest of these nine trials, was not big enough for statistically reliable subgroup analyses, but when all nine of these trials were taken together[8] they included a total of about 60,000 patients, half randomly allocated fibrinolytic and half not.

It might appear, from FIGURE 1, that there was no need for any more randomized evidence about fibrinolytic therapy, but this ignores the hazards of such treatment and the heterogeneity of patients. Those entering a coronary care unit with a diagnosis of suspected or definite acute MI range from patients who are already in cardiogenic shock, with low blood pressure and a fast pulse, half of whom will die rapidly, to those who have merely got a history of chest pain and no very definite ECG changes, only a few per cent of whom will die before discharge. Fibrinolytic therapy often causes a frightening blood pressure drop;

TABLE 2. Worldwide Vascular Mortality Patterns[12]

	Deaths Attributed to Ischemic Heart Disease or Stroke (millions/year)	
	Age 35–69	Age 70+
Developed countries	1.1	3.2
Less developed countries	2.3	3.1
	Total: 10 million/year	

should it be used in patients who are already hypotensive? It occasionally causes serious strokes; should it be used in patients who are elderly or hypertensive, and therefore already have a fairly high risk of stroke (or who have only slight changes on their ECG, and therefore have only a low risk of cardiac death)? Finally, if the coronary artery has been occluded for long enough, then the heart muscle that it supplies will have been irreversibly destroyed; how late after the heart attack starts is fibrinolytic treatment still worth risking—3 hours? 6 hours? 12 hours? 24 hours?

These questions need to be answered reliably before appropriate and generally accepted indications for, and against, such an immediately hazardous but potentially effective therapy can be devised. To address them, all fibrinolytic therapy trialists with studies that randomized more than 1000 patients between fibrinolytic and control have collaborated.[8] On review of these 60,000 randomized patients, some of the therapeutic questions were relatively easy to answer satisfactorily. For example, it appeared that most of those whose ECG was still fairly normal (or showed some other pattern that indicated only a **low** risk of death) might as well be left untreated, leaving open the option of starting fibrinolytic treatment urgently if their ECG changed suddenly for the worse over the next few hours— which, in general, it will not do. Conversely, among those who already had "high-risk" ECG changes when they were randomized, the absolute benefit of immediate fibrinolytic therapy was, if anything, slightly greater than is indicated by FIGURE 1, and age, sex, blood pressure, heart rate, diabetes, and previous history of MI could not identify reliably any group that would not, on average, have their chances of survival appreciably increased by treatment.

The longer that fibrinolytic treatment for such patients was delayed, however, the less benefit it seemed to produce. Among those whose ECG showed definite ST-segment elevation (ST ↑) or bundle branch block (BBB), the benefit was greatest (about 30 per 1000) among those randomized 0–6 hours after the onset of pain (FIG. 4). But, the mortality reduction was still substantial and significant (about 20 per 1000, $2P < 0.003$) when such patients were randomized 7–12 hours after onset of pain. Indeed, if they were randomized 13–18 hours after pain onset there still appeared to be some net reduction in mortality (about 10 per 1000, but not statistically significant). The regression line in FIGURE 4 reinforces, in a more reliable way, these separate subgroup analyses. Before these large trials, it was forcefully argued that such treatments could not possibly be of any worthwhile benefit if given more than a few hours after the onset of pain.

Such detailed inferences are difficult enough with large-scale, properly randomized evidence, and would be impossible without it; because of their unknowable biases (see below), non-randomized database analyses are simply not a viable alternative to large-scale randomized evidence. Nor, indeed, would randomization of "only" several thousand patients have been sufficient.

At first sight it might appear that the fibrinolytic mega-trials should not have been necessary, if only doctors had trusted the overview of 6000 patients in two dozen small trials that was already available ten years ago[13]: alternatively, it might appear that GISSI-1,[5] the first such mega-trial, should have been sufficient to produce the appropriate changes in cardiological practice without any further large trials. But, given the complexity of the evidence that is available now that 60,000 have been randomized (FTT Collaborative Group[8]: see also FIG. 4), it is clear that this would not have provided a sufficiently reliable basis for deciding which of the millions of heart attack patients who reach hospital each year should be treated, and which should merely be placed under close observation, sparing many patients the hazards of immediate fibrinolytic therapy.

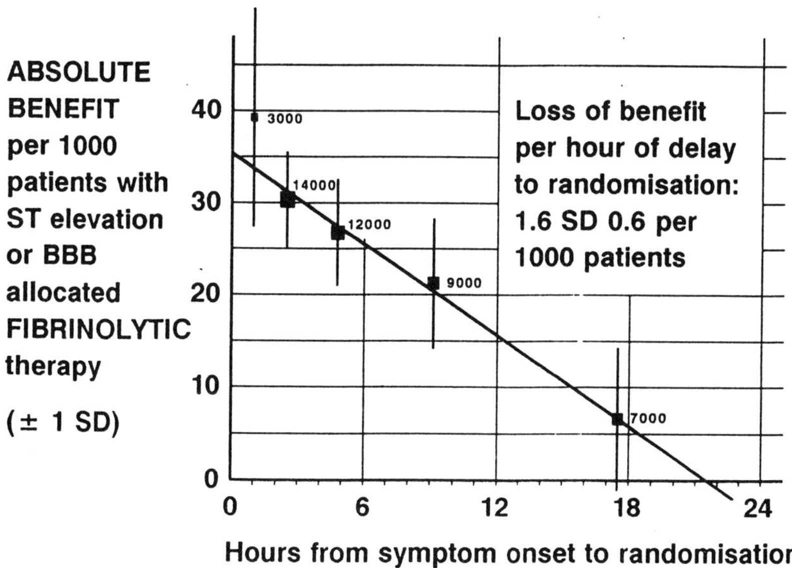

FIGURE 4. Benefit versus delay in the nine largest unconfounded randomized trials of fibrinolytic therapy versus control in patients with suspected acute myocardial infarction[8]: 1-month mortality results for the 45,000 patients with ST elevation or bundle branch block when randomized, showing the persistence of definite net benefit even for those randomized 7–12 hours after the onset of pain.

Indeed, in several important respects what is still needed is more, rather than less, randomized evidence about the effects of fibrinolytic therapy in various particular types of patient. First, it is still not clear whether patients who do have definite ECG changes such as ST ↑ or BBB but who present 12–18, or even 18–24, hours after onset of pain should be treated: more randomized evidence is still needed (FIG. 4). Second, for one particular poor-prognosis ECG category (ST depression), the 1-month mortality results still appear unpromising even when all currently available trials are combined (15% dead among those allocated fibrinolytic versus 14% among controls, based on 4000 patients[8]). Yet, analogy with the results in other high-risk categories suggests that this result for patients with ST depression may be a false negative. Perhaps it has arisen from unduly data-dependent emphasis on what may in retrospect prove to have been a misleadingly random irregularity in the results in one particular subgroup that included only a few thousand individuals with ST depression on their ECG. Again, more randomized evidence is needed.

Third Example: Lack of Significant Benefit of Magnesium Infusion in Suspected Acute MI (A Small Overview of Randomized Trials, Involving a Highly Significant (2p < 0.001) Mortality Reduction Based on Only a Few Thousand Patients, is Strongly Contradicted by Much More Reliable Evidence from a Large Randomized Trial)

Theory suggests that, in patients with suspected acute myocardial infarction, a 24-hour infusion of a magnesium salt might reduce early mortality. Several small

TABLE 3. Magnesium in Acute Myocardial Infarction: Contrast between the Results of the Smaller and the Larger Randomized Trials

	Number of Patients Randomized	1-month Mortality	
		Allocated Magnesium	Allocated Control
Seven small trials[14]	1000	38/637 (6.0%)	69/629 (11.0%)
LIMIT-2 trial[15]	2000	90/1159 (7.8%)	118/1157 (10.2%)
ISIS-4 trial (preliminary results)	58,000	Non-significantly adverse	
All trials	61,000	Non-significantly adverse	

NOTE: The results of ISIS-4 have not been published, but the 35-day mortality results, which were non-significantly adverse, have been presented at the 1993 American Heart Association meeting. There is highly significant heterogeneity ($p < 0.001$) between the group of seven small trials whose "hypothesis-generating" results led to the testing of magnesium in ISIS-4 and the pair of larger trials (ISIS-4 and LIMIT-2) that tested that hypothesis.

trials, involving between them a total of only 1000 patients, had addressed this question by 1990, and their aggregated results[14] indicated a statistically significant, but implausibly large, benefit (25/657 deaths among those allocated magnesium versus 53/644 among the controls; 2p = 0.001). Some argued that these results constituted proof beyond reasonable doubt that magnesium was of sufficient value to justify widespread usage without seeking further randomized evidence, but others remained sceptical, arguing that the apparent results were far too good to be true.

Two trials, one (LIMIT-2[15]) involving 2000 patients and one (ISIS-4[4]) involving 58,000, were therefore set up to test more reliably the possible effects of magnesium. The former yielded a moderately promising result (TABLE 3) indicating avoidance of about one-quarter of the early deaths (but with results that were statistically compatible with a true benefit that ranged from about zero to about a halving of early mortality). This, in combination with an update of the smaller trials, yielded an overview that was based on a few thousand randomized patients, which is still not enough to be reliable and which still indicated an implausibly large reduction of one-third in mortality (128 vs. 187 deaths: TABLE 3). The much larger ISIS-4 trial, however, has yielded a completely unpromising preliminary result, so the overall evidence, based on about 60,000 randomized patients, is now non-significantly adverse.

In view of the striking disparity between the apparent effects of magnesium before and after the ISIS-4 preliminary results had provided large-scale randomized evidence, it is of interest to recall some of the expert views that were expressed while ISIS-4 was in progress. One prominent specialist in the meta-analysis of randomized trials who was not directly involved with ISIS-4 nevertheless felt so strongly that magnesium was already of proven benefit (and hence that further randomization was unethical) that he lobbied the data monitoring committee to try to have the ISIS-4 study stopped early and all future patients given magnesium.

In contrast, the ISIS-4 steering committee was sufficiently sceptical to want large-scale randomized evidence.[4] They knew that there might well be a negligible benefit, or even a small net hazard, but they all thought it more likely that at least some net benefit would be seen. Even after the LIMIT-2 result[15] was available, they continued to hold these opinions, and thought that if there was any real benefit then this was likely to be somewhat less than LIMIT-2 had suggested (and hence very much less than the other small trials had suggested). Just before the preliminary ISIS-4 results were shown to them, the ISIS steering committee was asked to write down the effect of magnesium on 1-month mortality that they thought most likely, if the control mortality was 8%. The median of these "best guesses" was 7%, half of the other guesses lay between 7.2% and 6.8% (indicating a 10–15% proportional mortality reduction), a quarter lay between 7.6% and 7.2% (indicating a 5–10% proportional mortality reduction), and none lay above 7.6%.

The disappointment of even these moderate hopes by the subsequent large-scale randomized evidence (TABLE 3) illustrates two general principles: first, treatments that are hoped to be of substantial clinical value may in fact be of little or no value; and, second, treatment effects that differ from zero by "only" about two or three standard deviations in medium-sized randomized trials or medium-sized overviews, or meta-analyses, may well prove evanescent. For many questions, only large amounts of properly randomized evidence can suffice.

Fourth Example: Hormonal Adjuvant Treatments for Early Breast Cancer (Stages I/II) (Some Years of Postoperative "Adjuvant" Therapy with Tamoxifen or with Some Other Antiestrogenic Therapy) for Breast Cancer Patients in Whom the Only Detectable Disease Involved Resectable Deposits in the Breast Alone [Stage I] or in the Breast and Armpit [Stage II])

In "early" breast cancer all detectable deposits of disease are limited to the breast and the loco-regional lymph nodes, and can be removed surgically. But, experience shows that undetectably small deposits may remain elsewhere that eventually, perhaps after a delay of several years, cause clinical recurrence at a distant site, which is then usually followed by death from the disease. These "micrometastatic" deposits may, in the years before recurrence becomes detectable, have been stimulated by the body's own hormones. So, among women who have had the detectable deposits of breast cancer removed by surgery (or by surgery with radiotherapy) there have been many trials of treatments that either reduce the production of endogenous estrogens (e.g., various forms of ovarian ablation), or that block the access of those estrogens to the tumor cells (e.g., tamoxifen, which blocks the estrogen receptor protein in some breast cancer cells).

Taken separately, most of these adjuvant trials have been too small to provide reliable evidence about long-term survival. But, if the results of all of them are combined,[9] then both ovarian ablation and, particularly, tamoxifen produce very definite differences in 10-year survival (FIG. 5).

Among women with Stage II disease who were less than 50 years old (and, therefore, generally pre- or peri-menopausal), ovarian ablation appears to produce about a 10% absolute difference in survival (e.g., 50% vs. 40%), but because this finding is based on the analysis of only a few hundred deaths it is still not as reliable as might ideally be wished, and (where substantial uncertainty remains) much larger trials are now in progress. Among older women, ovarian ablation is unlikely to be of much relevance (since most of the endogenous estrogen at older ages comes from sources other than the ovaries) but, in aggregate, the randomized trials among such women have shown that a few years of tamoxifen likewise produces about a 10% absolute difference in 10-year survival. A smaller, but still

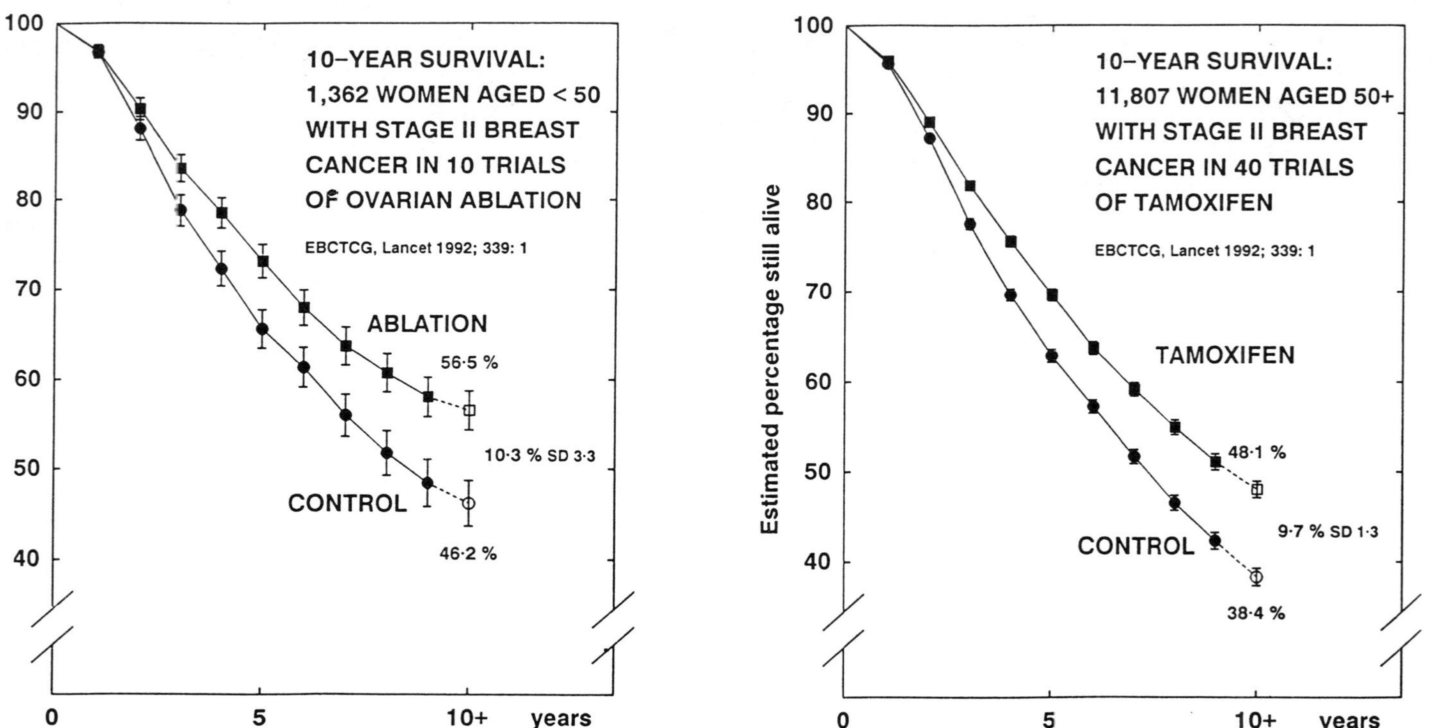

FIGURE 5. Hormcnal adjuvant treatments for early breast cancer: Effect on 10-year survival in a worldwide overview of randomized trials.[9]

highly significant, reduction in mortality by tamoxifen has now been seen[9] among the 10,000 randomized women with Stage I disease.

These tamoxifen results have already changed clinical practice substantially, and have re-directed research towards assessment of the effects of different durations of tamoxifen—should tamoxifen continue for 2 years, for 5 years, or indefinitely?—and towards assessment of the effects of tamoxifen in the primary prevention of breast cancer among high-risk women. Large randomized studies of the primary prevention of breast cancer by tamoxifen are only just getting going, but they have been encouraged by the results from the tamoxifen trials in patients with established cancer (Stage II or Stage I) in one breast, among whom there has been a highly significant reduction of one-third in the likelihood of development of contralateral breast cancer.[9] This degree of trustworthy detail would again not be attainable without large-scale randomized evidence.

PART II: STRATEGIC IMPLICATIONS

Two Fundamental Medical Assumptions

Apart from a general indication that large-scale randomized evidence can yield striking findings, the two fundamental medical assumptions that were to be illustrated by these real trial results were:

(1) the importance of reliably detecting or refuting MODERATE risk reductions, and;

(2) the idea that, for specific outcomes, the DIRECTIONS of the effect of treatment may be similar in many different categories of patient.

The former implies the need for large-scale randomized evidence, and the latter implies the practicability of getting it, and the wide generalizability of whatever overall findings it indicates.[16,17]

There are circumstances, of course, where one or other of these two assumptions is inappropriate, and then randomized trials may be unnecessary, or difficult to interpret. For example, randomization is not needed to show that cigarette smoking causes lung cancer: in middle-aged American men, for example, the disease is about twenty times more common among regular cigarette smokers than among those who have never smoked,[18] and although there may be other systematic differences (in, for example, alcohol intake, body weight, or occupation) between smokers and non-smokers, there are none that could plausibly account for such an extreme difference.[19] Extreme relative risks may be reliably demonstrable without large-scale randomization, but moderate relative risks may not be.

Reliable Detection or Refutation of Moderate Differences Requires Negligible Biases, and Small Random Errors

If moderate differences in outcome are to be detected or refuted reliably, then the errors in comparative assessments of the effects of treatment must obviously be much less than the difference between a moderate but worthwhile effect, and an effect that is too small to bother with. This in turn implies that moderate biases cannot be tolerated, and moderate random errors cannot be tolerated: in practice, this implies the need for methods that involve negligible biases and very small random errors. The only way to guarantee very small random errors is to study really large numbers, and these can be achieved in two main ways: make individual studies large, and combine information from as many studies as possible (TABLE 3). But, it is not much use having very small random errors if there may well be moderate biases, so even the very large sizes of some non-randomized analyses of medical records cannot guarantee statistically reliable results.

Avoiding Moderate Biases

The fundamental reason for randomization is to make possible the avoidance of moderate biases. Non-randomized methods, by contrast, cannot in general guarantee the avoidance of moderate bias. There are several reasons for this, some but not all of which might be circumvented. One particular problem in non-randomized comparisons of various treatment groups is to avoid systematic differences between those groups in some other potentially important aspects of patient management, or in the assessment of major outcomes. In principle this might be achievable, but in practice non-randomized comparisons, especially those that merely involve retrospective review of medical records, may well suffer uncorrectably from moderate biases due to such systematic differences.

An even more fundamental problem with non-randomized comparisons is the difficulty—or, in many cases, impossibility—of ensuring that the types of patient initially allocated to the study treatment do not differ systematically in any important way from the types of patient allocated to whatever other treatment(s) that study treatment is to be compared with. Moderate biases might well, for example, arise if the study treatment was fairly novel, and doctors were somewhat afraid to try it out on the most seriously ill patients (or, conversely, if they were more ready to try it out on those who were more seriously ill). There may also be other ways in which the seriousness of the condition differentially affects the likelihood of being included in different treatment groups.

It might at first sight appear that by collecting enough information about various prognostic features it would be possible to make some mathematical adjustments that would correct for any such differences between the types of patients who, in a non-randomized study, actually get given the different treatments that are to be compared. The hope with such statistical methods is that they might achieve comparability between those entering the different treatment groups, but in general they cannot be guaranteed to do so. One reason is that some important prognostic factors may be unrecorded. Second, some prognostic features may be intrinsically inaccurate (and, perhaps surprisingly, even completely unbiased inaccuracies in prognostic factors that differ systematically between two treatment groups can introduce a moderate bias into the statistically adjusted comparison between those treatments). Third, in a non-randomized comparison the care with which prognostic factors are recorded may differ between one treatment group and another—for example, doctors studying a new treatment may investigate their patients particularly carefully—and this too can introduce a moderate bias.

For example, among women with early breast cancer an unusually careful search of the axilla will sometimes result in tiny deposits of cancer cells being found that would normally have been overlooked. If such tiny deposits are found, then women who would have been classified as "Stage I" will get reclassified as "Stage II." The prognosis of these "down-staged" women is worse than that of those who remain as Stage I, but better than that of those already classified as Stage II. Paradoxically, therefore, such down-staging not only improves the average prognosis of Stage I breast cancer, but also improves the prognosis of Stage II breast cancer, biasing any non-randomized comparison with other studies of women with Stage I or Stage II disease in which the staging was less careful.[20]

By contrast, in randomized comparisons appropriate statistical procedures can easily avoid all such biases. But, even in a properly randomized trial, unnecessary biases could be introduced by inappropriate statistical analysis. A minor bias that is easily avoided is that caused by post-randomization exclusions, especially if these are more numerous in one treatment group than in another. The fundamental statistical analysis of a trial should, therefore, generally compare all those originally allocated one treatment (even though some of them may not have actually received it) with all those allocated the other treatment, that is, it should be an "intention-to-treat" analysis.[21]

The largest and most important bias that is still very commonly introduced during the statistical analysis of randomized trials is that produced by **unduly data-dependent emphasis on the results in particular subgroups**. If the trial treatment is in fact largely or wholly ineffective, then such subgroup analyses may well engender false positive results, while if the trial treatment is in fact moderately effective, then they may well engender false negative results (as, perhaps, in the example cited earlier of fibrinolytic therapy for patients with an acute heart attack whose ECG shows ST depression: FTT Collaborative Group, 1994). Hence, for the analysis of some specific outcome it is often the overall results of a trial that should chiefly be emphasized, with the effects in particular subgroups being estimated not directly, but indirectly, by semi-quantitative extrapolation of the overall findings for the entire trial to that one particular subgroup.[22]

When several trials have all addressed much the same therapeutic question, then the traditional procedure of choosing only a few of them for emphasis and fame may likewise be a source of serious bias, for chance fluctuations for or against treatment may affect which trials become famous: to avoid this, it is appropriate to base inference chiefly on an overview of all the results from all the trials that have addressed a particular question, not on some potentially biased subset of the trials.

In summary, to avoid moderate biases, four things are needed (TABLE 4): properly randomized evidence, an "intention-to-treat" analysis of all randomized patients, no unduly data-derived emphasis on particular subgroups, and, finally, an overview of all the relevant randomized trials (without unduly data-derived emphasis on the results from particular studies).

PART III: PRACTICAL ASPECTS OF OBTAINING LARGE-SCALE RANDOMIZED EVIDENCE FROM MEGA-TRIALS AND FROM SYSTEMATIC OVERVIEWS

Having decided that large-scale randomized evidence is important, the next question is how (if such evidence does not already exist) a worldwide overview of trials, or a new mega-trial, might be generated. What, in practice, are the main medical, statistical, and organizational pitfalls?

Overviews will be dealt with first, because before entering a major clinical trial it is helpful to have available a careful review of all previous or current trials.

TABLE 4. Requirements for Reliable Assessment of MODERATE Treatment Effects[16,17]

1. *Negligible Bias*
   (i.e., guaranteed avoidance of MODERATE biases)
   - Proper RANDOMIZATION (non-randomized methods cannot guarantee the avoidance of moderate biases)
   - Analysis by ALLOCATED treatment (i.e., an "intention-to-treat" analysis)
   - Chief emphasis on OVERALL results (with no unduly data-derived subgroup analysis)
   - Systematic OVERVIEW (or "meta-analysis") of all the relevant randomized trials (with no unduly data-dependent emphasis on the results from particular studies)

2. *Small Random Errors*
   (i.e., guaranteed avoidance of MODERATE random errors)
   - LARGE NUMBERS (since detailed statistical analyses of masses of data on prognostic features generally add little to the effective size of a trial)
   - Systematic OVERVIEW, or "meta-analysis," of all the relevant randomized trials.

The amount of work that goes into an overview depends how carefully the data from each trial are to be sought and checked. As a first step, the simplest approach is merely to collect and tabulate the published data from whatever trial reports can be found in the literature, and sometimes this may suffice. At the opposite extreme, extensive efforts may be made to locate every potentially relevant randomized trial, to collaborate closely with the trialists to seek individual data on each patient ever randomized into those trials, and then (after extensive checks and corrections of such data) to produce, in collaboration with those trialists, agreed analyses. Some of the largest such collaborations have already been described: the Antiplatelet Trialists' (APT) Collaboration,[7] the Fibrinolytic Therapy Trialists' (FTT) Collaborative Group,[8] and the Early Breast Cancer Trialists' Collaborative Group (EBCTCG).[9] The fullest account of the principles and methods that are appropriate for such fully collaborative overviews is that in the Methods section of the 1990 EBCTCG monograph,[22] and those sections are summarized below.

Overview Methodology, from EBCTCG Monograph[22]

There have already been several hundred randomized trials of various aspects of the treatment of early breast cancer. One aim of the EBCTCG was merely to make unbiased data available from all (or from an unbiased subset of all) these trials, to facilitate the construction of various different assessments of the trial evidence. In addition, even though the trials all differ from each other in various ways, an overview of the results from several trials can provide an unbiased test of whether some particular type of treatment is at all effective. For example, there are already several dozen randomized trials of adjuvant tamoxifen, but they are heterogeneous in their entry criteria, their treatment schedules, their follow-up procedures, and their methods of treating relapse. At one extreme each tamoxifen trial might be considered in virtual isolation from all others, while at the opposite extreme all might be considered together (as in FIGURE 3). Both of these extreme views have some merit, and the pursuit of each by different people may prove more illuminating than too definite an insistence on any one particular approach. This will be still more the case for the adjuvant chemotherapy trial results, since several very different regimens have been tested, ranging from just a few days of cyclophosphamide to some months or years of fairly intensive multiple-agent chemotherapy. Moreover, even chemotherapy regimens that nominally involve the same agents—cyclophosphamide, methotrexate and 5-fluorouracil (CMF), for example—may differ so substantially in intensity or duration that their main therapeutic effects are substantially different. These sources of heterogeneity are, however, merely arguments for careful interpretation of any overviews of different trial results, rather than arguments against any such overviews. For, whatever the difficulties of interpretation of overviews may be, without systematic overviews moderate biases cannot generally be avoided. But, the biases that might be introduced by selective exclusion of certain randomized trial results can be largely or wholly avoided by systematic review of all (or of an unbiased subset of all) the randomized trials ever undertaken.

Overviews that involve the detailed collaboration of the original trialists can also help avoid the biases that could be produced by post-randomization withdrawals or by failure to allocate treatment properly at random. If randomization was done properly in the first place, then post-randomization withdrawals can often be followed up and restored to the study for an appropriate "intention-to-treat" analysis, but if it was not, then the whole study may have to be excluded from any overview of trial results. In particular, knowledge of the next treatment allocation before patient entry is confirmed (for example, where randomization lists are publicly available, allowing foreknowledge, or where allocation is alternate, or based on odd/even dates or record numbers) can produce biases that are uncorrectable even if the original sequence of treatments was completely random. Trials that permit foreknowledge are not, in fact, properly randomized, though they are often mistakenly described as such, and need to be identified by correspondence about exact methods of randomization (backed up by knowledge of whether the main prognostic factors are non-randomly distributed between the treatment groups in a particular trial), so that such studies can be excluded from an overview of the properly randomized trials.

Subgroup Analyses

The treatment that is appropriate for one patient may be inappropriate for another. Ideally, therefore, what is wanted is not only an answer to the question "Is this treatment helpful on average for a wide range of patients?", but also an answer to the question "For which recognizable categories of patient is this treatment helpful?". This ideal is, however, difficult to attain, for the direct use of clinical trial results in particular subgroups of patients is surprisingly unreliable. Even if the real sizes of the treatment effect in specific subgroups are importantly different, standard subgroup analyses are so insensitive that they may well fail to demonstrate this difference. Conversely, even if there is a highly significant "interaction," that is, a difference between the **sizes** of the apparent therapeutic effects in different subgroups, and if, in addition, the results seem to suggest that treatment appears to work in some subgroups but not in others (i.e., giving the appearance of a "qualitative interaction"), then this may still not be good evidence for subgroup-specific treatment preferences. In general, clinical trials rarely provide a direct and reliable demonstration that treatment works in some subgroups,

TABLE 5. Real Trial (ISIS-2)[2]: False Negative Mortality Effect in a Subgroup Defined only by the Astrological "Birth Sign"

Astrological "Birth Sign"	No. of 1-month Deaths (aspirin vs. placebo) &	p value
Libra or Gemini	150 vs. 147	NS
All other signs	654 vs. 869	<0.000001
Any birth sign[a] (i.e., appropriate overall analysis)	804 vs. 1016	<0.000001

[a] 8587 were allocated active aspirin, and 8600 placebo.

but not in others, the one exception being that low absolute risk may well indicate low absolute benefit.

Questions about such "interactions" between patient characteristics and the effects of treatment are easy to ask, but surprisingly difficult to answer reliably. Striking-looking interactions can often be produced just by the play of chance, and these can mimic or obscure some of the moderate treatment effects that one might realistically expect. (For example, in the ISIS-2[2] trial, aspirin produced a highly significant reduction in 1-month mortality, but when these aspirin analyses were, absurdly, subdivided by the patients' astrological birth signs, aspirin appeared particularly effective for those born under Capricorn, and totally ineffective for those born under Libra or Gemini: TABLE 5.)

There are two main remedies for this unavoidable conflict between the reliable subgroup-specific conclusions that doctors want and the unreliable findings that direct subgroup analyses can usually offer. But, the extent to which these remedies are helpful in particular instances is one on which informed judgements differ. The first is to emphasize chiefly the overall results for particular outcomes as a guide (or at least a context for speculation) as to the qualitative results in various specific subgroups of patients, and to give proportionately less weight to the actual results in that subgroup than to extrapolation of the overall results.[23]

The second is to be influenced, in discussing the likely effects on mortality in specific subgroups, not only by the mortality analyses in these subgroups, but also by the analyses of recurrence-free survival or some other "surrogate" outcome. Since the overall results are more highly significant for recurrence-free survival than for mortality, subgroup analyses with respect to the former may be more stable.

Data Collection Methods

Trials in early breast cancer were to be included only if they started before a certain date and they contained some properly randomized comparison (without significant foreknowledge: see above). In practice, it may never be possible to identify absolutely all relevant randomized trials and to obtain absolutely all the data from such trials. So, the question to ask of an overview of many trials is not whether completeness can be guaranteed, but instead whether any biases due to missing trials or missing patients could reasonably be thought to be causing any serious problems of inference. Some may initially suppose that no valid inferences can be drawn from a review that is at all incomplete. This would be too rigid, however, for if taken literally it would mean that once some information from some randomized trial had been permanently lost then no amount of evidence from subsequent trials could ever suffice to answer the question of interest.

Clear evidence of benefit from an overview merely requires a result to have random errors small enough to make it highly significantly different not just from zero but also from the size of any selective bias that could plausibly be attributed to any incompleteness. Greater completeness therefore serves two complementary purposes: first, it generally reduces the size of selective bias that might plausibly be ascribed to incompleteness, and second, it somewhat reduces the purely random errors, by providing more data.

Multiple Sources of Information

Several avenues of enquiry were pursued to locate as many of the relevant randomized trials as possible, starting with review articles, discussions with trialists and with drug manufacturers, computer-aided searches, and scrutiny of the special lists of trials that are maintained by various organizations. Nevertheless, despite substantial, prolonged efforts, it took several years (and personal visits to several trial centers) before the lists of trials were reasonably complete.

Data on Each Patient

Brief data on the dates of birth, entry, follow-up, recurrence and death were sought, together with a few main prognostic features. This allowed the integrity of randomization and the unbiasedness of follow-up to be checked, and correspondence arising out of these checks reduced the incompleteness of the data from some particular studies.

Statistical Methods

The basic method is to calculate, for each trial, a simple "Observed minus Expected" (O-E) statistic and its variance, and then add these up, one from each trial, to see if their grand total (GT) differs significantly from zero. The variance (VT) of the grand total is obtained by simply summing the separate variances, one per trial. This method involves no unjustified assumptions about the sizes of the treatment effects being the same in each trial, so it should not be called a fixed effect model.

These simple statistical methods provide a valid, efficient, and assumption-free, test of the hypothesis that treatment does nothing in any trial.[22] The O-E value from each trial could be the "logrank"[21] O-E value, as in the EBCTCG overview,[9] or it could be, as in the APT[7] or FTT[8] overviews, the simple O-E value that is calculated from a table of outcome (Yes/No) versus allocated treatment.

These methods that are based on the simple summation of one O-E value per trial also provide a useful description of the average size of the treatment effect (since O-E divided by its variance approximately equals the "log odds ratio" for a particular trial, and GT/VT indicates it for an overview of many trials). The EBCTCG monograph[22] and APT review[7] provide more discussion of these methods.

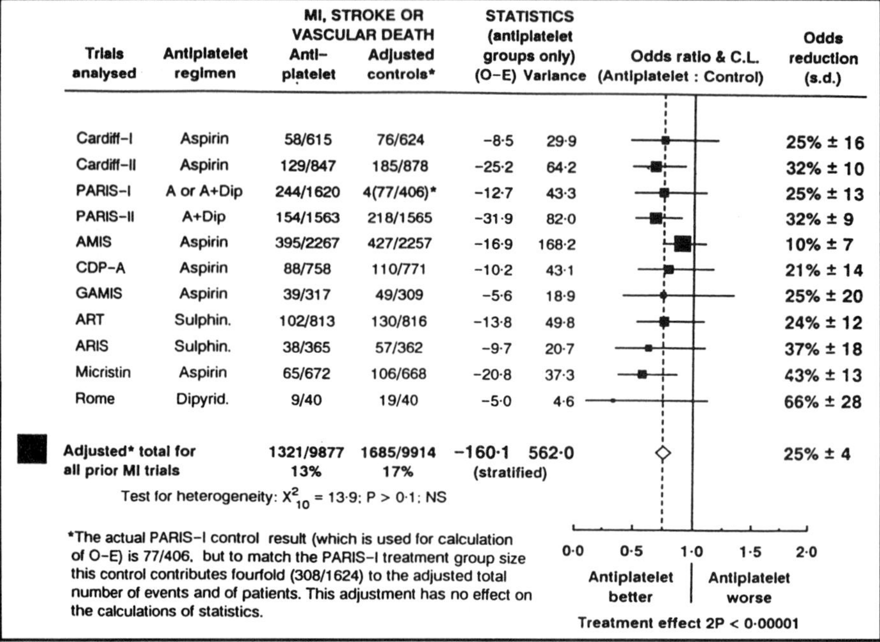

Trials analysed	Antiplatelet regimen	Anti-platelet	Adjusted controls*	(O–E)	Variance		Odds reduction (s.d.)
Cardiff–I	Aspirin	58/615	76/624	–8·5	29·9		25% ± 16
Cardiff–II	Aspirin	129/847	185/878	–25·2	64·2		32% ± 10
PARIS–I	A or A+Dip	244/1620	4(77/406)*	–12·7	43·3		25% ± 13
PARIS–II	A+Dip	154/1563	218/1565	–31·9	82·0		32% ± 9
AMIS	Aspirin	395/2267	427/2257	–16·9	168·2		10% ± 7
CDP–A	Aspirin	88/758	110/771	–10·2	43·1		21% ± 14
GAMIS	Aspirin	39/317	49/309	–5·6	18·9		25% ± 20
ART	Sulphin.	102/813	130/816	–13·8	49·8		24% ± 12
ARIS	Sulphin.	38/365	57/362	–9·7	20·7		37% ± 18
Micristin	Aspirin	65/672	106/668	–20·8	37·3		43% ± 13
Rome	Dipyrid.	9/40	19/40	–5·0	4·6		66% ± 28
Adjusted* total for all prior MI trials		1321/9877 13%	1685/9914 17%	–160·1 (stratified)	562·0		25% ± 4

Test for heterogeneity: X^2_{10} = 13·9; P > 0·1; NS

FIGURE 6. Proportional effects on vascular events (myocardial infarction, stroke, or vascular death) in 11 randomized trials of prolonged antiplatelet therapy (for 1 month or more) versus control in patients with prior myocardial infarction. O-E = Observed minus Expected; Asp = Aspirin; Dip = Dipyridamole; MI = Myocardial infarction.

FIGURE 6 provides an example of the use of these methods to combine data from the 11 randomized trials of a few months or years of antiplatelet therapy following myocardial infarction. The area of the square is proportional to the amount of statistical information that that study provides (as indicated by the variance of O-E), and the black lines represent 99% confidence limits for the individual trial results.

Practical Meaning of a Clear Effect of Treatment in One Large Trial or in an Overview

Suppose, hypothetically, that only one trial had ever addressed a particular therapeutic question, that the trial was extraordinarily large, and that it yielded a very definite 45% mortality reduction with very tight 99% confidence limits (e.g., 40–50%). What would the practical implications be? Although this strong result would still not imply that another very large trial of some approximately similar treatment for some approximately similar patients must also yield a 40–50% effect, it might well imply that such a trial should be expected to yield an effect in the same direction and of **approximately** similar size (e.g., a 30% reduction, or a 60% reduction, perhaps). Likewise, although the original trial result would not guarantee that attempts to use that treatment in the future would produce a 40–50% mortality reduction outside trials (since future patients could well differ in various ways from the previous trial patients and there could well be important differences between the care of patients in trials and out of trials), an **approximately** similar effect on mortality might be expected. In making sensible use of really clear results from a single clinical trial, the key assumption is merely that, in somewhat different medical circumstances, therapeutic effects in the same direction but of only approximately similar magnitude are still likely to exist. Extrapolation too far, of course, may lead to mistaken decisions about treatment, but so too may failure to extrapolate far enough. Thus, even for a single trial result, an estimated risk reduction with tight confidence limits implies only that similar, but not necessarily identical, treatment effects will be achieved in other circumstances.

Practical Meaning of a Clear Effect of Treatment in an Overview of Many Trials

Exactly the same is true of the "typical mortality reductions" and associated confidence limits derived from an overview of many trials. As with a single trial, the statistical calculations address the question "Given the studies that were undertaken, what range of results is statistically compatible with the actual data?" They do **not** involve saying "If different trials had been performed, what would have been seen?"

After calculation of the "typical mortality reduction" and its associated confidence limits, medical judgement—with its attendant uncertainties and disputes—is needed to help determine the circumstances to which that result is likely to be approximately relevant, just as was the case with a large single trial result. For practical purposes, therefore, it may make little difference whether large-scale randomized evidence was derived from one large unbiased trial or from a similarly large unbiased overview of many smaller trials.

Fixed-effect "Assumption-free" Methods and Random-effect "Assumed Representativeness" Methods

The general approach that has been described in the present report for analyzing and interpreting overviews is sometimes called the "fixed effects" method, because the overall result that it gets (by comparing like with like within each separate trial) is not directly influenced by any heterogeneity among the true effects of treatment in different trials. This terminology is, however, unsatisfactory, for it misleadingly suggests that any heterogeneity between the true effects of treatment in different trials is assumed to be zero in this general approach, whereas in fact no such unjustified assumptions are involved—indeed, the "assumption-free" method might be a better name.[22]

When several trials have addressed similar questions it might appear that formal statistical analyses of the heterogeneity of their findings (perhaps assessing it by the DerSimonian and Laird[24] method or some other "random effects" statistical method) are needed to augment the use of medical judgement in determining how far an overview of their results can be trusted. But, the statistical assumptions needed for such statistical methods to be of direct medical relevance are unlikely to be met. In particular, the different trial designs that were adopted would have to have been randomly selected from some underlying set of possibilities that includes the populations about which predictions are to be made. This is unlikely to be the case since trial designs are adopted for a variety of reasons, many of which depend in a complex way on the apparent results of earlier trials. Moreover, selective factors that are difficult to define may affect the types of patients in trials, and therapeutic factors that are also difficult to define may differ between trials, or between past trials and future medical practice. Finally, tests of the heterogeneity of the results of many trials may be biased by a tendency for trials with extreme results in either direction to stop recruitment early. Thus, whereas various "fixed effects" methods may actually be assumption-free, various "random effects" methods may unjustifiably assume representativeness. In view of these difficulties, such "assumed representativeness" (i.e., random-effects) methods should not generally be recommended.

Heterogeneity Tests

Formal statistical estimates of the degree of heterogeneity that exists are surprisingly insensitive, and may not help much in judging how far the overall results of an overview should be trusted. But, turning from statistical formulae to common sense, whatever formal heterogeneity tests may or may not indicate, it is obviously sensible to scrutinize thoughtfully any "outliers" in an overview of many trial results. It is also sensible, as long as appropriate caution is exercised (see above), to "subgroup" the trials and/or the patients in various medically meaningful ways—as, for example, with respect to the scheduled duration of tamoxifen in the early breast cancer trials[9] or the delay (FIG. 4) between onset of pain and randomization in the fibrinolytic trials.[8]

Mega-trials: How to Randomize Large Numbers

Turning from overviews to trials, the fundamental requirement of a good trial is that it should ask a good question and answer it reliably. The criteria for a good question are rather vague, and an overview of all the randomized trials ever done in a particular disease can be very helpful in choosing good questions for further study. In general, the most important questions are those that assess the effects of some **major outcome** of various **widely practicable** treatments for a **common disease**.

If the disease is common and the treatment widely practicable, then the trial could well be made very simple, involving randomization of as wide a range of patients as possible in as many centers as possible, without close monitoring of how treatment is given or outcome assessed. If the trial is kept really simple, then it might be possible to make it large—and, it may well need to be **extremely** large to monitor the modest differences in mortality or major morbidity that might be produced by widely practicable treatments for a common disease.

Any obstacle to simplicity is an obstacle to large size, so it is worth making great efforts to simplify the process of entering, treating and assessing patients. It is particularly necessary to simplify the entry of patients, for if this is made complicated then recruitment may be very seriously damaged. Most trials would be of much greater scientific value if they collected ten times less data, both at entry and during follow-up, and were therefore much larger. The modern fashions for complicated eligibility criteria, extensive "informed" consent, careful quality-of-life assessments and measurements of economic costs of treatment in trials are likewise often seriously inappropriate. Of course, the cost-effectiveness of treatments needs to be assessed, but that does not necessarily imply that costs should be assessed in the **same** studies in which effectiveness is to be assessed, especially if attempts to assess costs seriously damage attempts to assess the effects on mortality and major morbidity. (Also, what really matters is the cost of a treatment in routine practice, not its cost when given in the special circumstances of a randomized trial.) Likewise, of course, any important ways in which treatments affect the quality of life need to be assessed, but again that does not necessarily imply that the quality of life should be assessed in the same trials that assess the main effects of treatment. Indeed, if it takes 20,000 to assess reliably the effects of treatment on mortality and major morbidity, but would take only a few hundred to assess the main costs of treatment or the common side-effects (or other quality-of-life indices), then what should be a large, simple trial of efficacy should not be complicated by the measurement of such factors.

The Uncertainty Principle

For ethical reasons, patients cannot have their treatment chosen at random if they or their doctor are reasonably certain that they know what treatment to prefer. Hence, randomization can be offered only if both doctor and patient feel substantially uncertain which of the trial treatments is best. The question then arises: of those about whose treatment there is such uncertainty, which categories should be offered randomization? The obvious answer is all of them, welcoming the heterogeneity that this will produce. (For example, either the treatment of choice will turn out to be the same for male and female, in which case the trial might as well include both, or it will be different, in which case it is particularly important to study both sexes.) In trial design, homogeneity is generally a defect, while heterogeneity is generally a strength. Consider, for example, the fibrinolytic trials in FIGURE 4. Some homogeneous trials included only patients 0–6 hours after pain onset; those trials, however, contributed almost nothing to the key question of how late such treatment can be given. In contrast, heterogeneous trials that also included some patients with longer delays between pain onset and randomization have shown definite effects not only 0–6 but also 7–12 hours after pain onset (FIG. 4).

The "uncertainty principle" meets simultaneously the requirements of ethicality,[25] heterogeneity, maximal simplicity, and maximal size. It says that the sole eligibility criterion is that both patient and doctor should be substantially uncertain about the appropriateness for this particular patient of each of the trial treatments. The uncertainty principle (which defines eligibility not on medical but on mental criteria) is a minor design detail that has been used successfully to simplify, and thereby facilitate recruitment into, many trials, such as the ISIS studies[1-4] (FIG. 7) or the European Carotid Surgery Trial[26] (in which eligibility was greatly simplified by the uncertainty principle, making this the largest randomized trial of vascular surgery ever reported). With such uncertainty as the fundamental principle of eligibility, informed consent can also be simplified, as can the data monitoring committee's[4] terms of reference.

This is just one way to simplify trials, and there are many others. At present, trials often get tied down in a mass of wholly unnecessary traditional complexity. There is simply no serious scientific alternative to the generation of large-scale

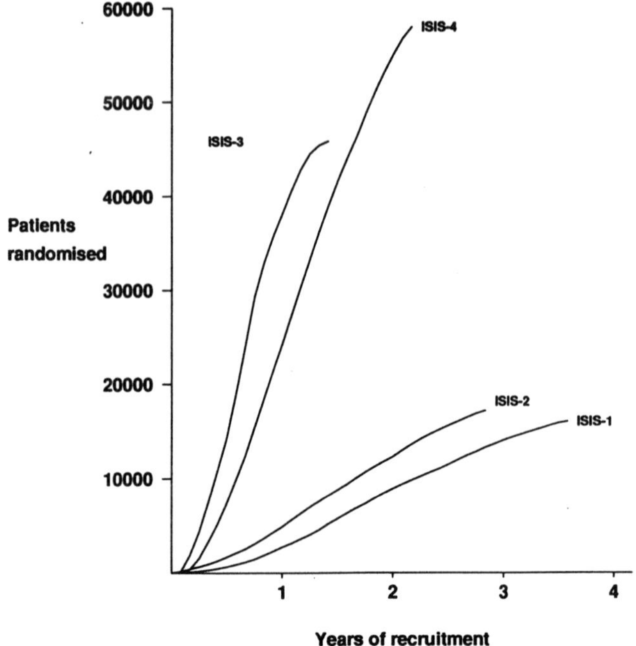

FIGURE 7. Rapidity of recruitment into the first four ISIS trials.[1-4]

randomized evidence. If trials can be vastly simplified, as has already been achieved in a few major diseases, and thereby made vastly larger, then they have a central role to play in the development of rational criteria for the planning of health care throughout the world.

REFERENCES

1. ISIS-1 (FIRST INTERNATIONAL STUDY OF INFARCT SURVIVAL) COLLABORATIVE GROUP. 1986. Randomised trial of intravenous atenolol among 16,027 cases of suspected acute myocardial infarction: ISIS-1. Lancet **ii:** 57–66.
2. ISIS-2 (SECOND INTERNATIONAL STUDY OF INFARCT SURVIVAL) COLLABORATIVE GROUP. 1988. Randomised trial of intravenous streptokinase, oral aspirin, both, or neither among 17,187 cases of suspected acute myocardial infarction: ISIS-2. Lancet **ii:** 349–360.
3. ISIS-3 (THIRD INTERNATIONAL STUDY OF INFARCT SURVIVAL) COLLABORATIVE GROUP. 1992. ISIS-3: A randomised trial of streptokinase *vs* tissue plasminogen activator *vs* anistreplase and of aspirin plus heparin *vs* aspirin alone among 41,299 cases of suspected acute myocardial infarction. Lancet **339:** 753–770.
4. ISIS-4 COLLABORATIVE GROUP. 1991. Fourth International Study of Infarct Survival: Protocol for a large, simple study of the effects of oral mononitrate, of oral captopril, and of intravenous magnesium. Am. J. Cardiol. **68:** 87D–100D.
5. GRUPPO ITALIANO PER LO STUDIO DELLA STREPTOCHINASI NELL'INFARTO MIOCARDICO (GISSI). 1986. Effectiveness of intravenous thrombolytic treatment in acute myocardial infarction. Lancet **i:** 397–402.

6. GRUPPO ITALIANO PER LO STUDIO DELLA STREPTOCHINASI NELL'INFARTO MIOCAR-
   DICO (GISSI). 1990. GISSI-2: A factorial randomized trial of alteplase versus streptokinase and heparin versus no heparin among 12490 patients with acute myocardial
   infarction. Lancet **336:** 65–71.
7. ANTIPLATELET TRIALISTS' COLLABORATION. 1994. Collaborative overview of randomized trials of antiplatelet therapy. I: Prevention of death, myocardial infarction, and
   stroke by prolonged antiplatelet therapy in various categories of patients. Br. Med.
   J. **308:** 81–106.
8. FIBRINOLYTIC THERAPY TRIALISTS' COLLABORATIVE GROUP. 1994. Indications for
   fibrinolytic therapy in suspected acute myocardial infarction: Collaborative overview
   of early mortality and major morbidity results from all randomized trials of more
   than 1000 patients. Lancet **343:** 311–322.
9. EARLY BREAST CANCER TRIALISTS' COLLABORATIVE GROUP. 1992. Systemic treatment
   of early breast cancer by hormonal, cytotoxic, or immune therapy: 133 randomized
   trials involving 31,000 recurrences and 24,000 deaths among 75,000 women. Lancet
   339: 1–15 (Part I) and 71–85 (Part II).
10. CHALMERS, I. The Cochrane Collaboration: Preparing, maintaining, and disseminating
    systematic reviews of the effects of health care. Ann. N.Y. Acad. Sci. **703:** 156–165
    [this volume].
11. COLLINS, R. & D. JULIAN. 1991. British Heart Foundation surveys (1987 and 1989) of
    United Kingdom treatment policies for acute myocardial infarction. Br. Heart J.
    66: 250–255.
12. MURRAY, C. J. & A. D. LOPEZ. 1994. Global causes of death patterns in 1990. Bull.
    WHO **72**(3): In press.
13. YUSUF, S., R. COLLINS, R. PETO, *et al.* 1985. Intravenous and intracoronary fibrinolytic
    therapy in acute myocardial infarction: Overview of results on mortality, reinfarction
    and side-effects from 33 randomized controls trials. Eur. Heart J. **6:** 556–585.
14. TEO, K. K., S. YUSUF, R. COLLINS, P. H. HELD & R. PETO. 1991. Effects of intravenous
    magnesium in suspected acute myocardial infarction: Overview of randomized trials.
    Br. Med. J. **303:** 1499–1503.
15. WOODS, K. L., S. FLETCHER, C. ROFFE & Y. HAIDER. 1992. Intravenous magnesium
    sulphate in suspected acute myocardial infarction: Results of the Second Leicester
    Intravenous Magnesium Intervention Trial (LIMIT-2). Lancet **339:** 1553–1558.
16. PETO, R. 1987. Why do we need systematic overviews of randomized trials? Stat.
    Med. **6:** 233–240.
17. YUSUF, S., R. COLLINS & R. PETO. 1984. Why do we need some large, simple random-
    ized trials? Stat. Med. **3:** 409–420.
18. PETO, R., A. J. LOPEZ, J. BOREHAM, M. THUN & C. HEATH, JR. 1992. Mortality from
    tobacco in developed countries: indirect estimation from national vital statistics.
    Lancet **339:** 1268–1278.
19. DOLL, R. & R. PETO. 1981. The causes of cancer: Quantitative estimates of avoidable
    risks of cancer in the United States today. J. Natl. Cancer Inst. **66:** 1191–1308.
20. FEINSTEIN, A. R., D. M. SOSIN & C. K. WELLS. 1985. The Will Rogers phenomenon.
    Stage migration and new diagnostic techniques as a source of misleading statistics
    for survival in cancer. N. Engl. J. Med. **312:** 1604–1608.
21. PETO, R., M. C. PIKE, P. ARMITAGE, N. E. BRESLOW, D. R. COX, S. V. HOWARD,
    N. MANTEL, K. MCPHERSON, J. PETO & P. G. SMITH. 1976 and 1977. Design and
    analysis of randomized clinical trials requiring prolonged observation of each patient.
    Part I: Introduction and design. Br. J. Cancer **34:** 585–612 (1976); Part II: Analysis
    and examples. Br. J. Cancer **35:** 1–39 (1977).
22. EARLY BREAST CANCER TRIALISTS' COLLABORATIVE GROUP. 1990. Treatment of early
    breast cancer, Vol. I: Worldwide Evidence, 1985–1990. Oxford University Press.
    Oxford and New York.
23. PETO, R. 1982. Statistical aspects of cancer trials. *In* Treatment of Cancer. K. E.
    Halnan, Ed.: 867–871. Chapman & Hall. London.
24. DERSIMONIAN, R. & N. LAIRD. 1986. Meta-analysis in clinical trials. Controlled Clinical
    Trials **7:** 177–188.

25. COLLINS, R., R. DOLL R. & R. PETO. 1992. Ethics of clinical trials. *In* Introducing New Treatments for Cancer: Practical, Ethical and Legal Problems. C. J. Williams, Ed.: 49–65. Wiley. London.
26. EUROPEAN CAROTID SURGERY TRIALISTS' COLLABORATIVE GROUP. 1991. MRC European Carotid Surgery Trial: Interim results for symptomatic patients with severe (70–99%) or with mild (0–29%) carotid stenosis. Lancet **337:** 1235–1243.

Index of Contributors

Altman, L. K., 200–209, *208, 209, 281*

Barry, J., *309*
Barry, M. J., 52–62
Brook, R. H., 74–85, *84, 85, 170–171, 235*
Buring, J. E., 18–24

Callahan, C. M., 86–95
Chalmers, I., *121,* 156–165, *163–164, 164–165, 241, 278–279, 279–280, 285, 302, 308*
Chalmers, T. C., *31, 32,* 96–106, *105–106, 122–123, 134, 154, 236, 238–239*
Chiasson, M. A., *281*
Clarke, J., *119, 170*
Clinton, J. J., 295–297, *299, 300–301, 302–303*
Collins, R., *117*
Cook, D. J., 25–32

Davis, K., 287–290, *299–300, 301–302*
Dickersin, K., *123,* 135–148, *146, 147, 148*
Doll, R., *31, 147, 208–209, 264,* 310–313

Ferguson, J. H., *118,* 180–199, *198, 199*
Feussner, J. R., 268–271, *280–281, 283, 284, 284–285*
Fletcher, S., *166–167, 171, 198*
Fowler, F. J., 52–62
Frenk, J., 250–254, *262–263, 266*
Freund, D. A., 86–95

Goyan, J. E., 275–277, *280, 283, 286*
Grant, A., 107–118, *117–118*
Greenberg, H., 41–43, *84, 224–225, 299*
Guyatt, G. H., 125–134

Haynes, R. B., *155,* 210–225, *225, 264–265*
Hennekens, C. H., 18–24, *24, 167–168, 172*
Hillis, A., *124, 147, 238, 278, 284*

Jacobs, J. J., 304–309, *308–309*
Johnson, K., *85, 147*

Kassirer, J. P., 173–179
Katz, B. P., 86–95, *94, 95, 122*

Lau, J., 96–106
Lawrence, R., *298*
Lebrón, M., *169–170, 172*
Lomas, J., *73,* 226–237, *235, 236, 237*
Lucey, J., *123–124, 146, 147, 168–169, 264, 280*

McNeil, B. J., 63–73, *72, 73, 94, 123*
Min, Y. I., 135–148
Morillo, A., 255–256, *265*
Morris, A., *24, 39, 50–51, 72–73, 94, 106, 118, 171–172, 198, 261–262, 282–283, 283–284, 301*
Mosteller, F., xi–xii, 12–17, *120, 123, 298*
Mulley, A., 52–62

O'Connor, G. T., 44–51, *51*
Orza, M., *39, 146, 263*
Oxman, A. D., 125–134, *133, 134*

Peto, R., *39–40, 72, 94–95, 119, 121–122, 124, 133–134, 147–148, 236–237, 240–241, 262, 300, 301,* 314–340
Plume, S. K., 44–51
Power, E., *235–236*

Roper, W. L., 33–40, *39, 40*

Sackett, D., 25–32, *31, 32, 84, 85, 119, 120, 198–199*
Sandercock, P., *120, 121,* 149–155, *155, 164*
Schoenbaum, S. C., 272–274, *278, 279*
Silverman, G., *122, 239–240*
Silverman, W. A., 5–11
Snider, D., *120, 134, 264*
Sox, H. C., Jr., 245–249, *262, 263, 265–266, 280, 285*
Stocking, B., 291–294

Thacker, S. B., 33–40

Walton, H., 242–244, *261, 262, 263, 264*
Warren, K., xi–xii, 1–4, *120, 238, 239, 240, 241, 265, 281–282, 308*
Wennberg, J. E., 44–51, 52–62, *164*
Wentz, D. K., 257–260, *266–267, 284*
White, L. J., 268–271